Health Promotion Settings
Principles and Practice

Edited by

Angela Scriven and Margaret Hodgins

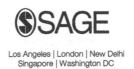

Los Angeles | London | New Delhi
Singapore | Washington DC

First published 2012

SAGE Publications Ltd
1 Oliver's Yard
55 City Road
London EC1Y 1SP

SAGE Publications Inc.
2455 Teller Road
Thousand Oaks, California 91320

SAGE Publications India Pvt Ltd
B 1/I 1 Mohan Cooperative Industrial Area
Mathura Road
New Delhi 110 044

SAGE Publications Asia-Pacific Pte Ltd
33 Pekin Street #02-01
Far East Square
Singapore 048763

Library of Congress Control Number: 2011926630

British Library Cataloguing in Publication data

A catalogue record for this book is available from the British Library

ISBN 978-0-85702-545-6
ISBN 978-0-85702-546-3 (pbk)

Typeset by C&M Digitals (P) Ltd, Chennai, India
Printed by MPG Books Group, Bodmin, Cornwall
Printed on paper from sustainable resources

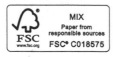

Health Promotion Settings

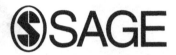

We wish to dedicate this book to all those health promoters globally who have worked and/or are working to promote health in settings.

Contents

List of Figures and Tables

Figures

Tables

About the Editors

Angela Scriven is Reader in Health Promotion at Brunel University in London, UK. She has been teaching and researching in the field of health promotion for over 25 years and has published widely, including authoring, editing or co-editing the following books: *Health Promotion Alliances: Theory and Practice* (1998), *Health Promotion: Professional Perspectives* (1996; 2001 2nd edn), *Promoting Health: Global Perspectives* (2005), *Health Promoting Practice: The Contribution of Nurses and Allied Health Professionals* (2005), *Public Health: Social Context and Action* (2007), *Promoting Health: A Practical Guide* (2010), *Health Promotion for Health Practitioners* (2010). Her research is centred on the relationship between health promotion policy and practice within specific contexts. She is a member of the International Union of Health Promotion and Education (IUHPE), is President Elect for the Institute of Health Promotion and Education (IHPE) and is a Fellow of the Royal Society for Public Health (RSPH).

Margaret Hodgins is a lecturer in Health Promotion at the National University of Ireland (NUI), Galway. She is the Programme Director for the MA in Health Promotion and the Postgraduate Diploma in Health Promotion. The programme is recognized by the Institute of Health Promotion and Education. She has extensive teaching experience and is an active researcher within the Health Promotion Research Centre at NUI Galway, a WHO collaborating centre for Health Promotion research. Her research interests include workplace health promotion and healthy ageing, and she has been principal investigator on 13 projects, leading to 21 peer-reviewed papers. She is a member of the International Union of Health Promotion and Education (IUHPE), a registered psychologist with the Psychological Society of Ireland, and is currently Chairperson of the Association for Health Promotion, Ireland.

About the Contributors

Susan Biddle is joint Head of Programme for Healthy Communities at Local Government Improvement and Development (LGID), UK. She leads the programme on behalf of LGID, providing strategic vision and direction and managing the interface with key public health stakeholders. Susan has worked with LGID for over 11 years, joining the newly formed IDeA in 1999 as Head of Workforce Development. Her work at LGID has included providing the professional lead on workforce development and designing a local government e-learning service. Susan's professional background is in organizational development and her expertise is in large programme design and delivery, and change management. She has an MA in Management Learning, a Diploma in Executive Coaching and a first degree in Art History. Susan has worked in local government for more than 25 years, in a variety of roles, is a parent and active in her local community as a parent governor and PTA chair.

Steven Boorman is Director of Health and Safety to Royal Mail Group, an experienced consultant occupational health physician with 20 years' experience working in one of the UK's largest employers. He also led the 2009 review of health and wellbeing of the NHS workforce, commissioned by the Secretary of State for Health. His career has involved developing practical and cost-effective workplace-based programmes to maintain and improve employee health. He holds appointments as Chief Examiner to the Faculty of Occupational Medicine's Diploma examination, Honorary Senior Clinical Lecturer, University of Birmingham, and is a past president of the Royal Society of Medicine's Occupational Medicine section.

Uwe Brandenburg is Head of Work Science/Strategies and Projects at Volkswagen AG, Central Health Division, Wolfsburg, Germany, and also Honorary Professor at the Technical University, Braunschweig. He has a degree in Business Studies and in Social Sciences. He has written more than 70 publications in the field of health prevention and health promotion on health management, workplace design, work organization, absenteeism, demographic change. His current research is centred on the relationship between leadership and health. He is President of the German Network Enterprise for Health and advises several private and public institutions.

Jennie Cawood is Coordinator of the UK Healthy Cities Network and the English Healthy Universities Network based in the Healthy Settings Development

Unit at the University of Central Lancashire. Previously, Jennie has worked in public health at a regional level, as Director of the Yorkshire and Humber Teaching Public Health Network and in various roles with the Yorkshire and Humber Regional Public Health Group. She has extensive experience of leading and developing public health networks and managing public health programmes.

Sharon Doherty is based in the Healthy Settings Development Unit, at the University of Central Lancashire in Preston. Her post combines the coordination of the University of Central Lancashire's Healthy University initiative with a wider development role, supporting the unit's generic work across settings and contributing to research, lecturing, evaluation, training and consultancy. She has experience of working in public health/health promotion for over 20 years. Previous posts include, Sexual Health Lead, Healthy School Coordinator and Health Promotion Specialist for Young People and Sexual Health. Her public health work has focused on sexual health, drugs issues, young people within the education setting. Sharon has previously worked as a further education lecturer in Communication and Media Studies and as an Arts Administrator/Project Manager with a community-based theatre company specializing in health work.

Mark Dooris is Director of the Healthy Settings Development Unit and Reader in Health and Sustainable Development at the University of Central Lancashire. Mark is engaged in research, evaluation, teaching, training and programme delivery and is currently project manager for the UK Healthy Cities Network and the English Network of Healthy Universities. Mark studied at Oxford University and Southbank Polytechnic, has completed the National Public Health Leadership Programme, undertook his Doctorate at Deakin University and is a Fellow of the Royal Society for Public Health and Visiting Professor in Wellbeing at London South Bank University. He has a background in health promotion, public health, community development and environmental policy and has worked in a range of local government, health service and voluntary sector roles, as well as being a consultant to WHO. Mark was co-chair of the UK Health for All Network from 1992 to 1994 and currently chairs the International Union of Health Promotion and Education's Global Working Group on Healthy Settings.

Katrin Engelhardt was a Technical Officer in the Health Promotion Unit, WHO Regional Office for the Western Pacific Region (WPRO), working on issues related to urbanization and health. Between 2003 and 2006 she was Adviser to the Seoul Metropolitan Government, Republic of Korea, working to help strengthen health promotion and establish a Healthy City programme within the city government and its districts; and as visiting research fellow at the Korean Institute for Health and Social Affairs (KIHASA). Prior to her employment in Korea she was project coordinator for a Healthy City Pilot Project in Vienna, Austria. Katrin also worked as study coordinator at the University of Munich where she coordinated the establishment of Masters Programmes in Public

Health and Epidemiology at the School of Public Health. She lectures on health promotion, community nutrition, evaluation and global public health as a part-time lecturer at various universities, including the Seoul National University and the University of Munich.

Sally Fawkes is currently Senior Lecturer in Health Promotion and Leadership at La Trobe University in Melbourne, Australia, and has worked as a practitioner, manager, educator and researcher in health promotion. In relation to healthy cities/urban health, she has worked at WHO (EURO) Healthy Cities Unit and for WHO (Western Pacific) on strengthening a regional healthy cities network across Asia and the Pacific. Recent research has focused on leadership for health, building foresight capacity in public health and healthcare, and reform of health services and systems. She is co-author (with Lin and Smith) of *Public Health Practice in Australia: The Organized Effort* (2007). Sally is an elected member of the Governance Board of the International Network of Health Promoting Hospitals and Health Services, Convenor of the Regional Coordinating Institution (Victoria-Australia) for the International HPH Network and Council Member of Women's Health Victoria. She is a member of the International Union of Health Promotion and Education (IUHPE) and an Associate Fellow of the Australian College of Health Service Executives.

Paul Fleming is Pro Vice-Chancellor (Science) at the University of Canterbury in New Zealand where he is also a professor in health promotion and population health. He has been involved in health promotion for over 30 years, mainly in the UK, as a health promotion specialist, lecturer and researcher. He established the Masters programme in health promotion at the University of Ulster and has particular research interests in workplace health, cancer education and men's health. In health promotion practice he has developed theory related to reflection in health promotion. His publications include a co-authored book *Impacting Health at Work,* several book chapters and a number of research papers and reports. He is a Fellow of the Royal Society for Public Health, a Member of the Institute of Health Promotion and Education, a Fellow of the Higher Education Academy and a member of the International Union of Health Promotion and Education.

Colin Fudge is Pro Vice-Chancellor and Vice-President of RMIT, Australia. He has worked in the University of Bristol (UK), the University of Cardiff (UK), Chalmers University and Royal Institute of Technology, Stockholm, and, in government, in the UK, European Commission, Sweden and Australia. Among his previous appointments are: Chair, European Union Expert Group on the Urban Environment; Founding Director of the WHO Collaborative Research Centre for Healthy Cities and Urban Policy; Chair, European Sustainable Cities and Towns Campaign; Chair, OECD International Urban Indicators Panel and member of the Commission for Architecture and the Built Environment (CABE) in England. Professor Fudge has contributed through interdisciplinary and transdisciplinary research on public policy formulation and implementation; cities, sustainable development and adaptation to climate change; public health; demographic change and urban design. This has been recognized through the awarding of the Royal Professorship of Environmental Science by the Swedish Academy of Sciences in 2002 and the award of an Honorary Fellowship of the Royal Institute of British Architects (RIBA). He was awarded an Honorary Doctorate in Bristol in 2009 for his work on public policy. Professor Fudge has written eight books, over 80 articles and reports, numerous book chapters and presented more than 120 conference papers.

John Griffiths has 24 years' experience in the development and implementation of health promotion programmes, and has worked for the Welsh Heart Programme (Heartbeat Wales), Health Promotion Wales and the Welsh Assembly Government. He led the development and implementation of the workplace health accreditation scheme, 'Health at Work: the Corporate Standard' and more recently the development of the Small Business Health Award. He was the principal author of the trainer's pack on alcohol and substance misuse in the workplace and is currently leading a Leonardo Life Long Learning Programme to equip line managers and supervisors in SMEs to deal with problematic use of alcohol and drugs among their staff. John has been closely involved in the development of the European Network for Workplace Health Promotion and is a technical adviser to the European Enterprise for Health Network. He is the external evaluator of two European mental health promotion programmes and is a Fellow of the Royal Society for Public Health (RSPH).

Trevor Hancock is a public health physician and population and public health consultant in Victoria, British Columbia, Canada. He has worked in public health and health promotion for more than 30 years, first for the City of Toronto and then as an independent consultant. He presented the 'Supportive Environments' theme paper at the Ottawa Charter conference in 1986 and was one of the pioneers of the Healthy Cities and Communities movement from its inception, also in 1986. He was a co-founder of the Canadian Association of Physicians for the Environment and the Canadian Coalition for Green Healthcare, and from 1998 to 2002 was a co-Principal of Planetree Canada (but has had no financial or other interest in Planetree since then). He has many publications to his credit and his honours include Life Membership in the Canadian Public Health Association (1990) and a Regent's Lectureship at UC Berkeley (2000).

Colin Noble is a senior adviser for behaviour and attendance within the National Strategies school improvement programme in England. He was previously a teacher, local education authority adviser and national coordinator of the National Healthy School Programme from 2004 to 2007. His published books include *Getting it Right for Boys ... and Girls* (1999), *The PSHE*

Coordinator's Handbook (2002) and *How to Raise Boys' Achievement* (2001) as well as a large number of articles and chapters in edited books. He is on the Editorial Advisory Committee of the journal *Health Education*.

Sue Powell is Head of the Academy for Health and Wellbeing, Manchester Metropolitan University, UK. She is engaged in research, workforce development and training in public health. She is the Chief Operating Officer for the Greater Manchester Health Innovation and Education Cluster and leads research projects in health at work, healthy universities, preventing gambling-related harm in higher education and promoting healthy weight in adults and children. Until March 2010, Sue was the Coordinator of the North West Teaching Public Health Network which focused on public health curriculum development and she regularly delivers workforce development programmes for the health service and voluntary sectors. Sue started her career as an environmental health officer in local government. She maintains her links with environmental health and chairs the Qualifications Board for the Chartered Institute of Environmental Health.

Martin Seymour is a Principal Consultant with the Local Government Improvement and Development Healthy Communities Programme with lead responsibility for work-streams on the social determinants of health and the role of local government and population mental health and wellbeing. Martin has previously worked with NHS Norfolk and in joint PCT and local authority roles with a broad remit around health inequalities, partnership working and community development. Martin came into public health from a career in local authority leisure and community services. He has recently completed an MSc with distinction in public health and health promotion and has undertaken research into whether local strategic partnerships provide collaborative advantage for health improvement. Martin is a director of East Anglia Food Link, co-chair of the UK Public Health Association (UKPHA) Health and Sustainable Environments Special Interest Group and is a Fellow of the Royal Society for Public Health (RSPH).

Jane South is a Reader in Health Promotion and Director of the Centre for Health Promotion Research, Leeds Metropolitan University. She has wide experience of research in community-based health promotion and has an interest in methodologies for evaluating health promotion. She is regularly involved in training practitioners around practical evaluation skills and is the author of *Evaluation: Key concepts for public health practice*. Her research interests are focused on community involvement in health and Jane was the lead investigator on the People in Public Health study, which looked at approaches to involve volunteers and lay health workers in delivering health improvement programmes. Her research has led to innovative tools for practice including evaluation and planning frameworks and a self assessment tool for community involvement.

Marilyn Toft is the cross-phase programme director for behaviour and attendance within the National Strategies School Improvement Programme in England. Previously a secondary school teacher with management responsibility, Marilyn worked as a research associate for the DES on HIV and Aids education in the mid 1980s, evaluating resources produced for schools. Subsequently, she worked at a senior level in a local authority, leading schools' professional development programmes, as well as the local Healthy Schools programme. In 1998, Marilyn was appointed to lead the development and implementation of a national scheme for schools that aligned education and health priorities. This resulted in the successful launch of the National Healthy School Programme the following year and the engagement of all local education and health authorities. During her career, Marilyn has contributed to several publications about health education including HIV and Aids, curriculum resources and advice documents for schools on improving behaviour and attendance.

Rob Whiting began his working life in engineering before embarking on a 20-year career in computing. In the late 1980s he changed direction and went into Facilities Management. It was while working in the printing industry that the opportunity to train in Health and Safety management arose. He took this opportunity and gained his NEBOSH certificate. In 2002 he moved to Williams Medical Supplies as Facilities/H&S Manager and added environmental management to his role. In 2006 he was part of the team that won Health at Work (Gold) and in 2009 he led the team that achieved OHSAS 18001 and ISO 14001.

James Woodall is a Lecturer in Health Promotion at Leeds Metropolitan University, UK. His PhD explored the health promoting prison and how values central to health promotion are applied to the context of imprisonment. James has published in a number of areas related to prison and offender health, including prisoners' lay views on health, the mental health of prisoners and young offenders and the role of prison visitors' centres in reducing health inequalities.

Acknowledgements

We would like to thank all the contributors for their enthusiasm and cooperation in supporting this book and all those whose work has helped with the
development of ideas in individual chapters. Particular thanks go to Alison
Poyner and Emma Milman and the production team at Sage.

Chapter 10 draws on research funded by the Higher Education Academy and
the Department of Health (Dooris and Doherty, 2009, 2010a, 2010b) and on
development work funded by the Higher Education Funding Council for
England as part of the Developing Leadership and Governance for Healthy
Universities Project.

Foreword

Since the development of principles and guidelines for health promoting settings in the mid-1980s there has been a great deal of progress and application in the field. *Health Promotion Settings: principles and practice* provides a twenty-first century perspective on the settings approach and its application to a broad range of contexts. Workplaces, schools, hospitals, universities, prisons, neighbourhoods and cities are discussed and useful real-life examples of work in these settings are provided. Further, the authors look critically and analytically at the settings approach and the social milieu in which it has developed. These considerations result in a work that successfully documents emerging thinking, frameworks and processes that are actively shaping contemporary health promotion.

Health promotion activity is divisible into three main areas of focus: the regulatory or policy level; the population or community level; and the individual level. At a time when a great deal of attention is being paid to national policy level, changes to address determinants of health and to individual behaviour change to address non-communicable diseases, it is refreshing to read of ways to re-engage communities in settings. In this book, settings are seen as a useful way to engage community members, build partnerships for sustainable health promotion and address determinants. The chapters lead us through the background and principles of healthy settings and then show us how these can be effectively utilized to make a difference. A case is also made for the use of settings as a way of connecting the work that is done on determinants and that which is focused on behaviour change.

Effective twenty-first century health promotion requires practitioners to be well informed, evidence based, analytical and up to date. The authors and editors have a wealth and breadth of experience in healthy settings that ensure the chapters are both academically rigorous and relevant to practitioners. This book is a welcomed and useful reference for those engaged in health promotion settings as well as those who are learning about them. Just as the settings profiled in this volume are broad-ranging, so too should be the readership. This text will appeal to workers in the health, health promotion and community development sectors but should also resonate with workers in fields as diverse as education, youth work, workplaces and local authorities.

Michael Sparks
President, IUHPE

Online Further Reading

The companion website for this book allows you to extend your reading with a range of relevant SAGE journal articles selected by the editors and authors of this book.

Visit www.sagepub.co.uk/scriven for free access to the following articles:

Chapter 1

Dooris, M (2009) 'Holistic and sustainable health improvement: the contribution of the settings-based approach to health promotion', *Perspectives in Public Health*, 129 (1): 29–36.

Chapter 2

Dooris, M. (2006) 'Editorial – Healthy settings: future directions', *Promotion and Education*, XIII (1): 4–6.
Dooris, M. (2009) 'Holistic and sustainable health improvement: the contribution of the settings-based approach to health promotion', *Perspectives in Public Health*, 129: 29–36.

Chapter 3

Naaldenberg, J., Vaandrager, L., Koelen, M., Wagemakers, A., Saan, H and de Hoog, K. (2009) 'Elaborating on systems thinking in health promotion practice', *Global Health Promotion*, 16 (39): 39–47.

Chapter 4

Halliday, G., Asthana, S.N.M. and Richardson, S. (2004) 'Evaluating partnership: the role of formal assessment tools', *Evaluation*, 10 (3): 285–303.

Chapter 5

Poland, B., Krupa, G. and McCall, D. (2009) 'Settings for health promotion: an analytic framework to guide intervention design and implementation', *Health Promotion Practice*, 10: 505–16.

Chapter 6

Douglas, J. (2007) 'Promoting the public health: continuity and change over two centuries', in J. Douglas, S. Earle, S. Handsley, C.E. Lloyd and S. Spur, *A Reader in Promoting Public Health, Challenge and Controversy*. London: Sage.

Semenza, J. and Krishnasamy, V. (2007) 'Design of a Health-promoting Neighbourhood Intervention', *Health Promotion Practice*, 8: 243–56.

Chapter 7

Kjellstrom, T. and Mercado, S. (2008) 'Towards action on social determinants for health equity in urban settings', *Environment and Urbanization*, 20: 551–75.

Chapter 8

Delobelle, P., Onya, H., Langa, C., Mashamba, J. and Depoorter, A. (2010) 'Advances in health promotion in Africa: promoting health through hospitals', *Global Health Promotion*, 17: 33-6.

Chapter 9

Barnekow Rasmussen, V. (2005) 'The European Network of Health-promoting Schools – from Iceland to Kyrgyzstan', *Promotion and Education*, 12: 169–72.

Chapter 10

Dooris, M. and Doherty, S. (2010) 'Healthy Universities: current activity and future directions – findings and reflections from a national-level qualitative research study', *Global Health Promotion*, 17 (3): 6-16.

Chapter 11

Condon, L., Hek, G.and Harris, F. (2008) 'Choosing health in prison: prisoners' views on making healthy choices in English prisons', *Health Education Journal*, 67: 155–66.

Woodall, J. (2007) 'Barriers to positive mental health in a Young Offenders Institution: a qualitative study', *Health Education Journal*, 66, 132–40.

Chapter 12

Moore, A.B., Parahoo, K. and Fleming, P. (2011) 'Managers' understanding of workplace health promotion within small and medium-sized enterprises: A phenomenological study', *Health Education Journal*, 70: 92–101.

Chapter 13

Hunt, M.K., Lederman, R., Stoddard, A.M., LaMontagne, A.D., McLellan, D., Combe, C., Barbeau, E. and Sorensen, G. (2005) 'Process evaluation of an integrated health promotion/occupational health model in WellWorks-2', *Health Education and Behaviour*, 32: 10–26.

Chapter 14

Lomas, L. and McLuskey, J. (2005) 'Pumping up the pressure: a qualitative evaluation of a workplace health promotion initiative for male employees', *Health Education Journal*, 64: 88–95.

Chapter 15

Hodgins, M., Battel-Kirk, B. and. Asgeirsdottir, A. (2010) 'Building capacity in workplace health promotion: the case of the Healthy Together e-learning project', *Global Health Promotion*, 17 (1): 60–8.

1

Health Promotion Settings: An Overview

Angela Scriven

Aims

- To provide an overview of the content of the book, outlining the context and structure
- To offer the rationale for a text on the settings approach to health promotion
- To identify the focus of each of the chapters in the book
- To introduce general themes and arguments that will be expanded on in the specific introductions to Parts I – III

Since the Ottawa Charter (WHO, 1986) highlighted the idea that health is created within the settings of people's everyday lives, where they learn, work, play and love, the settings approach has become an established component of the global health promotion agenda for action. The World Health Organization (WHO, 1998) has defined settings as the context in which people engage in daily activities and in which environmental, organizational and personal factors interact to affect health and wellbeing. The WHO definition also argues that normally, settings can be identified as having physical boundaries, a range of people with defined roles, and an organizational structure. Making these contexts the object of health promotion intervention and inquiry uses a wide range of processes and takes many different forms (Poland et al., 2009), but frequently involves some form of organizational development, including change to the physical environment and to the organizational structure (see Whitelaw et al., 2001 for a critical overview).

Settings can include those that have been coordinated at an international level by WHO, such as Healthy Cities, Villages, Municipalities and Healthy Islands projects, the networks of Health Promoting Schools and Health Promoting Hospitals, and the Healthy Marketplaces and Health Promoting Workplaces projects (Kickbusch, 1998). There are those that argue that twenty-first century settings should also include other more diffuse contexts, such as where people Google, shop and travel (Kickbusch, 2006). Currently healthy setting approaches have been implemented in many different ways in multiple areas. A list of all existing WHO coordinated Healthy Settings projects, including initiatives and documented activities, can be found on the WHO web pages at www.who.int/healthy_settings/types/en/index.html. The list cites:

- Cities
- Villages
- Municipalities and Communities
- Schools
- Workplaces
- Markets
- Homes
- Islands
- Hospitals
- Prisons
- Universities
- Ageing

Each setting on the list above has a web link which provides a description of the approach, outlines the fundamental theory of the programme and provides information on implementation, existing networks and available resources for each application. The website, therefore, is an invaluable resource for those working in settings.

The important point to note, however, is that planned, comprehensive and multisectoral settings approaches to health promotion action are now well established and an essential component of the twenty-first century health promotion agenda (Dooris, 2009), with the settings approach delivered locally and in many cases coordinated nationally and internationally by organizations such as WHO. The overall purpose of this book is to provide a detailed account of the principles on which a settings approach is based and to highlight some of the settings listed above. The book will combine a theoretical discourse of the settings approach with real-life examples of the settings, covering a wide range and including workplaces, schools, neighbourhoods, cities and prisons. Thinking, frameworks and processes that are actively shaping health promotion in settings in the twenty-first century are documented and the ideas and research covered will provide a vital set of materials for those who promote health in settings. The examination of health promotion through a settings approach is covered in three discrete parts, as outlined in Box 1.1.

Box 1.1 *Health Promotion Settings* **in three parts**

The book is divided in to three distinctive parts. Each part has not only a discrete focus but also a synergistic relationship.

Part I concentrates on theoretical principles, policy and the practical processes underpinning the settings approach to health promotion. The focus of the contributors will be on the history, concepts, values, principles, planning and evaluation that are fundamental elements to health promotion action in settings, covering, for example, partnership working.

Part II will offer examples of the broad range of settings, including schools, neighbourhoods, cities, prisons.

Part III provides an in-depth examination of workplace settings and will act as a major case study of a settings approach. A critical overview of the workplace context is offered alongside evidence and examples of practice covering a range of workplaces, including manufacturing and small and medium-sized enterprises (SMEs).

Each part of the book has an introduction which summarizes the key themes. There is cross-referencing between the three parts in order to locate theoretical, conceptual, process and policy issues within each setting.

There are a number of reasons for devoting a whole section to the workplace setting. Firstly, it is important to understand both the breadth and depth of the settings approach to health promotion. The workplace is a substantial setting and has been identified as one of the priority areas for health promotion into the twenty-first century (WHO, 2010). The significance of the workplace in terms of influencing the determinants of health is an important motive for the WHO prioritizing this setting. The nature of employment is a major contributing factor to health, directly influencing the physical, psychosocial and economic wellbeing of the population. Changing the overall conditions of work is recommended in terms of global action on the social determinants of health (WHO, 2008) and preventing accidents and illness at work can result in significant population health gain. The International Labour Organization (ILO) estimates that within the world's 2.7 billion workers, at least 2 million deaths have occupational causes (Rosenstock et al., 2006). The relationship between adverse working conditions and negative health outcomes displays a strong social class gradient, with higher risk for accident and illness clustering in low status occupations (WHO, 2008), suggesting that improving working conditions might contribute significantly to reducing health inequities. Further, settings-based workplace health promotion has the potential not just to protect but to improve health through creating positive and health enhancing social environments and work cultures. The global labour force participation rate is 65% (ILO, 2008), demonstrating the extensive reach of the workplace setting and making it an ideal setting and infrastructure to support the promotion of health to large audiences. Using the modes of communication already in place in a workplace can be an effective means of encouraging participation in programmes and follow up with employees (Naidoo and Wills, 2009). Moreover, the workplace gives access to target groups not easily reached in other ways, for example, younger men. Finally, the reach of the workplace as a setting can also extend beyond employees, having indirect influences on families and communities, such as work–life balance policy and practice.

The workplace can be considered an overarching setting insofar as other well-established settings – schools, universities, prisons and hospitals – are also workplaces. To take just one illustration of this, the health sector is a major employer, estimated to employ 1.3 million people in the UK alone. Links need to be made, therefore, between hospitals, schools, prisons and university settings in Part II, which are workplaces, and the more specific examples of workplace settings in Part III. See Figure 1.1 for a figurative explanation of how the settings discussed in this book relate and Chapter 2 for a discussion of the link between the different health promoting settings.

Because the settings approach is universal and many of the settings, such as health promoting schools, are linked to global initiatives, all of the issues and

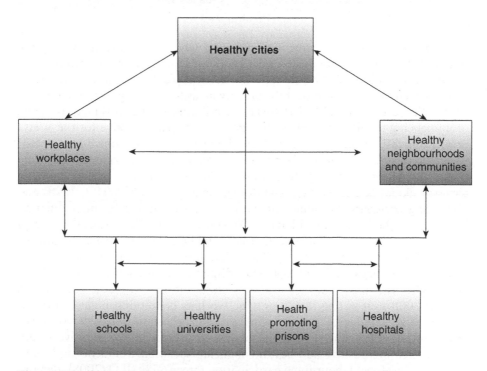

Figure 1.1 Connections between different health promotion settings

ideas addressed in this book will have international applicability, with international examples and comparisons used where applicable or appropriate.

> ## Box 1.2 *Health Promotion Settings* offers:
>
> - Reference to relevant and recent settings interventions, research, policies and evidence informed practice.
> - Ideas, debates, issues linked, where appropriate, to international examples and global policies.
> - Identification of principles, contemporary trends and viewpoints on developing health promotion initiatives in settings.

Part I opens with a chapter containing a detailed analysis of the origins, history, evolution and challenges of health promoting settings. The review of the theoretical and conceptual base, including outlining frameworks and typologies, of the settings approach highlights its ecological perspective, presenting an understanding of settings as dynamic open systems and with a primary focus on whole system organizations, development and change. The benefits of settings as foci of health promotion are debated and questions are asked about the challenges that health promoters face when working in settings. Key challenges are discussed and these include the difficulties relating to the construction of the evidence base, the diversity of conceptual understandings and practice, and the complexity of evaluating whole system approaches. The chapter concludes by exploring key issues: funding evaluation within and across settings; ensuring links between evidence, policy and practice; and clarifying and articulating the theories that underpin the settings approach generically and inform the approach within particular settings.

This broad opening introduction is followed in Chapter 3 by an examination of one of the introductory themes, a whole systems approach to working in settings. Settings are complex dynamic systems, set within and interacting with, larger systems, such as the political or economic environment. This view of settings as systems is consistent with the core principles and theory of health promotion. While it is often the case that problems seen in systems are addressed by isolating and attending to specific elements or parts of the system, for example the teachers in a school, or the canteen in a workplace, systems thinking advocates that change within a system can best be achieved by considering how the parts relate to one another and working with the system as a whole. Further, a healthy settings approach can take an organization beyond problem solving, contributing to a bigger picture of systems development and evolution. These ideas are discussed in this chapter with special reference to successful healthy settings work, the Management Standards Approach to work-related stress and the Bullying Prevention programme for schools. The overview of the Management Standards Approach demonstrates how at an organizational rather than individual level, workplaces need to engage both management and workers in joint problem solving to develop actions to address gaps between organizational practice and evidence informed standards. The Bullying Prevention programme relates to a comprehensive, school-wide programme designed for use in secondary level schools, for pupils aged 11–18 years of age. Its goals are to reduce and prevent bullying problems among school children and to improve peer relations at school. The programme comprises parent, school, classroom and community elements and has been evaluated extensively. Both initiatives are examples of how to draw on a systems approach in settings with a view to improving health.

Partnership working is a fundamental principle and prerequisite to work within settings. Chapter 4 begins by arguing that enabling and encouraging people to participate in the process of defining and promoting their collective needs and concerns in relation to health are key aims in health promotion and fundamentally important to a healthy settings approach. The difference between collaboration, participation and partnerships will be outlined and critiqued, and recommendations made for how professionals working in settings can fully engage in collaborative, participatory and partnership working with individuals, groups and other professionals.

Planning and evaluating health promotion in settings is multifaceted because of their inherent complexity. Chapter 5 examines the principles of health promotion programme planning and evaluation and their application within a settings approach. The assessment of health needs within settings underpins effective planning, and sources of evidence, including lay knowledge, need to inform the design of interventions. A simple planning framework will be utilized to demonstrate how health goals can be met in the context of settings through establishing realistic objectives, choosing appropriate methods and mobilizing professional and community resources within the setting. The chapter also explores how evaluation can be built into projects and interventions, and lead to enhanced learning across settings. Measurement of change at both individual and within the broader parameters of the setting is critically examined with reference to wider methodological debates on the significance of evaluation in health promotion. It is argued that an understanding of the range of health outcomes enables the selection of appropriate indicators and evaluation methods. Issues pertaining to health promotion evaluation, including the merits of wider stakeholder engagement, are explored, with examples drawn from different settings. The chapter concludes by arguing that clear articulation of health goals, attention to processes and strengthening evaluation within the planning cycle are crucial to a settings approach.

Having covered the fundamental principles that guide work in settings, Part II illustrates the settings themselves and begins with a chapter on healthy neighbourhoods and communities. Neighbourhoods and communities are important settings for health promotion because health inequality and social exclusion derive from poor social and physical environments. Multiagency approaches in partnership with communities appear to hold the key to closing the health gap and delivering health improvements. Many influences on health operate at the community and neighbourhood level, among them culture, religion, housing and environment. Working at the community level opens up opportunities for health empowerment and building up the capacity of communities to participate in meeting their health needs. The Healthy Communities Programme is an example of how this can work. The programme aims to build the capacity of local authorities working within their communities to tackle local health inequalities, to provide leadership to promote wellbeing, and to foster a joined up approach to health improvement across local government itself and through Local Strategic Partnerships (LSPs) and Local Area Agreements (LAAs). The chapter critically considers the various approaches taken to advance the community as a setting for health, locating the approach in policy and practice agendas.

Communities and neighbourhoods reside within larger conglomerations. So, the next chapter considers cities as settings through the Healthy Cities programme. The health of people living in towns and cities is strongly determined by their living and working conditions, the quality of their physical and socioeconomic environment and the quality and accessibility of care services. While the WHO Healthy Cities approach can offer comprehensive policy and planning solutions to urban health problems across a setting as large as a city, there needs to be engagement with local government and governance, through a process of political commitment, institutional changes, capacity building, partnerships and other actions. National and international examples are used to good effect to demonstrate that urban poverty, the needs of vulnerable groups, the social, economic and environmental root causes of ill health, and the positioning of health considerations in the centre of economic regeneration and urban development efforts are potential outcomes of a Healthy Cities settings approach. The principles and values of the Healthy Cities Project (2009–13) are outlined.

Healthy cities contain within them a plethora of other settings, so the chapter on healthy cities is followed by some of these smaller, more contained settings. Although healthcare institutions would seem to be the most obvious setting for the promotion of health it can be argued that structures, policies and processes in these institutions are antithetical to the principles of health promotion and the settings approach. In this context the WHO Health Promoting Hospitals (HPH) movement was developed in 1990 with a number of specific aims relating to health gain for patients, visitors, staff and community. The work of Health Promoting Hospitals is integral to the fifth action of the Ottawa Charter, reorienting health services (WHO, 1986). A healthy hospital is described as one that creates a healthy environment for patients and a healthy workplace for staff. It is healthy both because of the way it is designed and because of the way it operates. In Chapter 8 the work of the Health Promoting Hospitals movement is outlined and key projects explored in the four focus areas of patients, staff, community and organization. The potential for linking the work in this setting with quality management is discussed.

The question of how effective schools are as a setting for health promotion is dealt with in Chapter 9. Schools are generally regarded as important settings in which to promote children's and young people's health. The Healthy Schools programme is designed to make a difference to both the health and academic achievement of school children. The initiative is growing, with global networks that span countries and continents. In England, for example, nine out of ten schools are trying to meet the National Healthy Schools Programme criteria to become an accredited Healthy School. Seven out of ten have already achieved Healthy School status. The National Healthy Schools Programme has been running for over 10 years and is coordinated jointly by the Department of Health and the Department for Education. It has a network of 150 local programmes, which are supported by partnerships between local authorities and primary care trusts. The current development of this Healthy Schools movement is discussed and suggestions made for ways forward. Key principles are examined, including taking a whole school perspective, ensuring ownership and responsiveness to particular needs, looking at mental and social as well as physical health, and including the role of the school within its community.

From schools to another educational setting, universities. The Healthy Universities approach reflects a broad understanding of health and wellbeing and applies a whole system perspective, aiming to create healthy and sustainable working, learning and living environments for students, staff and visitors. Another goal is to increase the profile of health in teaching, research and knowledge exchange and contribute to the health and sustainability of the wider community. The chapter on healthy universities outlines the challenges involved in introducing and integrating health within a sector that does not have this as its central aim, is experiencing resource constraints and comprises fiercely autonomous and often competitive institutions. A key point is that a system-based approach has significant added value for universities offering the potential to address health in a coherent and integrated way and to forge connections to both health-related targets and core drivers within higher education.

The Health Promoting Prisons (HPP) project (also called the Health in Prisons Project, HIPP) began in 1995 in the WHO EURO region, in view of the recognition of inequality between general population health and prisoner health. Prisoners tend to have poorer health in comparison to the general public due to common prison issues, like bullying, mobbing and boredom. Prisons provide a unique opportunity for accessing the hard to reach with important aspects of health promotion, health education and disease prevention. Chapter 11 provides an overview of the settings approach to promoting health in prisons and draws on prison policies that promote health, a prison environment that is supportive of health, and health promotion initiatives specific to individual prisons. While more than 30 Member States of the WHO European Region participate in HPP to various degrees, the chapter debates why the HPP movement seems to be the least popular of all the settings-based environments. The problems encountered are assessed, including underfunding, poor support and over-crowding. These challenges to the success of the HPP movement are discussed in full and examples offered of good practice, with recommendations made for further development of prisons as a setting for health improvement.

Part III of the book has a detailed focus on workplaces as a setting for health promotion. Exemplars of good practice in workplace health promotion are offered to provide decision makers in companies and organizations with knowledge on how workplace health promotion programmes can be successfully implemented. Models of healthy workplaces are required for a range of workplaces, since although basic principles of health promotion programme planning apply universally, specific contexts present different challenges in respect of implementation. For example, a small rural enterprise will be unlikely to consider the experiences of a large multinational to be of relevance to their situation. For this reason, three chapters provide detailed case studies of good practice in workplace health promotion for a large multinational private sector company (Volkswagen), a large public sector organization (Royal Mail, UK) and a small enterprise (Williams Medical Supplies).

Prior to the three workplace case studies there is an overview chapter on workplace health promotion. Workplaces are a key setting through which to improve health and reduce health inequalities. The Healthy Workplace initiative encapsulates a new approach to the problems of health at work. There is an examination of what constitutes a healthy workplace and the World Health Organization Healthy Workplace initiative is examined, as are examples of good practice at a UK and international level. The philosophy underpinning the initiative and the precise nature of workplaces as a setting is examined and an assessment made of the benefits it affords to achieving public health targets and confronting the social determinants of health. A critique of the partnership approach is offered, with business (employers and employees), trade unions and other organizations at international, national and local level, and the case is argued for the economic expediency of health promoting workplaces.

From this general introduction to workplace health promotion follows a case study of a multinational manufacturing company, Volkswagen. Volkswagen AG is a large multinational automobile manufacturer which employs in excess of 350,000 employees across sites in 15 countries. Volkswagen's approach to the workplace as a setting for health improvement is comprehensive and includes both prevention and occupational health. A series of concrete measures has been drawn up in close cooperation with Volkswagen Health Services. These are outlined and an overview of some of the programmes and prevention schemes for workers are described, demonstrating Volkswagen's preventive approach to illness and injuries. The Check Up scheme providing personalized preventive advice and information, and a number of rehabilitation and reintegration programmes are used as examples of good practice. Finally, Volkswagen's approach to creating health throughout the chain of supplier, producer and dealership is described.

Chapter 14 offers a case study on Royal Mail, UK and illustrates a culture that supports health and wellbeing. The Royal Mail employs around 190,000 people in a diversity of tasks, providing a frontline public service on a daily basis. The organization has secured awards for occupational health management and for the promotion of gender equity and diversity in the workplace. A wide range of specific occupational and health promotion services are available including driver medicals, health screening, vaccinations service, an employee and family helpline, a bullying and harassment confidential helpline and an in-house gym. However, beyond services, the Royal Mail takes a fully integrated approach to workplace health, aiming to creating a workplace culture where employees consider themselves valued, supported and respected. Health clinics assist employees in returning to work successfully after illness or injury. A public health qualification is available to staff using a cascade model which focuses on both health and safety. This chapter provides an overview of projects and outcomes, in addition to exploring new initiatives such as the Royal Mail's Corporate and Social Responsibility programme, and a partnership project with occupational healthcare providers to build managerial awareness of early indicators of workplace stress.

The final chapter describes workplace health promotion in SMEs, providing an example of good practice. Small and medium-sized enterprises (SMEs) make up a very significant proportion of the global economy, employing about 77 million people and representing approximately 66% of the workforce. However, their situation with respect to health and safety is less favourable than that of larger enterprises with work-related ill health risk increasing as enterprise size decreases. In this chapter some of the difficulties SMEs encounter in promoting workplace health are explored, along with an example of good practice in a small enterprise in Wales – Williams Medical Supplies (WMS). WMS employs 160 people and is the largest supplier to general practice in the United Kingdom. It was voted a Sunday Times Best 100 Small Companies to Work For and has been recognized as an Investors in People (IiP) Company since 2000. Workplace health promotion at WMS has been facilitated by their involvement with a national workplace health promotion accreditation programme, based from the outset on a whole company approach. At the centre of this is the high value that the company places on its staff, recognizing that their wellbeing is central to the company's performance.

In summary, the 15 chapters that make up this text range from those that offer an element of critical review and theoretical overview to those that bring together a range of perspectives and case studies on current settings. The combination of contributions gives a detailed introduction and coverage of settings-based work, highlighting the history, frameworks, principles and interventions that make up a settings approach. The factors that influence the ability of health promoters to effectively deliver interventions are considered and those with a responsibility to promote health in settings should find the contributions invaluable as a guide to practice.

Summary points

- The settings approach to health promotion as evidenced in this book is a dynamic feature of twenty-first century health promotion.
- Settings are diverse and wide ranging, from discrete organizational units such as schools to large diffuse settings such as cities.
- There are discrete settings within settings, so schools are within communities which are within cities.
- The workplace as a setting is also represented within many other settings, so schools, prisons and hospitals are also workplace settings.

Online Further Reading

Dooris, M (2009) 'Holistic and sustainable health improvement: the contribution of the settings-based approach to health promotion', *Perspectives in Public Health*, 129 (1): 29–36.

In addition to Dooris's contributions to this book (see Chapter 2 and Chapter 10), this article offers an introductory glimpse of the issues linked to working in a settings approach, giving an overview of current practice both internationally and nationally and exploring future developments of settings-based health promotion in relation to three key issues: inequalities and inclusion, place-shaping and systems-based responses to complex problems.

References

Dooris, M. (2009) 'Holistic and sustainable health improvement: the contribution of the settings-based approach to health promotion', *Perspectives in Public Health*, 129 (1): 29–36.

ILO (International Labour Organization) (2008) *Declaration on Social Justice for a Fair Globalization*. Geneva: ILO.

Kickbusch, I. (1998) 'Foreword' to WHO (1998) *Health Promotion Glossary*. Geneva: WHO.

Kickbusch, I. (2006) PowerPoint presentation given to UK Academic Network. London.

Naidoo, J. and Wills, J. (2009) *Foundations for Health Promotion*. London: Elsevier.

Poland, B., Krupa, G. and McCall, D. (2009) 'Settings for health promotion: an analytic framework to guide intervention design and implementation', *Health Promotion Practice*, 10 (4): 505–16.

Rosenstock, L., Cullen, M. and Fingerhut, M. (2006) *Disease Control Priorities in Developing Countries*, 2nd edn. New York: Oxford University Press.

Whitelaw, S., Baxendale, A., Bryce, C., MacHardy, L., Young, I. and Witney, E. (2001) 'Settings-based health promotion: a review', *Health Promotion International*, 16 (4): 339–53.

WHO (World Health Organization) (1986) *Ottawa Charter for Health Promotion*. Geneva: WHO.

WHO (World Health Organization) (1998) *Health Promotion Glossary*. Geneva: WHO.

WHO (World Health Organization) (2008) Closing the Gap in a Generation. Report of the Commission on the Social Determinants. Geneva: WHO.

WHO (World Health Organization) (2010) *Occupational Health and Workplace Health Promotion*. Available at: www.who.int/occupational_health/topics/workplace/en/index2.html (accessed 9 March 2010).

Part 1

Health Promotion Principles and the Settings Approach

Introduction to Part I

Principles and practice in a settings approach

Angela Scriven

This first part of the book critically examines a range of theoretical issues and ideas that are central to informing the promotion of health using a settings approach and, as such, creates the context for what follows in the remaining two parts. It is evident from the chapters that make up this part and elsewhere (see Whitelaw et al., cited in Chapter 1) that the settings approach has emerged from a rejection of individualistic approaches to health promotion. In addition to the fundamental values and principles that underpin health promotion, those working in settings draw on a number of disciplinary perspectives, such as organizational sociology. These perspectives and standpoints are embedded in the discourse and themes of Part I.

The history, evolution and rationale of the settings approach is covered in depth in the first chapter. Dooris, who has been a significant figure both in the UK and internationally in the development of thinking and conceptual frameworks that have formed the paradigm shift from a focus on the individual to work within settings, raises highly pertinent considerations for those responsible for promoting health within and across settings. This chapter forms an excellent introduction to the philosophy of settings and highlights a number of note-worthy questions which are invaluable in developing a more critical view of the settings described in Parts II and III. One interesting conundrum is the concern that is raised that promoting health through settings could serve to exacerbate health inequalities, particularly amongst marginalized groups. This is a curious dilemma given that settings are designed to reach people in the context of their everyday lives. The argument focuses on those who are unemployed, homeless or excluded from schools, so the healthy workplaces, healthy schools and healthy communities that make up a significant part of the settings momentum would have no impact on these groups (see Part II for detailed accounts of healthy schools in Chapter 9, healthy cities in Chapter 7, healthy communities and neighbourhoods in Chapter 6 and for workplaces, see Part III). While there are strong arguments for how some settings are able to access vulnerable and hard-to-reach groups (see the chapter on health promoting prisons, Part II, Chapter 11) those promoting health in settings need to be cognisant of this problem and appraise how their actions might impact on inequalities.

Another important point made by Dooris is the synergy and interrelationship between the various settings resulting in individuals and groups frequently strad-dling more than one (Chapter 1 also offers an indication of this synergistic con-nection, as represented in Figure 1.1). The problem with this interconnection is that unless there is efficient and effective coordination across settings then population groups might suffer from health promotion overload and/or there could be a duplication of effort and waste of resources and/or stakeholders could be overburdened in terms of participatory and partnership efforts.

Dooris makes cogent links between settings thinking and whole systems the-ory. This association is continued by Hodgins and Griffiths, who provide a detailed exploration of the connection between the principles of systems theory and the settings approach to health promotion. The fundamental premise is that while health promoters need to adopt the values of systems theory, examples of health promotion interventions that focus only on parts rather than holistically remain too plentiful. The conclusion here is that practitioners find it difficult to adopt a systems perspective. One argument for this is that a continued dominant focus on the individual and individualistic approaches is resulting in an under-developed application of systems theory to settings. This is surprising, given that the paradigmatic shift from reductionism to systems is mirrored in health promo-tion in the shift from focusing on individual behaviour to the entire setting. Moreover, the settings methodology clearly recognizes wholeness and the need to consider interrelationships within settings, rather than elemental parts. It is the inherent unpredictability and messiness of complex systems which, the authors argue, is presenting a challenge to practitioners. Tolerance of complexity and unpredictability is therefore seen as a necessary skill for whole systems thinking.

The issue of complexity is revisited by Scriven in Chapter 4, when the argu-ment is posed that partnerships in settings can be thwarted by a range of com-plexities. One of these complexities is the plethora of terminology used and misused within partnership discourse. Definitions are offered for some of this terminology but, it is contended, confusion around meaning still abounds. Nonetheless, an essential premise of the chapter is that partnership working is a fundamental principle on which settings work should be established. The opportunities for collaborative, cooperative and partnership working have to be embraced in order to advance settings. In turn, it is argued that settings provide the structure and the milieu in which partnerships are formed and maintained. There is, therefore, a synergistic and co-dependent relationship between settings and partnerships. A major problem is the lack of evidence for this synergy, or indeed for the benefits that are said to be imparted from partnership engagement. There is a rallying call for evaluation and recommendations made to establish both the process and outcome indicators of success.

The theme of evaluation is the focus of the last chapters in this part of the book. Because of the complexity of settings as systems as identified by all of the authors, there are numerous pitfalls to planning and implementation, a point argued by South and Woodall in their chapter on planning and evaluating health promotion (Chapter 5). Complexity can lead to some settings-based projects resulting in unanticipated outcomes that need to be captured in evaluation and the authors recommend collaborative and developmental evaluation in these settings. The problem is compounded, the authors argue, because the multifariousness of settings precludes the use of experimental design on both pragmatic and methodological grounds.

Another challenge is that the emphasis embedded within settings calls for less service delivery for people, to more health outcomes with people. This requires robust programme planning processes and wider stakeholder participation to ensure that plans are relevant. Planning and evaluation in settings therefore, like partnership working, demands collaborative and developmental approaches. These approaches must take account of and capture added value of whole systems working as well as assessing the effectiveness of individual programmes and projects, with the interrelationships, interactions and synergies with and between settings taken into account.

As in other chapters, the weak evidence base is not only alluded to but critiqued. The argument is that settings are legitimized through an act of faith rather than through robust research and evaluation. The conceptual variances, pragmatic influences and differences in the size and type of setting are identified as a major inhibitor of evidence informed practice. Building a substantive view of what works in settings is challenging. Planning and evaluation are said to be informed by an ecological model that recognizes that health is determined by various environmental, organizational and personal factors. The focus for planning is therefore on supporting system change through policy development, participation and partnership working.

Conclusions

The dearth of generic frameworks that support practitioners to plan and design settings work has arguably created a gap between the theory of settings approaches and the implementation in practice. No two settings are alike, which makes the transferability of what works problematic. A major difficulty is that the whole system philosophy of the settings approach demands consideration of all those who interact with or are part of the setting.

Some interesting insights are offered about the theoretical underpinning of settings approaches in different contexts that will underpin the chapters in Part II. A number of conundrums are presented that those promoting health in settings must address. Through the examination of these fundamental issues, the chapters in this section represent an important conceptual foundation for the rest of the book. The authors move beyond simply describing basic principles to making recommendations based on their assessment of current and future trends in settings.

Those professionals with a responsibility to promote health are undoubtedly facing challenges within settings. Confronting these challenges will require concerted efforts, systems thinking and innovatory and outward looking, rather than insular, ways of working. This must include effective, collaborative, long term planning and the combining of resources between different statutory and non-statutory agencies. Health partnerships within settings should be wide ranging and are necessary because progress both within and between settings will only be achieved through the wider participation of all stakeholders.

The overriding deduction is that there is much to be done in the development of settings as key forums to promote health. There is no room for rhetoric or complacency. There are serious, praxis and theoretical matters that need to be addressed. Health promoters will have a key role in arguing for a shift of focus from measuring individual actions in settings to capturing system change in relation to wider determinants. These are daunting challenges that require enhanced workforce capacity and capability if system thinking is to permeate at a practice level within settings. The concerns over a questionable evidence base is discussed in a number of chapters, but it is clear that if this is to be advanced then innovative evaluation methods have to be developed and delivered.

Finally, a fundamental conclusion to this part of the book is that while there are many challenges still to be overcome, the settings approach is at the heart of health promotion, as a radical alternative to earlier technical approaches to health education. The chapters offer pragmatic solutions and fundamental understandings that will enable health promoters to engage with settings work in a way that enables these challenges to be addressed.

2

The Settings Approach: Looking Back, Looking Forward

Mark Dooris

Aims

- To provide an overview of the history and evolution of the settings approach
- To outline its conceptual development
- To discuss key contemporary challenges for the settings approach
- To propose opportunities for addressing these challenges and ensuring continued relevance for twenty-first century practice

---

Health promotion has long recognized the value of utilizing settings such as healthcare, workplaces and schools as influential channels for reaching defined populations (Mullen et al., 1995). In this way, settings, alongside population groups and health topics or problems, make up the traditional three-dimensional matrix used to organize health promotion programmes, particularly those concerned with individual behaviour change. However, what has become known as the settings approach moves beyond this mechanistic view of delivering interventions in a setting, appreciating that the places in which people live their lives are themselves crucially important in determining health (Dooris et al., 2007). A number of terms have been used in relation to this focus on context. These include 'settings for health', 'the settings approach', 'the settings-based approach', 'health promoting settings' and 'healthy settings'. While it is possible to identify semantic differences, the terms have increasingly been used interchangeably, with a dual focus on context and methods (Dooris, 2006).

The history and evolution of the settings approach

The settings approach has its origins within the World Health Organization (WHO) Health for All movement (WHO, 1980, 1981), which was instrumental in the development of the new public health, with its focus on how physical, social, economic and political environments affect health and wellbeing. Within this context, the Ottawa Charter (WHO, 1986) presented a framework for health promotion with an explicit focus on settings. Describing health promotion as the process of enabling people to increase control over and improve their health, the Charter stated:

> Health is created and lived by people within the settings of their everyday life; where they learn, work, play and love. Health is created by caring for oneself and others, by being able to take decisions and have control over one's life circumstances, and by ensuring that the society one lives in creates conditions that allow the attainment of health by all its members. Caring, holism and ecology are essential issues in developing strategies for health promotion. (WHO, 1986: 3–4)

From the late 1980s, the settings approach emerged across Europe and globally. Launched by WHO in 1987 as a small European project, Healthy Cities rapidly grew to become a global movement (Tsouros, 1991). Drawing on this experience, developments took place at the European level within settings such as schools, prisons, hospitals and universities (Barnekow et al., 2000; Squires and Strobl, 1996; Tsouros, 1993; Tsouros et al., 1998). In parallel, similar developments took place elsewhere, the WHO Western Pacific Region developing Healthy Islands and Healthy Marketplaces (Galea et al., 2000; WHO, 2004); the WHO South-East Asia Region promoting a Healthy District programme as an umbrella for smaller settings projects (WHO, 2002); and Canada launching a Healthy Communities network (O'Neill et al., 2000).

Subsequent international health promotion conferences served to legitimize further the settings approach. The Sundsvall Statement argued that a call for the creation of supportive environments is a practical proposal for public health action at the local level, with a focus on settings for health that allow for broad community involvement and control (WHO, 1991: 4), while the Jakarta Declaration asserted that settings for health contribute an important infrastructure for health promotion and comprehensive approaches to health development are the most effective suggesting that particular settings offer practical opportunities for the implementation of comprehensive strategies (WHO, 1997: 3).

By the millennium, there were national and international programmes and networks covering settings as diverse as regions, cities, islands, districts, schools, hospitals, marketplaces, workplaces, prisons and universities. This provided legitimacy for the inclusion of 'settings for health' within the WHO Health Promotion Glossary (WHO, 1998a) as well as within WHO regional policy frameworks. For instance, Target 13 of the European Health 21 publication stated that 'by the year 2015, people in the region should have greater opportunities to live in healthy physical and social environments at home, at school, at the workplace and in the local community' (WHO, 1998b: 100). While the Bangkok Charter (WHO, 2005) and Nairobi Call to Action (WHO, 2009) both highlighted the role of settings, neither gave as high profile an endorsement as had the Ottawa Charter or Jakarta Declaration. By way of contrast, Shaping the Future of Health Promotion (IUHPE/CCHPR, 2007) reflected on the success of the approach and called for its reach to be extended.

The settings approach: conceptual development

As highlighted above, the Ottawa Charter represented an important catalyst for the settings approach. Kickbusch (1996: 5) has suggested that its holistic socio-ecological model of health led to the settings approach becoming the starting point for WHO's lead health promotion programmes, by 'shifting the focus from the deficit model of disease to the health potentials inherent in the social and institutional settings of everyday life ... [and] pioneer[ing] strategies that strengthened both sense of place and sense of self'.

The rationale for the settings approach is based on an appreciation that health is determined not only by individual lifestyles and so-called health services, but by wider social, economic, environmental, organizational and cultural circumstances. The approach has the potential to increase effectiveness by focusing on settings not only as channels for delivering interventions, but also as contexts which in themselves influence wellbeing directly and indirectly through social rules, norms, values and interrelationships (Dooris et al., 2007; Poland et al., 2009). More specifically, it views health as both an asset for and outcome of effectively functioning settings (Dooris et al., 1998) and represents a response to the realization that many risk factors are interrelated and can be best tackled through comprehensive, integrated programmes in appropriate settings where people live, work and interact (Department of Health, Social Services and Public Safety, 2002). Figure 2.1

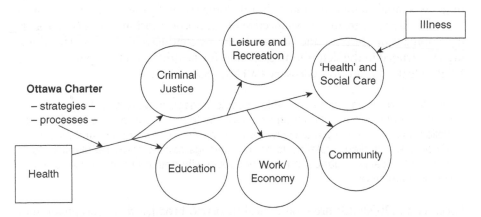

Figure 2.1 Putting 'health' into settings (reproduced with permission from Dooris (2004) *Critical Public Health*, www.tandf.co.uk/journals, adapted from Grossman and Scala, 1993, with permission from WHO)

applies this thinking, showing how health needs to be integrated into settings and social systems of everyday life.

Conceptualizing healthy settings

The 1990s saw increasing attempts to conceptualize the settings approach. Influenced by organization and management theory and drawing on the early experience of Health Promoting Hospitals, Barić (1993, 1994) emphasized the relationship between environmental and personal factors within settings. Arguing that the shift from a problem-based to a settings-based approach required a shift of emphasis from a medical to an organizational model, Barić articulated his understanding of the hospital setting as a system with an input (clients), a production process (care and treatment) and an output (health gain of clients). His framework has provided the basis for many subsequent developments in relation to healthy settings, suggesting that the approach requires a threefold commitment to: creating a healthy working and living environment; integrating health promotion into the daily activities of the setting; and reaching out into the community in the form of healthy alliances. Around the same time, Grossman and Scala (1993) argued the case for the settings approach in terms of intervening in social systems to bring about organizational change, emphasizing competencies required for this new health promotion approach and advocating project management as the key instrument for introducing and facilitating change.

Wenzel (1997) responded to this European based body of work, and in particular to that of Barić by questioning its theoretical integrity. He suggested that despite drawing a distinction between carrying out health promotion activities within a setting and developing as a health promoting setting, the literature perpetuated the mechanistic view of health promotion as primarily concerned with individual behaviour change. Emphasizing the connections between people and their environment and suggesting that settings can be understood in terms of the relationship between context and patterns of action, Wenzel defined settings as spatial, temporal and cultural domains of face-to-face interaction in everyday life that, from the perspective of health promotion, are crucial for the development of lifestyles and living conditions conducive to health. This thinking was echoed in the definition of 'settings for health' that later appeared in the WHO Health Promotion Glossary (WHO, 1998a: 19):

> The place or social context in which people engage in daily activities in which environmental, organizational and personal factors interact to affect health and wellbeing ... where people actively use and shape the environment and thus create or solve problems relating to health. Settings can normally be identified as having physical boundaries, a range of people with defined roles, and an organizational structure.

Green et al. (2000: 23) drew on critical theory to broaden this conceptualization and similarly argue against an instrumental view of settings as vehicles for delivering interventions. They also implicitly challenged the WHO definition by emphasizing that most settings do not have health as their raison d'être, suggesting that they are not only physically bounded space-times in which people come together to perform specific tasks, usually orientated to goals other than health, but also arenas of sustained interaction, with pre-existing structures, policies, characteristics, institutional values, and both formal and informal sanctions on behaviours.

While Wenzel was criticized for what was seen as his provocative and unduly harsh stance (Mittelmark, 1997), his pioneering role in critically exploring the concept of settings is widely acknowledged. Significantly, he drew extensively on Bronfenbrenner (1979, 1994), whose work in the field of ecological psychology contends that human development occurs in nested settings within a number of interconnected layers. In doing so, he intimated the importance of moving beyond a simplistic conceptualization of settings as discrete and homogenous, emphasizing their interconnectedness and specificity.

Typologies of healthy settings practice

Closely linked to advances in conceptualization, a number of writers have attempted to categorize healthy settings practice. Recognizing that there continues to be significant variation within the field of healthy settings, Whitelaw et al. (2001) have identified a range of problems involved in the development and application of settings-based models. These included the homogenization of practice, where divergent activities are unhelpfully brought under a single settings banner, the consequent sense of failure when practice does not live up to the theoretical ideal and the use of the settings label for traditional health promotion concerned only with individual behaviour change. They responded by formulating a typology distinguishing different forms of settings-based practice. Acknowledging that there are not only different models of health promotion and different analyses of the problem and solution in terms of individual and organizational focus, but also different organizational contexts with different degrees of opportunity and constraint, they identified five types of practice (see Table 2.1):

- the **passive model**, in which the problem and solution are understood to depend on the individual
- the **active model**, in which the problem is understood to rest with the individual, and the solution is understood to depend on action at the level of both the individual and the setting (that the setting can help shape individual behaviour)
- the **vehicle model**, in which the problem is seen to lie primarily within the system, and the solution is understood to be dependent on learning from individually focused topic-based projects
- the **organic model**, in which the problem is understood to lie within the setting, and the solution is seen to comprise the actions of a collection of individual actions
- the **comprehensive model**, in which the setting is viewed as an entity beyond the individuals within it, and both the problem and the solution are seen to lie within the system.

While, on the one hand, they present what is essentially a representational typology of different models of settings activity and caution against a one-size-fits-all

Table 2.1 Five types of settings-based health promotion

Type/model	Core perspective/ analysis of problem-solution	Relationship between the health promotion and the setting	Practical focus of activity
Passive	The problem and solution rest within the behaviour and action of individuals	Setting is passive: only provides access to participants and medium for intervention; health promotion occurs in setting independent of settings features	Mass media and communication, individual education
Active	The problem lies within the behaviour of individuals, some of the solution lies in the setting	Setting provides 'active' and comprehensive resources to fulfil health promotion goals; health promotion utilizes setting resources	Mass media and communication, individual education plus complementary work on policy development and structural change around the specific topic area
Vehicle	The problem lies within the setting, the solution is learning from individually-based projects	Health promotion initiatives provide an appropriate means for highlighting the need for broader setting development; health promotion seen as a vehicle for setting change	Principal focus on developing policies and bringing about structural change using feeder activity from mass media and communication, individual education
Organic	The problem lies within the setting, the solution in the actions of individuals	Organic setting processes involving communication and participation are inherently linked to health and are thus 'health promoting'	Facilitating and strengthening collective/ community action
Comprehensive/ Structural	The problem and the solution lie in the setting	Broad setting structures and cultures inherently linked to health and are thus 'health promoting'; health promotion as central component of comprehensive setting development	Focus on developing policies and bringing about structural change

Source: Adapted from Whitelaw et al. (2001), reproduced with permission from Oxford University Press, http://heapro.oxfordjournals.org

approach, they also go beyond description to argue that those who deploy a settings model need to ensure that their work is more than simply a repackaging of traditional individualistic health education in a particular setting (Whitelaw et al., 2001: 348).

This view has been reinforced by Johnson and Baum (2001) in relation to work on Health Promoting Hospitals. Drawing on a review of literature and practice, they proposed a typology based on degree of organizational commitment and types of health promotion activities undertaken, identifying four distinct approaches: doing a health promotion project; delegating health promotion to the role of a specific division, department or staff; being a health promotion setting; being a health promotion setting and improving the health of the community. They concluded by suggesting that the latter two forms of practice represent a more comprehensive understanding and application of the settings approach.

Towards a conceptual framework for healthy settings

The early twenty-first century has seen attempts to synthesize this earlier thinking. Although it would be premature to suggest that there is a widely accepted healthy settings theory, Dooris (2005) has proposed a conceptual framework that emphasizes the application of underpinning values such as equity, participation, empowerment, partnership and sustainability, and contends that the settings approach has three key characteristics:

ECOLOGICAL MODEL OF HEALTH PROMOTION
The settings approach is based on an ecological model, whereby health is understood to be determined by a complex interplay of environmental, organizational and personal factors. This understanding has shaped the settings approach as a framework for health promotion, reflecting a change of focus from the individual to the population within a setting, from pathogenesis to salutogenesis (Antonovsky, 1987, 1996), and from a reductionist emphasis on single issues, risk factors and linear causality towards an holistic concern to develop supportive contexts in the places that people live their lives (Kickbusch, 1996, 2003). This understanding also emphasizes the interaction between people and their environment, or agency and structure, as highlighted by both Wenzel (1997) and Green et al. (2000).

SYSTEMS PERSPECTIVE
Reflecting this ecological thinking and drawing also on organizational theory, the approach understands settings as complex dynamic systems with inputs, throughputs and outputs (Paton et al., 2005). A systems perspective recognizes the interconnectedness, interrelationships, interdependencies and synergy between different components and looks not only at these different parts of the whole, but also at the spaces between them (Capra, 1983; French and Bell, 1999). To quote Senge (1990: 68), 'Systems thinking is a

discipline for seeing wholes. It is a framework for seeing interrelationships rather than things, for seeing patterns of change rather than static "snap-shots"'. Systems thinking also acknowledges that settings do not function as trivial machines (Grossman and Scala, 1993), but as complex systems that are at times unpredictable. This complexity becomes even more apparent when it is recognized that each setting functions as an open system with permeable boundaries, interacting with the wider environment and, within this, other settings (Green et al., 2000), a perspective that echoes the work of Bronfenbrenner (1979, 1994).

WHOLE SYSTEM DEVELOPMENT AND CHANGE FOCUS

Thirdly, informed by this ecological understanding and systems perspective, the approach uses organization development and/or community development to introduce and manage change within the setting in its totality, applying 'whole system thinking' (Pratt et al., 1999). Reflecting on the absence of a health system in most developed countries, Dooris and Hunter (2007) have suggested that 'health promotion can be viewed as an intervention in social and organizational systems to improve health [whereby] health ... becomes an integrative goal'. Developing thinking first articulated by Barić (1993, 1994), it is significant that the approach uses multiple, interconnected interventions and programmes to integrate health within the culture, routine life and mainstream business of a specific setting; ensure living and working environments that promote greater health and productivity; and engage with and promote the health of the wider community. Exploring how emerging theory can be meaningfully translated into practice and facilitate whole system change, Dooris has proposed the Question of Balance Model (Dooris, 2004; Dooris et al., 2007). This emphasizes core underpinning values and the importance of drawing on and utilizing a wide range of different methods, the choice dependent on the particular focus and context of the work. It goes on to highlight three key balancing acts pivotal to the success of the settings approach in achieving whole system change (see Figure 2.2):

- It is necessary to keep health high on the agenda through high profile projects and initiatives, while also working to embed a long term commitment to health within the setting's ethos, culture and policy and planning processes.
- It is important to enable wide-ranging stakeholder involvement in prioritizing needs and planning and delivering action, while securing high level commitment, advocacy and corporate responsibility for health, wellbeing and sustainable development.
- It is essential to respond to the public health agenda and ensure that the setting is at the forefront of action to address key issues pertaining to its population, while simultaneously mapping health challenges against key drivers relating to the particular setting's core business and demonstrating the contribution that the settings approach can make.

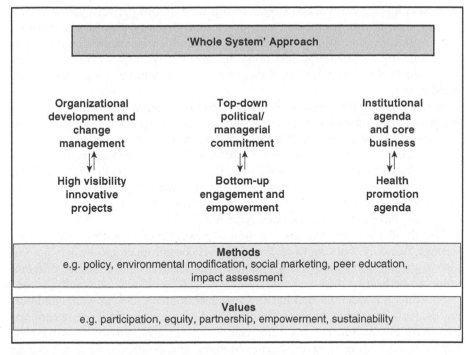

Figure 2.2 A model for conceptualizing and operationalizing the health promoting settings approach (adapted from Dooris (2004), reproduced with permission from *Critical Public Health*, www.tandf.co.uk/journals

Identifying and responding to key contemporary challenges

Having outlined the origins, history and evolution of the settings approach and explored its conceptual development, it is important to highlight key contemporary challenges and consider opportunities to effectively address these, thereby helping to ensure continued relevance for twenty-first century practice.

Ensuring that the settings approach tackles inequalities

Concern that the settings approach could serve to exacerbate health inequalities has been highlighted by writers such as Kickbusch (1995, 1997), Galbally (1997) and Green et al. (2000). They have contended that its focus on formal settings inevitably leaves out many of the most marginalized and disenfranchised individuals and groups within society, such as the homeless, the unemployed and children who are excluded from school. A further issue concerns the relationship of settings initiatives to macro-policy, one criticism being that the approach might divert attention from underlying determinants of health that are often outwith the control of any one setting. Green et al. (2000: 24) have also highlighted concerns related to power in and between settings, suggesting that health promotion may have inadvertently played into existing power relations and alliances by aligning itself with management and thereby marginalizing or alienating less powerful groups (such as workers, students or patients). In responding to these challenges, a number of points can be highlighted.

Firstly, it is valuable to strengthen and learn from programmes that are already explicitly engaging with issues of exclusion and inequality, such as Healthy Cities (Ritsatakis, 2009), Healthy Prisons (Baybutt et al., 2006), Healthy Care for Looked After Children (National Children's Bureau, 2005), Healthy Sports Stadia (Ratinckx and Crabb, 2005) and Healthy Nightlife (Bellis et al., 2002).

Secondly, it is important to extend the reach of the settings approach to non-traditional, non-institutional and informal settings where people shop, get their hair done, have a drink, go out and have fun (Kickbusch, 1997: 433).

Thirdly, it is important to take account of power relations within and between settings, not only working to secure high level commitment and leadership, but also engaging and empowering multiple stakeholders and enabling different voices to be heard.

Fourthly, it is essential that healthy settings initiatives look upwards and outwards, focusing on the structures, policies and practices that will create supportive environments and make a difference (St Leger, 1997) and at the same time explicitly addressing broader social, economic and political contextual factors (Baum, 2002).

Lastly, as recommended by the Commission on Social Determinants of Health (2008), it is important to build evidence by evaluating the health equity impacts of different settings programmes.

Joining up settings

Despite a growing appreciation in the literature that settings should be viewed as interrelated open systems, there is a continuing tendency for different settings programmes to operate independently and without reference to each other. It is therefore important to encourage them to network horizontally, making links with other settings, seeking to understand more fully the synergies or contradictions between them, and maximizing their potential contribution to public health beyond their own boundaries by exploring joined up delivery through wider partnership mechanisms (Dooris, 2004). In responding effectively to this challenge, a number of points can be highlighted.

Firstly, health issues do not respect organizational or geographical boundaries. In order to tackle complex issues, it is therefore important to recognize that a problem made manifest in one setting may have its roots in a different setting (for example, bullying in schools may have its roots in neighbourhood relationships).

Secondly, people's lives straddle various settings, both concurrently (for instance, someone's time might be divided between their workplace, a place of study, leisure and home) and consecutively (such as an offender who moves from a community into prison and subsequently undergoes resettlement into a community). Effective health promotion therefore requires a holistic perspective that appreciates these interconnections.

Thirdly, settings function at multiple levels and may be located within the context of another (a school, for example, may be located within a neighbourhood, within a city, within a region). Viewed in this way, it is essential to map and understand the influences that different settings exert and to consider how initiatives in elemental settings such as healthy schools or healthy workplaces can contribute to the goals of initiatives in contextual settings such as healthy cities (Galea et al., 2000).

Connecting agendas: towards healthy and sustainable settings

A third key challenge is to move beyond the boundaries of traditional health promotion and forge connections to parallel agendas. Specifically, the importance of connecting health and sustainable development has been highlighted over recent years (Griffiths and Stewart, 2008; Griffiths et al., 2009). As Orme and Dooris (2010) contend, these agendas are closely interlinked in a number of ways: the concept of sustainable development embraces environmental, social and economic dimensions and aspires to health-enhancing communities, societies and environments; it is widely recognized that health is determined by a range of environmental, social and economic influences and that the health of people, places and the planet are interdependent; and the causes and manifestations of unsustainable development and poor health are interrelated and frequently pose further interconnected challenges. In particular, there has been growing recognition of the long term public health benefits of carbon reduction and climate change mitigation alongside an appreciation that action in relation to key issues such as transport and food offers the potential to achieve both environmental and health goals (Griffiths et al., 2009).

With regard to settings programmes, a number of writers have highlighted the challenge of aligning and integrating agendas, pointing to a vision of healthy and sustainable settings (Bentley 2007; Davis and Cooke, 2007; Dooris, 1999; Orme and Dooris, 2010). In responding to this challenge, a number of points can be made.

Firstly, those working within healthy settings programmes need to be proactive in forging alliances with parallel programmes, finding new and innovative ways to coordinate, integrate and enhance synergy between public health and sustainable development and when necessary daring to let go of the explicit language of health (Dooris, 2006).

Secondly, it is important to assert and translate into practice the whole system ecological perspective that underpins the settings approach. By so doing, there will be a natural focus on the interconnections between the health of people, the health of their environments and the health of the planet , as discussed by Poland

and Dooris (2010), who also highlight five other principles for progressive practice as a means of effectively grounding an integrated healthy and sustainable settings approach: starting where people are; rooting practice in place; deepening the sociopolitical analysis; building on strengths and successes; and building resilience.

Thirdly, as discussed by Orme and Dooris (2010) in relation to universities, many settings have considerable leverage for change at institutional and sectoral levels. It is therefore essential that we seek opportunities for the settings approach to be a catalyst for corporate social responsibility, developing settings as corporate citizens that contribute simultaneously to public health and sustainable development and demonstrate the role of low carbon living in improving population health.

Evidence and evaluation

In terms of effectiveness, the settings approach is widely seen to have a range of benefits, its whole system ecological approach contributing a richness and coherence that can make health promotion more relevant, appropriate and effective than narrowly focused topic-based and disease-specific interventions (Dooris et al., 2007). However, although a number of reviews point to the effectiveness of healthy settings programmes (see, for example, IUHPE, 2000; Rootman et al., 2001; Stewart-Brown, 2006), there is still much truth in the observation of St Leger (1997: 100) that the settings approach has been legitimated more through an act of faith than through rigorous research and evaluation studies and much more attention needs to be given to building the evidence and learning from it.

Reflecting on this, it has been argued that there are three interrelated challenges facing those who seek to build a convincing evidence base for the settings approach (Dooris, 2005; Dooris et al., 2007). The first is that the diversity of both conceptual understandings and real-life practice brought together under the banner of healthy settings makes it difficult to generate a substantive body of research allowing comparability and transferability. Second, the established evidence system for public health continues to retain a primary focus on specific diseases/problems and single risk factor interventions rather than multiple interventions and settings. While a few evidence reviews have looked specifically at programmes such as Health Promoting Schools and drawn promising conclusions regarding the value of a whole system approach (for example, Lister-Sharp et al., 1999; Stewart-Brown, 2006), most reviews that consider a particular setting are primarily concerned to assess the value of discrete interventions designed to impact on one specific risk factor. Third, it is very complex to evaluate the settings approach, characterized as it is by an ecological perspective, systems thinking and a concern to integrate health and wellbeing within routine life and core business. This complexity has reinforced a tendency to evaluate only discrete projects in settings, and mitigated against the generation of credible evidence of effectiveness for the settings approach as a whole. In responding effectively to these challenges, a number of points can be highlighted:

Firstly, it is important to develop and strengthen theory while at the same time acknowledging and clarifying similarity and difference within and across categories of settings (Dooris, 2005). Such a focus is important not only for supporting policy and practice, but also for enabling more appropriate evaluation and contributing to the generation of evidence. There is an increasing body of work on theory-based evaluation and its use in relation to complex initiatives (see, for example, Birckmayer and Weiss, 2000; de Leeuw and Skovgaard, 2005; Pawson and Tilley, 1997). Specifically, Dooris et al. (2007) have discussed the value of engaging with critical realism and realist evaluation, suggesting that it offers the potential to unpack the mechanism of how complex programmes work (or why they fail) in particular contexts and settings (Pawson et al., 2004: 1).

Secondly, if evaluation is to capture the added value of whole system working and help generate evidence of effectiveness for the settings approach, it must do more than focus separately on each intervention operating within the context of a settings initiative. Instead, it must look at the whole and attempt to map and understand interrelationships, interactions and synergies with regard to different groups of the population, components of the system and 'health' issues (Dooris, 2005). This means moving beyond conventional evaluation approaches that are both linear and reductionist, and engaging with complexity theory (Dooris et al., 2007; Keshavarz et al., 2010; Rowling and Jeffreys, 2006).

Finally, if the settings approach is to retain integrity and fulfil its potential, it is essential that it is not hijacked by proponents of individually focused behaviour change and reduced to health promotion in a setting. Following Syme (1996) and Kickbusch (1996, 1997, 2003), it is crucial to reassert that most health risks and the determinants of health are systemic and located within complex, dynamic and interactive social relationships which themselves are determined by social institutions and organizations, including families, communities, schools and workplaces (Dooris and Hunter, 2007).

Summary points

- As discussed above, it will be necessary to extend the reach of the settings approach into non-traditional settings. In so doing, it will be important to explore where virtual settings fit into the picture. Of particular relevance is the growing influence of information technology and the consequent challenges and opportunities (Kickbusch, 1997; Poland et al., 2009). It is clear that developments are increasingly testing a simplistic understanding of settings as places involving face-to-face interaction, through impacts such as distance learning, online healthcare and Internet chatrooms. At the same time, the influence of Internet-based advertising and marketing creates new challenges and opportunities for public health, with particular implications for certain settings.

- With its holistic focus, systems perspective and explicit commitment to moving beyond reductionist linear thinking, the settings approach has obvious relevance

(Continued)

(Continued)

and resonance to the challenges involved in tackling the 'wicked problems' that characterize our globalized twenty-first century world. Recent analyses of problems such as obesity and climate change emphasize the centrality of systems thinking and the importance of harnessing the influence of settings to achieve meaningful change (Butland et al., 2007; Griffiths et al., 2009).

- Linked to this, it will be important for health promotion, and within this, the settings approach, to position itself as we approach a future characterized by converging crises of climate change, peak oil and environmental degradation. Poland and Dooris (2010) contend that, while there have been attempts to green settings-related practice, more radical action will be required if we are to face up to the future. Commenting on the balance between these interconnected crises and the economic, social and health benefits of relocalization, they suggest that 'it is increasingly apparent that helping midwife the emergence of a new post-carbon society is perhaps the most important health promotion project of modern human history'.

Online Further Reading

Dooris, M. (2006) 'Editorial – Healthy settings: future directions', *Promotion and Education*, XIII (1): 4–6.

This paper provides a succinct overview of the settings approach, suggesting that it can make a valuable contribution to planning and delivering health and wellbeing in ways that take account of complexity, within the places that people live their lives. In looking to the future, it focuses on three key challenges – clarifying the theoretical base, staying with the bigger picture and developing the evidence base.

Dooris, M. (2009) 'Holistic and sustainable health improvement: the contribution of the settings-based approach to health promotion', *Perspectives in Public Health*, 129: 29–36.

This paper reviews the origins, history and conceptualization of the settings approach. It then takes stock of current practice both internationally and nationally, noting its continuing importance worldwide and its inconsistent profile and utilization across the four UK countries. It goes on to explore its applicability and future development in relation to three key issues – inequalities and inclusion, place-shaping and systems-based responses to complex problems – arguing that it offers an important contribution to holistic and sustainable health improvement.

References

Antonovsky, A. (1987) *Unraveling the Mystery of Health*. San Francisco: Jossey-Bass.
Antonovsky, A. (1996) 'The salutogenic model as a theory to guide health promotion', *Health Promotion International*, 11: 11–18.

Barić, L. (1993) 'The settings approach – implications for policy and strategy', *Journal of the Institute of Health Education*, 31: 17–24.

Barić, L. (1994) *Health Promotion and Health Education in Practice. Module 2: The Organizational Model.* Altrincham: Barns Publications.

Barnekow Rasmussen, V. and Rivett, D. (2000) The European Network of Health Promoting Schools – an alliance of health, education and democracy. *Health Education*, 100: 61–7.

Baum, F. (2002) *The New Public Health*, 2nd edn, Oxford: Oxford University Press.

Baybutt, M., Hayton, P. and Dooris, M. (2006) 'Prisons in England and Wales: an important public health opportunity?', in J. Douglas, S. Earle, S. Handsley, C. Lloyd and S. Spurr (eds), *A Reader in Promoting Public Health: Challenge and Controversy*. London: Sage/Milton Keynes: Open University.

Bellis, M.A., Hughes, K. and Lowey, H. (2002) 'Healthy nightclubs and recreational substance use: from a harm minimisation to healthy settings approach', *Addictive Behaviors*, 27: 1025–35.

Bentley, M. (2007) 'Healthy Cities, local environmental action and climate change', *Health Promotion International*, 22: 246–53.

Birckmayer, J. and Weiss, C. (2000) 'Theory-based evaluation in practice. What do we learn?', *Evaluation Review*, 24: 407–31.

Bronfenbrenner, U. (1979) *The Ecology of Human Development. Experiments by Nature and Design.* Cambridge, MA: Harvard University Press.

Bronfenbrenner, U. (1994). 'Ecological models of human development', in T. Husen and T. Postlethwaite (eds), *International Encyclopedia of Education*, 2nd edn, vol. 3. Oxford: Elsevier, pp. 1643–7.

Butland, B., Jebb, S., Kopelman, P., McPherson, K., Thomas, S., Mardell, J. and Parry, J. (2007) *Tackling Obesities: Future Choices – Project Report.* London: Foresight Programme, Government Office for Science.

Capra, F. (1983) *The Turning Point: Science, Society and the Rising Culture.* London: Flamingo.

Commission on Social Determinants of Health (2008) *Closing the Gap in a Generation: Health Equity through Action on the Social Determinants of Health.* Final Report of the Commission on Social Determinants of Health. Geneva: World Health Organization.

Davis, J. and Cooke, S. (2007) 'Educating for a healthy, sustainable world: an argument for integrating Health Promoting Schools and Sustainable Schools', *Health Promotion International*, 22: 346–53.

Department of Health, Social Services and Public Safety (2002) *Investing for Health*. Belfast: DHSSPH.

Dooris, M. (1999) 'Healthy cities and local agenda 21: The UK experience – challenges for the new millennium', *Health Promotion International*, 14: 365–75.

Dooris, M. (2004) 'Joining up settings for health: a valuable investment for strategic partnerships?', *Critical Public Health*, 14: 49–61.

Dooris, M. (2005) 'Healthy settings: challenges to generating evidence of effectiveness', *Health Promotion International*, 21: 55–65.

Dooris, M. (2006) 'Editorial – Healthy settings: future directions', *Promotion and Education*, XIII (1): 1–5.

Dooris, M. and Hunter, D. (2007) 'Organizations and settings for promoting public health', in C. Lloyd, S. Handsley, J. Douglas, S. Earle and S. Spurr (eds), *Policy and Practice in Promoting Public Health*. London: Sage/Milton Keynes: Open University.

Dooris, M., Dowding, G., Thompson, J. and Wynne, C. (1998) 'The settings-based approach to health promotion', in A. Tsouros, G. Dowding, J. Thompson and M. Dooris (eds), *Health Promoting Universities: Concept, Experience and Framework for Action*. Copenhagen: WHO Regional Office for Europe.

Dooris, M., Poland, B., Kolbe, L., de Leeuw, E., McCall, D. and Wharf-Higgins, J. (2007) 'Healthy settings: building evidence for the effectiveness of whole system health promotion – challenges and future directions', in D.V. McQueen and C.M. Jones (eds), *Global Perspectives on Health Promotion Effectiveness*. New York: Springer Science and Business Media.

French, W. and Bell, C. (1999) *Organization Development: Behavioural Science Interventions for Organization Improvement*. Englewood Cliffs, NJ: Prentice Hall.

Galbally, R. (1997) 'Health-promoting environments: who will miss out?', *Australian and New Zealand Journal of Public Health*, 21: 429–30.

Galea, G., Powis, B. and Tamplin, S. (2000) 'Healthy islands in the Western Pacific – international settings development', *Health Promotion International*, 15: 169–78.

Green, L., Poland, B. and Rootman, I. (2000) 'The settings approach to health promotion', in B. Poland, L. Green and I. Rootman (eds), *Settings for Health Promotion: Linking Theory and Practice*. Sage: London.

Griffiths, J. and Stewart, L. (2008) *Sustaining a Healthy Future*. London: Faculty of Public Health.

Griffiths, J., Rao, M., Adshead, F. and Thorpe, A. (eds) (2009) *The Health Practitioner's Guide to Climate Change. Diagnosis and Cure*. London: Earthscan.

Grossman, R. and Scala, K. (1993) *Health Promotion and Organizational Development: Developing Settings for Health*. Copenhagen: WHO Regional Office for Europe.

IUHPE (International Union for Health Promotion and Education) (2000) *The Evidence of Health Promotion Effectiveness. Shaping Public Health in a New Europe. Part Two: Evidence Book*. ECSC-EC-EAEC: Brussels.

IUHPE/CCHPR (International Union for Health Promotion and Education/ Canadian Consortium for Health Promotion Research) (2007) *Shaping the Future of Health Promotion*. Paris: IUHPE/Victoria, BC: CCHPR.

Johnson, A. and Baum, F. (2001) Health promoting hospitals: a typology of different organizational approaches to health promotion. *Health Promotion International*, 16: 281–7.

Keshavarz, N., Nutbeam, D., Rowling, L. and Khavarpour, F. (2010) 'Schools as social complex adaptive systems: a new way to understand the challenges of introducing the health promoting schools concept', *Social Science and Medicine*, 70: 1467–74.

Kickbusch, I. (1995) 'An overview to the settings-based approach to health promotion', in T. Theaker and J. Thompson (eds), *The Settings-based Approach to Health Promotion*. Conference Report. Welwyn Garden City: Hertfordshire Health Promotion.

Kickbusch, I. (1996) 'Tribute to Aaron Antonovsky – "what creates health"?', *Health Promotion International*, 11: 5–6.

Kickbusch, I. (1997) 'Health-promoting environments: the next steps', *Australian and New Zealand Journal of Public Health*, 21: 431–4.

Kickbusch, I. (2003) ,The contribution of the World Health Organization to a new public health and health promotion', *American Journal of Public Health*, 93: 383–8.

de Leeuw, E. and Skovgaard, T. (2005) 'Utility-driven evidence for healthy cities: problems with evidence generation and application', *Social Science and Medicine*, 61: 1331–41.

Lister-Sharp, D., Chapman, S., Stewart-Brown, S. and Soden, A. (1999) 'Health promoting schools and health promotion in school: Two systematic reviews', *Health Technology Assessment*, 3 (22):1–207.

Mittelmark, M. (1997) 'Editorial – Health promotion settings', *Internet Journal of Health Promotion*. Available at: http://rhpeo.net/ijhp-articles/1997/2/index.htm (accessed 2 November 2010).

Mullen, P., Evans, D., Forster, J., Gottlieb, N., Kreuter, M., Moon, R., O'Rourke, T. and Stretcher, V. (1995) Settings as an important dimension in health education/promotion policy, programs and research. *Health Education Quarterly*, 22: 329–45.

National Children's Bureau (2005) *Healthy Care Programme Handbook*. London: National Children's Bureau.

O'Neill, M., Pederson, A. and Rootman, I. (2000) 'Health promotion in Canada: declining or transforming?', *Health Promotion International*, 15: 135–41.

Orme, J. and Dooris, M. (2010) 'Integrating health and sustainability: the Higher Education sector as a timely catalyst', *Health Education Research*, 25: 425–37.

Paton, K., Sengupta, S. and Hassan, L. (2005) 'Settings, systems and organization development: the Healthy Living and Working Model', *Health Promotion International*, 20: 81–9.

Pawson, R. and Tilley, N. (1997) *Realistic Evaluation*. London: Sage.

Pawson, R., Greenhalgh, T., Harvey, G. and Walshe, K. (2004) *Realist Synthesis: An Introduction*. RMP Methods Paper 2/2004. Manchester: ESRC Research Methods Programme, University of Manchester.

Poland, B. and Dooris, M. (2010) 'A green and healthy future: a settings approach to building health, equity and sustainability', *Critical Public Health*, 20: 281–98.

Poland, B., Grupa, G. and McCall, D. (2009) 'Settings for health promotion: an analytic framework to guide intervention design and implementation', *Health Promotion Practice*, 10: 505–16.

Pratt, J., Gordon, P. and Plamping, D. (1999) *Working Whole Systems: Putting Theory into Practice in Organisations*. London: King's Fund.

Ratinckx, L. and Crabb, J. (2005) *The Healthy Stadia Toolkit. Developing Sustainable Partnerships for Local Health Improvement Strategies*. Preston: Healthy Settings Development Unit, University of Central Lancashire.

Ritsatakis, A. (2009) 'Equity and social determinants of health at a city level', *Health Promotion International*, 24: i81–i90.

Rootman, I., Goodstadt, M., Hyndman, B., McQueen, D., Potvin, L., Springett, J. and Ziglio, E. (eds) (2001) *Evaluation in Health Promotion: Principles and Perspectives*. Copenhagen: WHO Regional Office for Europe.

Rowling, L. and Jeffreys, V. (2006) 'Capturing complexity: integrating health and education research to inform health-promoting schools policy and practice', *Health Education Research*, 21: 705–18.

Senge, P. (1990) *The Fifth Discipline: The Art and Practice of the Learning Organization*. London: Random House.

Squires, N. and Strobl, J. (eds) (1996) *Healthy Prisons – A Vision for the Future*. Report of the First International Conference on Healthy Prisons, Liverpool, 24–27 March 1996. Liverpool: University of Liverpool.

St Leger, L. (1997) 'Health promoting settings: from Ottawa to Jakarta', *Health Promotion International*, 12: 99–101.

Stewart-Brown, S. (2006) *What Is the Evidence on School Health Promotion in Improving Health or Preventing Disease and, Specifically, What is the Effectiveness of the Health Promoting Schools Approach?* Health Evidence Network Report. Copenhagen: WHO Regional Office for Europe. Available at: www.euro.who.int/_data/assets/pdf_file/0007/74653/E88185.pdf (accessed 2 November 2010).

Syme, S.L. (1996) 'To prevent disease: the need for a new approach', in D. Blane, E. Brunner and R. Wilkinson (eds), *Health and Social Organization: Towards a Health Policy for the 21st Century.* London: Routledge.

Tsouros, A. (ed.) (1991) *World Health Organization Healthy Cities Project: A Project Becomes a Movement. Review of Progress 1987–1990.* Copenhagen: FADL Publishers/Milan: SOGESS.

Tsouros, A. (1993) 'Health Promoting Hospitals: European Perspectives', in Health Education Authority (ed.), *Health Promoting Hospitals: Principles and Practice.* London: Health Education Authority.

Tsouros, A., Dowding, G., Thompson, J. and Dooris, M. (eds) (1998) *Health Promoting Universities: Concept, Experience and Framework for Action.* Copenhagen: WHO Regional Office for Europe.

Wenzel, E. (1997) 'A comment on settings in health promotion', *Internet Journal of Health Promotion.* Available at: http://rhpeo.net/ijhp-articles/1997/1/index.htm (accessed 2 November 2010).

Whitelaw, S., Baxendale, A., Bryce, C., MacHardy, L., Young, I. and Witney, E. (2001) 'Settings based health promotion: a review', *Health Promotion International*, 16: 339–53.

WHO (World Health Organization) (1980) *European Regional Strategy for Health for All by the Year 2000.* Copenhagen: WHO Regional Office for Europe.

WHO (World Health Organization) (1981) *Global Strategy for Health for All by the Year 2000.* Geneva: WHO.

WHO (World Health Organization) (1986) *Ottawa Charter for Health Promotion.* Geneva: WHO.

WHO (World Health Organization) (1991) *Sundsvall Statement on Supportive Environments for Health.* Geneva: WHO.

WHO (World Health Organization) (1997) *Jakarta Declaration on Health Promotion into the 21st Century.* Geneva: WHO.

WHO (World Health Organization) (1998a) *Health Promotion Glossary.* Geneva: WHO.

WHO (World Health Organization) (1998b) *Health21 – The Health for All Policy for the WHO European Region – 21 Targets for the 21st Century.* Copenhagen: WHO Regional Office for Europe.

WHO (World Health Organization) (2002) *Integrated Management of Healthy Settings at the District Level. Report of an Intercountry Consultation.* Gurgaon, India, 7–11 May 2001. New Delhi: WHO Regional Office for South-East Asia.

WHO (World Health Organization) (2004) *Healthy Marketplaces in the Western Pacific: Guiding Future Action. Applying a Settings Approach to the Promotion of Health in Marketplaces.* Manila: WHO Regional Office for the Western Pacific.

WHO (World Health Organization) (2005) *Bangkok Charter for Health Promotion in a Globalized World.* Geneva: WHO.

WHO (World Health Organization) (2009) *Nairobi Call to Action for Closing the Implementation Gap in Health Promotion.* Geneva: WHO.

3

A Whole Systems Approach to Working in Settings

Margaret Hodgins and John Griffiths

Aims

- To link the paradigmatic shift from reductionism to a whole systems approach in scientific thinking generally, to the shift from individual behaviours to settings within health promotion
- To explore key elements of systems thinking in the context of the settings approach within health promotion
- To outline examples of successful healthy settings work employing a whole systems approach: the Management Standards Approach to work-related stress and the Bullying Prevention programme for schools
- To explore challenges and opportunities in adopting a whole systems approach to settings

---

Settings are complex dynamic systems, set within and interacting with larger systems such as the political or economic environment. This view of settings as systems is consistent with the core principles and theory of health promotion. While it is often the case that health problems or issues seen in systems are addressed by isolating and attending to specific elements or part of the system, for example the teachers in a school, or the canteen in a workplace, systems thinking advocates that change within a system can best be achieved by considering how the parts relate to one another and working with the system as a whole.

Paradigmatic shift

In the late 1800s Fredrick Winslow Taylor made a brave attempt to apply scientific principles to management in order to improve productivity in the steel industry in Philadelphia. Taylor, apparently appalled by the inefficiency of industrial practice, developed a science of work, in which he tried to standardize and simplify work by breaking down every job on the production line to specific elements. Having carefully measured sizes of tools, height and strength of workers, and time taken to move limbs, he selected workers and incentivized them through a piece-work system of pay. Taylor provided specification to managers on this basis in order to improve efficiency (Buchanan and Huczynski, 1985).

Taylor's unit of analysis was the individual worker and he seemingly disregarded the role of broader factors such as workers' relationships with other employees, management practices, organizational culture and the prevalent economic climate. Although Taylor's ideas may seem somewhat ridiculous today, his theory of efficiency was influential and was underpinned by an essential plank of scientific thought at that time: the principle of reductionism. Reductionism refers to our attempts to understand the nature of complex things by reducing them to their components or parts. Described as a machine model (French and Bell, 1998), it is summed up succinctly below:

> A machine has a designer who specifies the parts and how these interact. Only the designer needs to know how the whole works. The machine needs engineers to maintain it ... machines do not organize and maintain themselves, they do not naturally adapt to changing environments ... the parts of a machine are generally responsive rather then initiating action. They are expected to 'play their part' no more, no less. The machine works predominantly in sequence. It works as a whole because the relationships between the parts are designed in. (Pratt et al., 2005: 6)

Reductionism assumes that a system can be broken down into its individual components and understood by analysing the properties of each component, how it connects to the next component, and so on, along a linear type sequence. Reductionism has played a central role in many endeavours and while it has served science well in some respects, it has been challenged as a general paradigm. As a way of understanding the world it is seen to have limits and increasingly scientists (see for example, Manson, 2001) have moved to exploring the notion that we need to look at the whole system, rather than at a breakdown of its parts.

General systems theory (GST), the wellspring of systems thinking, is attributed to biologist von Bertalanffy. Von Bertalanffy (1968) proposed that there were principles of dynamic wholeness in systems that applied across many scientific disciplines, thus rejecting the notion that phenomena could be understood by reducing them to units. A system is characterized by the interdependence of interactions of the parts. The parts can only be understood in relation to the whole. Von Bertalanffy hoped to unify science with systems theory, perhaps an unrealistic goal. However, the idea was so important it is frequently described as a significant paradigm shift in scientific thinking. Systems theory can be summed up in the phrase 'the whole is greater than the sum of the parts', highlighting the need to consider the whole system over and above the constituent parts.

Systems theory has been seized by theorists and commentators in many disciplines, attesting to Von Bertalanffy's contention that the principles are not discipline-specific. It has proponents in life sciences, social sciences and management science, demonstrating the potency and utility of its core ideas. Later discussions of systems theory offer advances on earlier ideas in respect of the complexity of systems, the self-organizing capacity of systems and the unpredictability of systems. These advances are sometimes cast as a rejection of systems theory in favour of complexity theory (see, for example, Manson, 2001) or as a revision of earlier GST (Walby, 2007).

The healthy setting as a system

There is a strong correspondence between the principles of systems theory and the settings approach to health promotion (Dooris 2005, 2006; Dooris et al., 2007; Paton et al., 2005; Poland, 2007). Indeed, taking a systems perspective is one of the three interconnecting dimensions of the settings approach, as outlined by Dooris (2006). Clearly, settings are also systems. While acknowledging that a diversity of understandings and practice combine under the health promoting settings banner (Dooris, 2006: 4), the most ambitious and comprehensive of these describes the setting 'as an entity above the individuals in it', with Whitelaw et al. (2001: 344) unambiguously casting a setting as a system.

While some systems are theoretically considered closed systems, where interactions only occur among the system components and not the external environment, most systems are open systems that interact with the external environment. Open systems are described as having goals (existing for a purpose) and having inputs (people, resources, information) that are changed or transformed in some way and returned to the environment as outputs (Dooris, 2005). Systems theory also maintains that systems are predisposed to becoming increasingly differentiated and specialized over time (Paton et al., 2005). Health promotion settings that are also organizations comply with the features of open systems. Schools must work within the broader educational policy systems (see Part II, Chapter 9), prisons within the justice system (see Part II, Chapter 11) and workplaces within the economic and labour market environment (see Part III). However, while some settings (for example, schools, workplaces, prisons) have goals and tend to be specialized, settings such as cities (see Part II, Chapter 7) or neighbourhoods (see Part II, Chapter 6) are not organizations, they are clearly open, complex and provide intersecting contexts. All settings are inherently complex systems.

Three key dimensions of the paradigmatic shift between reductionism and systems theory are: (a) a shift from a focus on parts and objects to a focus on wholeness; (b) a shift from objective knowledge to contextual knowledge; and (c) a shift from an acceptance that parts have linear, predictable relationships with one another to an acknowledgment that systems are adaptive, with non-linear relationships and emergent properties. The following section will explore how these shifts are also required within health promotion in order to enable effective settings-based practice.

Refocusing from parts to whole systems thinking in healthy settings

The paradigmatic shift from reductionism to systems thinking in science is mirrored in the paradigmatic shift from the focus on individuals, health problems and risk factors to systems, organizations and environments in health promotion. The settings approach embodies this refocusing, its essence being the recognition that individuals cannot be treated in isolation from the larger social units in which they live (Green et al., 2000) and that these social units, living and working conditions, must be the target of health promotion interventions rather than individual behaviour. In this way, it can be argued that the settings approach is not an optional extra, but is in fact at the heart of health promotion, as a radical alternative to earlier technical approaches to health education.

Unfortunately, examples of health promotion interventions that focus only on parts remain plentiful, indicating the difficulty practitioners have adopting the systems perspective that underpins settings-based work. Indeed, some interventions in health promotion could be said to resemble Taylorism. Because of the dominant focus on the individual, the opportunities for pursuing the application of systems theory to settings is underdeveloped (Paton et al., 2005). For example, in relation to the prison setting, Caraher et al. (2002) found, following a survey of 120 prisons in the UK, that the focus of much work falling under the health promotion banner was specific, topic-based health education and rarely focused on creating a supportive environment (see Part II, Chapter 11 for a critical examination of the prison setting). Similarly, studies of farm health tend to focus on individual farmers, as opposed to the farm environment (Thurston and Blundell-Gosselin, 2005). Health promotion in workplaces is frequently characterized by interventions that target individuals (Dugdill and Springett, 2001); most evaluated workplace interventions address clinical risk factors or behavioural risk factors for coronary heart disease (Harden et al., 1999), or in the case of occupational stress, lifestyle-orientated strategies (Noblett, 2003) (see Part III for detailed case studies on the workplace setting).

The settings approach clearly recognizes wholeness and the need to consider interrelationships within settings, rather than elemental parts. Health promotion practitioners, in adopting the settings approach, need to ensure they are conversant with systems thinking. Two examples of good practice of systems thinking within settings are outlined in Box 3.1 and Box 3.2.

Box 3.1   Management standards for stress

Work-related stress affects 22% of workers through the European Union (EFIWLC, 2007). In 2005/6 work-related stress, depression and anxiety cost Great Britain in excess of £530 million. The number of workers who had sought medical advice for what they believed to be work-related stress increased by 110,000 to an estimated 530,000 (Health and Safety Executive,

2007) and stress is consistently in the top three causes of sickness absence for all types of worker. The reduction of stress and its consequences (sickness absence rates, business costs including the loss of performance and productivity, the threat to the wellbeing of the employee), has thus become a priority for government and employers alike.

In 2002 the Health and Safety Executive (HSE) undertook a major study of UK employees in order to determine the causes of work-related stress and to identify ways of reducing it. The study led to the identification of six work-related causes of stress:

- *Demands* – Issues such as workload, work patterns and the work environment.
- *Control* – How much say the person has in the way they do their work.
- *Role* – Whether people understand their role within the organization and whether the organization ensures that they do not have conflicting roles.
- *Relationships* – This includes promoting positive working to avoid conflict and dealing with unacceptable behaviour.
- *Change* – How organizational change (large or small) is managed and communicated in the organization.
- *Support* – This includes the encouragement, sponsorship and resources provided by the organization, line management and colleagues.

HSE also categorized organizational responses to stress in three ways. The most common organizational response is through the provision of counselling services, a tertiary level response as defined by the HSE. Here a person has a stress-related problem and treatment is provided. The fix, however, is focused on the individual rather than the organization and has little impact on the prevention of the problem. Secondary level responses include the provision of training for managers and staff and the development of corporate policies that address mental health and wellbeing.

Primary prevention is very much orientated towards a whole system, corporate approach. The Management Standards approach is a primary prevention strategy. Here employers work with their staff to first identify and then address the causes of work-related stress. In essence this means identifying situations where pressure becomes excessive. In terms of prevention of stress at work the HSE advises the adoption of a comprehensive corporate approach based on the identification and assessment of risk and the development of managerial competency. To assist organizations in the development of this approach guidance has been provided and an online stress audit tool based on the six causes identified in the study has been created to help managers assess their competences. Within this approach meeting the needs of individual employees whose work is leading them to experience excessive pressure and stress remains central. However, in developing this preventative approach HSE is leading employers away from a reactionary, 'we have a problem so we will treat it' approach, to a proactive, 'let's prevent, so far as possible' stress within this organization (Health and Safety Executive, 2007).

Box 3.2 School Bullying Prevention Programme

The Health Behaviour in School Children (HBSC) survey, in which 40 countries and 202,056 adolescents participated in 2006, revealed that overall, 12.6% of children between ages 11 and 15 report being bullied (Craig et al., 2009). The adverse health outcomes from school bullying include psychological maladjustment, psychosomatic problems and physical injury (Molcho et al., 2009). Children who are targets not only experience poorer self worth at the time but also are at greater risk for depression as adults. A range of interventions have been developed to address this problem, including curriculum-based strategies, social skills training, mentoring and social worker support (Vreeman and Carroll, 2007). Of interest here is the systemic whole school approach originally developed by Olweus (2001), following a survey of 130,000 Norwegian students. It is described as a comprehensive, school-wide programme designed to improve peer relations and make schools safer, more positive places for students to learn and develop, through reducing existing bullying and preventing new bullying problems emerging. The programme is underpinned by the assumption that the school environment is the appropriate target for intervention and teachers, parents and children are all key players in this environment. The programme aims to restructure the school environment, striving for the creation of an environment characterized by warmth, positive interest and involvement from adults, but balanced by the articulation of firm limits on unacceptable behaviour, with consistently applied sanctions for breaches of this code. These core principles are translated into a number of specific measures at the level of the school, the classroom and the individuals. The programme has been successfully implemented in schools across Norway involving at least 6,000 students, and in a number of school settings in other countries (Olweus, 2001). Evaluations typically include self report measures of bullying, measures of other aggressive or antisocial behaviours and in some cases implementation measures. Evaluations in Norwegian schools have consistently reported very positive results; data from 2,500 students across 42 schools demonstrated marked reductions – up to 50% in bully/victim problems, for both boys and girls and across all grades. Other antisocial behaviours were also reduced and an improved social climate registered (Olweus, 1991, 1997, 2005a, 2005b). Positive, although more modest, results have been reported from interventions in other countries. Bullying incident density decreased by 45% over 4 years of programme implementation across six American schools (Black and Jackson, 2007), and reduced by 4% over control schools along with significant decreases in antisocial behaviour in six American rural school districts (Melton at al., 1998). Reviews and meta-analyses (Ttofi et al., 2008) have also drawn favourable conclusions in respect of whole school programmes to address school bullying. The success of the programme has been attributed to system factors such as the balance between opportunity and reward structures (Olweus, 2001) and the multiple component aspect (Ttofi et al., 2008) (see Part II, Chapter 9 for a detailed account of the schools setting).

Shifting from objective knowledge to contextual knowledge in settings

Reductionism seeks to isolate parts, people and their behaviours from context (Poland, 2007), while systems thinking focuses on relationships and context. Capra (2008) claims that in order to understand complex systems it is insufficient to focus on the objective content of the system, instead the focus must be on relationships, the mapping of relationships and the relational context of the system. It is not about what is in the system, it is about how things and people relate and connect to each other.

Again, the parallel with health promotion settings is evident. Capra claims that systems thinking is always contextual thinking (Capra, 2008), a view shared by Dooris, who states unequivocally that context is fundamental to health promotion (Dooris et al., 2007: 330). Poland et al. (2009) also argue strongly for an appreciation of contextual knowledge in settings-based work:

> Interventions wither or thrive based on complex interactions between key personalities, circumstances, and coincidences. These include, but are not limited to, timely funding opportunities, changes in leadership, ideas whose time is right, organizational constraint, available resources, and local history of management–labour relations.
> (Poland et al., 2009: 505)

Poland (2007) suggests that contextual knowledge be addressed in terms of the target of the intervention, the intervention itself and the evaluation of the intervention (see Part I, Chapter 5 for a full discussion of evaluating health promotion in settings). In order to understand, and therefore implement change in a given setting, an understanding will be required of the relationships between relevant agencies, groups and sectors. In workplaces for example, relations between management and workers, the role and strength of unions, and the history of the organization's role with customers, suppliers and competitors must be appreciated. With regard to a healthy city or island project, community organizations and statutory agencies do not always enter into partnerships in a vacuum. They have historical relationships with other partners, sometimes collaborative, sometimes conflicted. Community organizations may have had to compete with each other for funding prior to entering partnerships and may anticipate that this situation will not change, even in partnership. The opportunities for promoting health in a hospital setting must be considered in the context of the overall structure of the health services and historical relationships between occupational groups. An example of use of contextual knowledge in settings-based health promotion is outlined in Box 3.3.

Box 3.3   Contextual factors in a primary health care setting

The primary health care (PHC) project for Irish Travellers offers a good example of a successful initiative in the primary care setting, based on recognition of contextual factors. Irish Travellers are an ethnically distinct minority, and although

(Continued)

(Continued)

indigenous to Ireland, their situation is applicable to many other ethnic minority groups. Travellers have a nomadic tradition, and many adults are pre-literate. They experience significantly poorer health status than the general population, particularly in respect of infant morbidity and mortality.

At the commencement of the PHC project, Traveller engagement with health services was characterized by high levels of utilization of emergency services, low uptake of other hospital-based and preventive services (such as post-natal, immunization), and difficulties with accessing consistent services in primary care (Department of Health, 1995). The context of health service delivery was one of hostility, cultural insensitivity and perceived discrimination.

A highly successful initiative involved Traveller women undertaking training as peer health workers, leading to their employment as Community Health Workers. Other outcomes of the project include targeted family planning and well woman clinics and the development of culturally appropriate education materials for topics of particular relevance to Travellers. The success of the project is attributed to many factors, but chief among these is the attention to contextual factors at the outset and throughout the project (McCabe and Keys, 2005). In the pilot project Traveller women were trained to collect baseline data on health matters in their community. This gave context to their own understanding of health and structural determinants. As the project unfolded, various statutory agencies were included. Education took place, of both Travellers and of service providers regarding Traveller culture and needs. In this project, relationships were extremely important, given the levels of misinformation, distrust and prejudice on either side. The project has led not only to a change in primary care service provision, but to greater inclusion of Travellers in health policy forums, genuine improvement in partnerships between voluntary and statutory agencies and much greater awareness of the barriers Travellers experience in respect of health and access to health care (Pavee Point, 2000; McCabe and Keys, 2005).

Emergent properties of systems and the unanticipated outcomes in settings

One of the most important aspects of whole systems thinking is the understanding it offers for the nature of change in a system, or more specifically the interdependent nature of movement within the system. The systems that constitute settings are complex with important features that have implications for settings-based work. Complex systems, for example are adaptive.

Complex systems, left to their own devices, will adapt and evolve. They can deal with novel situations. The parts and actors work together to shape the system and its outcomes, demonstrating flexibility and plasticity (Capra, 2008). In this way complex systems have emergent, self-organizing properties (Manson, 2001; Poland, 2007). Emergent properties can be unexpected structures, patterns or processes in a self-organizing system. This is a significant advance on thinking of a system in terms of the parts with designed-in connections.

Examples are legion: systems within the human body, for instance, adapt to pathogens; cities and communities grow and differentiate; universities evolve over time and develop new features and functions; organizations adapt and change to pressures in the environment such as labour markets or changes in supply and demand chains. The emergent qualities are not analytically tractable from the parts (Manson, 2001). Health promotion projects, such as those outlined in Part III, Chapters 13 and 14, emerge within the organization in response to the concerns and needs of staff.

The behaviour in complex systems is non-linear and whole systems are sensitive to small changes. The science of complexity acknowledges that the potential for interconnections and relationships within a complex system is infinite and thus, even knowing all the parts of a system, it is impossible to foresee or predict all interactions and their outcomes. Minor events can have greater consequences, consequences that cannot be predicted from the original event (Manson, 2001). As summed up by Plsek and Greenhalgh (2001: 627) the only way to know exactly what a complex system will do is to observe it. It is not a question of a better understanding of the agents, of better models, or of more analysis.

Many settings-based projects demonstrate unanticipated outcomes. In evaluating a health promoting hospitals project it was found that the project improved the image of the hospital in the community and the perception of working conditions, neither of which was an explicit objective (Tountas et al., 2004). A settings-based initiative in a youth work setting, the Health Quality Mark (HQM), found that the HQM was not only perceived to raise awareness of health and to validate and extend good practice but was also seen to bring health promotion centre stage, and provide a renewed focus for the work of the youth organization (Hodgins and Swinburne, 2008).

Taking a whole complex systems approach implies that practitioners should keep intervention specifications to a minimum and build vision as interventions develop, rather than detailed top-down planning of health promotion interventions (Poland, 2007). Progress to goals may be better met through establishing minimum specifications rather than detailed, target-driven standards (Pslek and Wilson, 2001). Minimum specifications provide space for innovation and encourage shared action. Examples are provided in the work of Lowe (2010) who finds that healthy work organizations are built through gradual and cumulative change, and that top-down, management-driven initiatives are rarely successful. Since individual workplaces are at different points on a healthy organization trajectory, Lowe contends that highly specified prescriptions are not useful, recommending that practitioners work with the organization from their particular position on the trajectory, modifying tools to fit the organization, and using language that works for the organization (Lowe, 2010).

Challenges and opportunities to a whole systems approach in healthy settings

The science of complex adaptive systems provides challenges in respect of levering change for health improvement in settings, including organizations and larger supra-organizational systems. In applying a whole systems approach the unpredictability of systems and the difficulties harnessing complex systems for evaluation are two key challenges. However, the whole systems approach challenges practitioners to work with, rather than side-step power structures in settings that potentially may improve health at a number of levels, as power itself can be construed as a determinant of health.

With many (and changing) parts, actors and groups, non-linear relationships, emergent properties and sensitivity to small changes, the detailed behaviour of any complex system is fundamentally unpredictable over time (Lorenz, 1993). The inherent unpredictability and messiness of complex systems presents a challenge to practitioners (Dooris et al., 2007). Furthermore, the health promotion practitioner is part of the system too. When they cannot predict with accuracy what will happen when, for example, they create a Healthy Action Committee in a workplace, or a Quality of Working Life project in a university, practitioners may balk at entering such uncharted territory, perhaps as a result of grounding in disciplines that value precision and prediction over context and organic processes, and approaches that screen or control for variation rather than embrace it. Westley et al. (2007) recommend that those who wish to facilitate innovative change need to be able to acknowledge their lack of control and the inherent uncertainties in any given system.

Training practitioners in tolerance of complexity and unpredictability is a necessary skill for whole systems thinking. Interestingly, it does not appear to be captured in the various public health or health promotion competency frameworks. However, a useful place to start meeting this challenge might be the inclusion of modules on basic complexity science on public health and health promotion educational programmes, and a focus in practice placements on the complexity of organizations.

Evaluation of whole systems approaches remains a challenge. Dooris (2006) recommends the application of theory-based evaluation, which explores links between activities, outcomes and contexts and takes account of relationships between people, echoing Capra's contention that whole systems thinking requires mapping as opposed to measurement of relationships (Capra, 2008). An example can be found in the STAR method (Guimarães, 2004) which has been used to map the degree of and potency of interagency relationship in Healthy Cities projects. Westley et al. (2007) argue that clear specific measurable outcomes, often specified by funding or statutory agencies, are appropriate when problems are well understood and solutions are known. Step-by-step specifications for project work that dictate inputs, activities and outputs assume knowledge of how things will unfold and actions take their course. While this can be said of some health problems in settings, it certainly cannot be said of all. Innovative health promotion activities in highly emergent settings will require more flexible approaches to evaluation (see Part I, Chapter 5).

It is clear that comprehensive evaluations, employing a range of methods are required if we are to capture the nature of change within complex systems. Process evaluation in particular is central to whole systems approaches, and within this the employment of qualitative methods such as the use of narratives which can offer significant insights in the complicated unfolding of events in complex systems.

Power has a very important place in the theory and practice of health promotion. Empowerment, the process through which people gain control over action and decisions affecting their health (WHO, 1998) is central to the practice of health promotion. Despite this, however, empowerment often takes the form of lip service rather than practice (Tones and Green, 2004) and debates on power, politics and ideology are largely absent from mainstream health promotion discourse (Bambra et al., 2007). Power exists within the contexts of relationships between people and is central therefore to the context of any health promotion setting. Children are the primary beneficiaries of health promotion in school settings yet principals and teachers and parents are invested with power over children in almost all matters. Prisoners are dramatically powerless in prisons, as are marginalized communities in cities (for further discussion on this see Part I, Chapter 2). In health service settings, service users not only have less power than healthcare professionals in society but also can be disempowered in the receipt of service by health professionals. Within workplaces the nature of the employer relationship is inherently and unavoidably inequitable. Where people within a system experience poorer health than others, this may because of the power others exercise over them. Yet in health promotion we continue to devise interventions, often under the banner of a settings approach, that unthinkingly ignore the realities of power relations. Interventions that press patients to remind their doctors to wash their hands, or address workplace stress interventions that offer employees programmes to better manage their time when in fact they have no control over their workload, ignore the realities of power relations.

Workplace bullying is a particular case in point. The most common response in workplaces is to devise an anti-bullying policy which typically requires the victim to lodge a complaint about the bully, which then triggers an investigation, culminating in either the bully being issued with a reprimand or not. The failure of this approach is evident; targets of workplace bullying have been reported to display high exit rates (Ironside and Seifert, 2003), and employees see such policies as only leading to further exposure of the victim while not addressing bullying within the organization (Hodgins, 2008). Bullies are usually in positions of superiority over targets (Zapf et al., 2003), making power and the exercise of it central to any understanding of bullying and intimidation. As long as workers are economically dependent on work, they are in a weaker position than their employer, and are likely to feel compromised if bullied by management or even if reporting bullying to management. Anti-bullying procedures that place the responsibility on the individual to report bullying and prove that it is happening cannot hope to address workplace bullying (Collins and Thompson, 2006). Understanding and addressing bullying in the workplace is more likely to occur when the whole system is considered, and power differentials are exposed. The focus on the whole system will permit the identification of the powerful levers in the system, which must be employed to bring about real change in the system (Whitelaw et al., 2001).

Summary points

- The paradigmatic shift from reductionism to systems is mirrored in health promotion in the shift from focusing on individual behaviour to the entire setting.
- The settings approach within health promotion is a systems approach. Settings are systems and the characteristics and laws that govern systems behaviour and change apply to the setting.
- In particular, in undertaking settings-based work, health promotion practitioners need to accommodate and embrace the unpredictability of the behaviour of the setting, both in terms of interventions and in terms of evaluation.
- A whole systems approach, in providing a focus on relationships, offers an opportunity to address issues of power and control in settings as relationships are where power or the abuse of it finds expression.

Online Further Reading

Naaldenberg, J., Vaandrager, L., Koelen, M., Wagemakers, A., Saan, H and de Hoog, K. (2009) 'Elaborating on systems thinking in health promotion practice', *Global Health Promotion*, 16 (39): 39–47.

This paper explores systems thinking in the context of health promotion practice. Three concepts: the structure of the system, the meaning attached to actions and the power relations between actors are identified as key concepts for the practical application of a systems perspective. A health promotion partnership in the Netherlands is described as a way of illustrating how using these concepts to apply a systems perspective can facilitate the processes of social learning and innovation, both of which are central to health promotion.

References

Bambra, C., Fox, D. and Scott-Samuel, A. (2007) 'Towards a politics of health', in J. Douglas, S. Earle, S. Handsley, C.E. Lloyd and S. Spurr (eds), *A Reader in Promoting Public Health: Challenge and Controversy*. London: Sage.

Black, S. and Jackson, E. (2007) 'Using bullying incident density to evaluate the Olweus Bullying Prevention programme', *School Psychology International*, 23 (5): 623–38.

Buchanan, D. and Huczynski, A. (1985) *Organizational Behaviour: An Introductory Text*. Englewood Cliffs, NJ: Prentice–Hall.

Capra, F. (2008) 'The new facts of life', www.ecoliteracy.org/essays/new-facts-life (accessed 26 August 2010).

Caraher, M., Dixon, P., Hayton, P., Carr-Hill, R., McGough, H. and Bird, L. (2002) 'Are health-promoting prisons an impossibility? Lessons from England and Wales', *Health Education*, 102 (5): 219–29.

Collins, J. and Thompson, K. (2006) The role of text in legitimising bullying in the risk society. Paper presented at 5th International Conference on Bullying and Harassment in the Workplace, Dublin, June 2006.

Craig, W., Harel-Fisch, Y., Fogel-Grinvald, H., Dostler, S., Hetland, J., Simons-Morton, S., Molcho, M., deMato, M., Overpeck, M., Due, P. and Pickett, W. (2009) 'A cross-national profile of bullying and victimisation among adolescents in 40 countries', *International Journal of Public Health*, 54: S216–S224.

Department of Health (1995) *Report of the Task Force on the Travelling Community*. Dublin: Government Publications.

Dooris, M. (2005) 'Healthy settings: challenges to generating evidence of effectiveness', *Health Promotion International*, 21 (1): 55–65.

Dooris, M. (2006) 'Health promoting settings: future directions', *Promotion and Education*, XIII (1): 4–6.

Dooris, M., Poland, B., Kolbe, L., De Leeuw, E., McCall, D.S. and Wharf-Higgins, J. (2007) 'Healthy settings: building evidence for the effectiveness of whole system health promotion – challenges and future directions', in D.V. McQueen and C.M. Jones (eds), *Global Perspectives on Health Promotion Effectiveness*. New York: Springer.

Dugdill, L. and Springett, J. (2001) 'Evaluating health promotion programmes in the workplace', in I. Rootman, M. Goodstadt, B. Hyndman, D. McQueen, L. Potvin, J. Springett and E. Ziglio (eds), *Evaluation in Health Promotion Principles and Perspectives*. Denmark: WHO Regional Publications European Series, No. 92.

EFIWLC (European Foundation for the Improvement of Working and Living Conditions) (2007) *Fourth European Working Conditions Survey*. Dublin: Eurofound.

French, W.L. and Bell, C.H. (1998) *Organizational Development: Behavior Science Interventions for Organizational Improvement*, 6th edn Englewood Cliffs, NJ: Prentice–Hall.

Green, L., Poland, B. and Rootman, I. (2000) 'The settings approach to health promotion', in B. Poland, L. Green and I. Rootman, *Settings for Health Promotion: Linking Theory and Practice*. London: Sage.

Guimarães, R. (2004) 'STAR, a qualitative evaluation process of the Healthy Cities', *Terrae*, 1 (1): 52–9.

Health and Safety Executive (2007) www.hse.gov.uk/press/2007/c07021.htm (accessed 25 September 2010).

Harden, A., Peersman, G., Oliver, S. Mauthner, M. and Oakley, A. (1999) 'A systematic review of the effectiveness of health promotion interventions in the workplace', *Occupational Medicine*, 49 (8): 540–8.

Hodgins, M. (2008) 'Taking a health promotion approach to the problem of bullying', *International Journal of Psychology and Psychological Therapy*, 8 (1): 13–23.

Hodgins, M. and Swinburne, L. (2008) '"It sort of widens the health word": Evaluation of a health promotion intervention in the youth work setting', *Youth Studies Ireland*, 3 (1): 30–44.

Ironside, M. and Seifert, R. (2003) 'Tackling bullying in the workplace: the collective dimension', in S. Einarsen, H. Hoel, D. Zapf, and C. Cooper (eds), *Bullying and Emotional Abuse in the Workplace*. London: Taylor and Francis.

Lorenz, E. (1993) *The Essence of Chaos*. Seattle, WA: University of Washington Press.

Lowe, G. (2010) *Creating Healthy Organizations*. Toronto: University of Toronto Press.

Manson, S.M. (2001) 'Simplifying complexity: a review of complexity theory', *Geoforum*, 32: 405–14.

McCabe, C. and Keys, F. (2005) *A Review of Travellers' Health using Primary Care as a Model of Good Practice*. Dublin: Pavee Point Travellers Centre.

Melton, G.B., Limber, S.P., Cunningham, P., Osgood, D.W., Chambers, J., Flerx, V., Henggeler, S. and Nation, M. (1998) Violence among Rural Youth. Final report to the United States Office of Juvenile Justice and Delinquency Prevention.

Molcho, M., Craig, W., Due, P., Pickett, W. and Overpeck, M. (2009) 'Cross-national time trends in bullying behaviour 1994–2006: findings from Europe and North America', *International Journal of Public Health*, 54: S1–S10.

Noblett, A. (2003) 'Building health promoting work settings: identifying the relationship between work characteristics and occupational stress in Australia', *Health Promotion International*, 18 (4): 351–9.

Nutbeam, D. (1998) 'Evaluating health promotion – progress, problems and solutions', *Health Promotion International*, 13: 27–44.

Olweus, D. (1991) 'Bully/victim problems among schoolchildren: basic facts and effects of a school based intervention program', in D. Pepler and K.H. Rubin (eds), *The Development and Treatment of Childhood Aggression*. Hillsdale, NJ: Erlbaum.

Olweus, D. (1997) 'Bully/victim problems in school: facts and intervention', *European Journal of Psychology of Education*, 12: 495–510.

Olweus, D. (2001) 'Bully/victim problems in school', in S. Einarsen, H. Hoel, D. Zapf and C. Cooper (eds), *Bullying and Emotional Abuse in the Workplace*. London: Taylor and Francis.

Olweus, D. (2005a) 'A useful evaluation design, and effects of the Olweus Bullying Prevention Program', *Psychology, Crime and Law*, 11: 389–402.

Olweus, D. (2005b) New Positive Results with the Olweus Bullying Prevention Program in 37 Oslo Schools. Report. Bergen, Norway: Research Centre for Health Promotion, University of Bergen.

Paton, K., Sengupta, S. and Hassan, L. (2005) 'Settings, systems and organizational development: the Healthy Living and Working Model', *Health Promotion International*, 20 (1): 81–9.

Poland, B. (2007) Settings for Health Promotion: promising directions in unpacking and addressing how place matters. Presented at Canada/International Symposium on Settings for Health and Learning, 2–4 June, University of Victoria, BC.

Poland, B., Krupa, G. and McCall, D. (2009) 'Settings for health promotion: an analytic framework to guide intervention design and implementation', *Health Promotion Practice*, 10: 505–16.

Pavee Point (2000) *Primary Health Care for Travellers Project Implementation Report 1996–1999*. Dublin: Pavee Point Publications.

Pslek, P. and Greenhalgh, T. (2001) 'The challenge of complexity in health care', *British Medical Journal*, 323: 625–722.

Plsek, P.E. and Wilson, T. (2001) 'Complexity, leadership and management in health care organizations', *British Medical Journal*, 323: 746–56.

Pratt, J., Gordon, P. and Plampling, D. (2005) *Working Whole Systems. Putting Theory into Practice in Organizations*. Oxford: Radcliffe Publishing.

Tones, K. and Green, J. (2004) *Health Promotion: Planning and Strategies*. London: Sage.

Tountas, Y., Pavi, E., Tsamandouraki, K., Arkadopoulos, and Triantafyllou, D. (2004) 'Evaluation of the participation of Aretaieion Hospital, Greece in the

WHO Pilot Project of Health Promoting Hospitals', *Health Promotion International*, 19 (4): 453–62.

Ttofi, M.M., Farrington, D.P. and Baldry, A.C. (2008) *Effectiveness of Programmes to Reduce School Bullying*. Swedish National Council for Crime Prevention.

Thurston, W. and Blundell-Gosselin, H.J. (2005) 'The farm as a setting for health promotion: results of a needs assessment in South Central Alberta', *Health and Place*, 11 (1): 31–43.

Von Bertalanffy, L. (1968) *General Systems Theory: Foundation, Developments, Application*. New York: Braziller.

Vreeman, R.C. and Carroll, A.E. (2007) 'A systematic review of school-based interventions to prevent bullying', *Archives of Paediatric and Adolescent Medicine*, 161: 78–88.

Walby, S. (2007) 'Complexity theory, systems theory and multiple intersecting social inequalities', *Philosophy of Social Sciences*, 37: 449–70.

Westley, F., Zimmerman, B. and Patton, M.Q. (2007) *Getting to Maybe*. Toronto: Random House Canada.

Whitelaw, S., Baxendale, A., Bryce, C., MacHardy, L., Young, I. and Whitney, E. (2001) '"Settings"-based health promotion: a review', *Health Promotion International*, 16 (4): 339–53.

WHO (1998) *Health Promotion Glossary*, WHO/HPR/HEP/98.1. Geneva: WHO.

Zapf, D., Einarsen, S., Hoel, H. and Vartia, M. (2003) 'Empirical findings on bullying in the workplace', in S. Einarsen, H. Hoel, D. Zapf and C. Cooper (eds), *Bullying and Emotional Abuse in the Workplace*. London: Taylor and Francis.

4

Partnership, Collaboration and Participation: Fundamental Principles in a Settings Approach to Health Promotion

Angela Scriven

Aims

- To highlight the policy imperatives linked to enabling and empowering people to collaborate, participate and engage in partnerships to promote their health
- To offer an overview of why and how stakeholders involved in settings can effectively engage with each other through partnerships to define health needs and plan and provide health promoting services
- To identify the different types of partnerships for health within and between settings and the key elements to effective partnership working
- To explore the complexities, challenges and opportunities for participatory and partnership working within settings

---

Enabling and empowering individuals and groups to participate in the process of taking control of and improving their health is a fundamental principle in health promotion. If health promoters are to fully engage population groups in this process they must understand the procedures for, and be fully competent in, participatory and partnership methods. There are many imperatives for partnerships for health (Scriven, 2007, 2010) and much has been said on the need for participation and partnerships working in the health promotion declarations and charters that have emerged over the past two decades. As early as 1978, the full participation of population groups in the multidimensional work of health improvement became one of the pillars of the Health for All movement, launched at the Alma Ata conference (WHO, 1978). This was further developed in 1986 when the Ottawa Charter (WHO, 1986) emphasized the mediation role of health promoters and the notion that the prerequisites and prospects for health could not be ensured by the health sector alone. Implicit within this was the case for partnerships to ensure coordinated action by all concerned with health development: by governments, by health and other social and economic sectors, by nongovernmental and voluntary organizations, by local authorities, by industry, the media and by people from all walks of life as individuals, families and communities (WHO, 1986). In a technical background paper at the WHO sixth Global Conference on Health Promotion from which the Bangkok Charter emerged (WHO, 2005) (see below), the centrality to health promotion effectiveness of interorganizational partnerships at all levels was confirmed (Jackson et al., 2006).

By the late 1990s, the WHO, in the Jakarta Declaration (WHO, 1997), had crafted a specific objective centred on the consolidation and expansion of partnerships, reiterating the necessity for partnerships for health between the different sectors at all levels of governance and society. Moreover, the Declaration called for existing partnerships to be strengthened and the potential for new partnerships explored. One reason given for this recommended expansion of partnership working is that the new health challenges that health promoters are confronted with in the twenty-first century mean that different and diverse partnerships need to be created. Such partnerships, it is proposed, should provide mutual assistance both within and among countries and facilitate the exchange of evidence information about which health promotion strategies have proved effective and in which settings.

The most recent international declaration from the WHO, the Bangkok Charter (WHO, 2005), prioritizes local partnerships and calls for the strengthening of the capacity of civil society and decision makers to act collectively to exert control over the factors that influence health. The Charter asserts that active participation, especially by the community, is essential for the sustainability of health promotion efforts. The challenge is clearly laid out for health promoters, it is to make a reality the commitment to engage and empower people. The formation of partnerships with public, private and nongovernmental organizations (NGOs) was prioritized and is designed to create sustainable actions across sectors to address the determinants of health (WHO, 2005). One argument given for the greater need for partnership working in the twenty-first century is to manage the challenges and opportunities of globalization at global and national levels. Tang et al. (2005) propose that collaboration and engagement of all sectors of society are required to ensure that the benefits for health from globalization are maximized and the negative effects are minimized and mitigated. Internationally, it is clear therefore, that the WHO has consistently promoted collaboration, participation and partnership approaches through their health promotion Charters and Declarations. This endorsement of partnership approaches is also supported by the International Union for Health Promotion and Education (IUHPE) who contend that partnerships carry significant effects for health promotion interventions, in terms of sustainability and community empowerment (IUHPE, 2011).

Partnership working and UK policy

Nationally, government health and welfare policy within the UK has demonstrated a similar impetus for participatory and partnership working. Jupp (2000) provided some evidence of this by pointing to the growth in the use of the term 'partnership' in parliament, documenting an increase from a total of 38 times in 1989 to 6,197 times in 1999. The current policy directives have led Knight et al. (2001) to argue that partnership engagement is no longer simply an option for some health and social services, it is a requirement. The evidence to support this argument is clearly set out in the policies of the last decade which have consistently advocated a move to partnership working. For example, *Our Health, Our Care, Our Say* (Department of Health, 2006) has strengthened the drive for partnership between people and public services. This directive was followed by *Health Challenge England* (Department of Health, 2007) in which the then Minister for Health, Caroline Flint, talks of new national alliances for good health and wellbeing across government and with industry and voluntary organizations and locally between public services, business and third sector partners (see Table 4.1 for definitions of the third sector and other terms used in this chapter).

The Partnerships for Better Health report (Department of Health, 2007) highlights the UK government's role in influencing non-statutory, commercial and not-for-profit sectors in securing public health goals. Throughout this report, by highlighting case studies and best practice tips, the government is encouraging the greater use of such partnerships for health at a local level and also emphasizing that (a) good health and wellbeing are everyone's responsibility and that (b) future healthcare will be underpinned by partnerships between individuals, communities, business, voluntary organizations, public services and government. An important statement in this publication is that a key role for government is to work with partners to positively influence people's lifestyle decisions and improve the nation's health. For further updates on the implications for local partnership working of the UK Coalition Government's plans, see Local Government Improvement and Development (2011a, 2011b).

The general policy consensus therefore, as indicated in the examples above, is that working in partnership is crucial to the current process of modernization under way in UK health and welfare services and across a range of policy arenas. The demand for partnership working for health promotion came to the forefront in the White Paper *The Health of the Nation* (Department of Health, 1994), where the term 'healthy alliances' was introduced and was to dominate terminology for a number of years. Healthy alliances referred to partnerships established specifically to achieve health gain. The WHO in their Glossary subsequently defined a health alliance as follows:

An alliance for health promotion is a *partnership* between two or more parties that pursue a set of agreed upon goals in *health promotion* ... Alliance building will often involve some form of *mediation* between the different partners in the definition of goals and ethical ground rules, joint action areas, and agreement on the form of cooperation which is reflected in the alliance. (WHO, 1998: 5)

What this definition identifies are some of the prerequisites for establishing a partnership for health, including the ground rules and ethical and professional behaviour required to initiate and sustain effective partnerships. These are discussed more fully later in this chapter.

The term 'health alliances' to describe partnership arrangements is still prevailing in some of the UK policy agendas, particularly in Wales, where the concept of Local Health Alliances has been developed as a means for bringing together all those who have a part to play in influencing the health of communities in Wales. At the time of writing Local Health Alliances exist in most local authority areas across Wales and the term is also used for other health-related groups. For example, Welsh Tobacco Control Alliance (WTCA) is a project developed by Action against Smoking and Health (ASH) Wales to enable all third sector organizations involved with tackling tobacco in Wales to inform and influence policy development and implementation, at both a UK and Wales level (ASH Wales, 2011).

Some alliances are health topic-orientated and often have specific aims, such as policy development. For example, the Scottish Physical Activity and Health Alliance (PAHA) is a multisector partnership that engages a variety of people from different sectors and professions who are involved in the promotion of physical activity and health in Scotland. Its purpose is to inform people, connect people with others and to aid policy development and implementation (PAHA, 2011). Another is the Food & Health Alliance, which is managed by NHS Health Scotland and supported by the Scottish Government and Food Standards Agency Scotland. The Alliance is a partnership of key stakeholders involved in implementing a multisector food and health strategy. Membership includes a broad range of sectors such as national and local government, NHS health boards and Community Healthcare Partnerships, community planning, voluntary and community organizations, national governance organizations, research and academia, media, local enterprise companies and all food chain organizations (Health Scotland, 2011).

It is generally the case, however, that the term 'partnerships' is now more likely to be used than 'alliances' and as already argued, there is a consensus that partnership working is essential in terms of creating the synergy required to accomplish the goals of health promotion (see Corbin and Mittelmark, 2008). This is even more likely to be the case in settings.

Partnership working and the settings approach

There are a number of strongly articulated points in the WHO Charters and Declaration and UK policy directives discussed above about the need for partnership working. Alongside this, the international and national policy arena has emphasized settings as the ecological and holistic approach to health gain (see Part I, Chapter 2 for a detailed discussion of this point). The Jakarta Declaration (WHO, 1997), for example, argues that settings provide the organizational base and the infrastructure for health promotion. By inference, therefore, settings provide the structure and the milieu in which partnerships are formed and maintained. In support of this, the WHO in listing the key principles for healthy settings highlights the need for community participation and partnership (WHO, 2011). It has also been suggested by Dooris (2004) that healthy settings have the potential to provide a tangible delivery route for local strategic partnerships (for more on local strategic partnerships see Department of the Environment, Transport and the Regions, 2001) thereby maximizing their contribution to public health. There appears to be, therefore, general agreement that partnership working and settings approaches are concomitant. It is crucial therefore, to develop understanding and competences in partnership working to enable the synergy required to achieve health gain in settings.

Working in partnership in a healthy setting

A first step is to be cognisant with the terms associated with participatory and partnership approaches. Some specific terms are commonly used and sometimes misinterpreted when working collaboratively within and across settings. For example, while some people actually use the term 'collaboration' interchangeably with 'partnership', others may mean 'cooperation' when they say 'partnership' (HealthKnowledge, 2011). Table 4.1 offers explanations of some of the most commonly used terminology. The similarity in some of these definitions has resulted in some confusion in the discourse around partnership engagement. (See also Scriven (2007) and Scriven (in press) for a fuller discussion on the different meanings and levels of collaborative, cooperative and partnership working.)

Table 4.1 Terms used in partnership working within and across settings

Term	Definition
Agency	Synonymous with organization; in practice usually used to refer to public sector organizations
Organization	A body constituted to enable it to conduct business (either profit-making or non-profit)
Private sector	All profit-making organizations
Public sector (Statutory sector)	All non-profit-making organizations constituted to conduct business directly on behalf of, and funded by, central and/or local government. Also called the statutory sector

Term	Definition
Voluntary sector	Non-profit-making organizations that are constituted charities. There is a level of overlap between the voluntary and community sectors: some community sector groups see themselves as part of the voluntary sector
Community sector	Non-profit-making organizations and groups that are not constituted charities
Third sector	Voluntary or non-profit sector (could also include community groups) where private energy can be deployed for public good, sometimes called tertiary sector
Service user	The general public who are the potential recipients of health promotion/ public health programmes within settings, could specifically include patients; unpaid carers; parents/guardians; users of health services; disabled people and interested community members and groups
Stakeholder	A person, group, or organization that has direct or indirect stake in a health promotion partnership because it can affect or be affected by the partnerships, objectives and actions. Stakeholding is usually self-legitimizing (those who judge themselves to be stakeholders are stakeholders), but in some partnerships the stakeholders are not equal
Partnership	A formally constituted group which can include representatives/ stakeholders from service users, the public sector, the voluntary and community sector and the private sector
Health Alliance	Similar to or the same as the definition for partnership above
Participation	A process by which people are enabled to become actively and genuinely involved in defining the issues of concern to them, in making decisions about factors that affect their lives, in formulating and implementing policies, in planning, developing and delivering services and in taking action to achieve change (WHO, 2002: 10)
Cooperation	Informal relationships that exist without any commonly defined mission, structure or planning effort; where information is shared and authority retained by each organization, with separate resources and rewards
Coordination	Formal relationship with understanding of compatible missions, some planning and division of roles and established communication channels. Authority rests with organizations, resources available to participants and rewards mutually acknowledged
Collaboration	Group of autonomous stakeholders who share a specific problem domain and engage in interactive processes, using shared rules, norms and structures, to act or decide on issues related to that domain
Subgroup	A small group made up of some members of a partnership and perhaps some external members. Subgroups may come together once to perform a specific task, such as draw up a job description, or they may have a longer lifetime, perhaps to oversee the rolling review of policies, procedures and protocols. In either case it is useful for the subgroup to have a clear statement of the task(s) it is intended to perform. In the latter case, the sub-group should also have written terms of reference

(Continued)

Table 4.1   (Continued)

Term	Definition
Interagency working	Joint working (see below) between two or more agencies or organizations
Joint working	Different organizations and public sectors working together irrespective of the boundaries to achieve a common goal
Multiagency working	Joint working between three or more agencies or organizations
Interdisciplinary working	Joint working between two different types of professional. This is not necessarily interagency. For example, school nurses and teachers employed by the same education authority and working together would be doing interdisciplinary working in a school setting
Multidisciplinary working	Joint working between three or more different types of professional. This is still not necessarily interagency or multiagency: for example, community psychiatric nurses, midwives and health visitors, employed by the same primary care trust and working together, would be doing multidisciplinary working
Inter-partnership working	Joint working between two partnerships
Multi-partnership working	Joint working between three or more partnerships
Intersectoral action	A coalition of two or more parties who agree on common objectives and work collaboratively
Local Strategic Partnership (LSPs)	LSPs bring together local councils, other public sector agencies, the business sector, and the third sector, voluntary and community organizations. They are non-statutory partnerships, established over the past decade in each local authority area in England. Their role has developed significantly since 2006 (see Local Government Improvement and Development, 2011b)
Terms of reference	A written document setting out guidelines for the working practices of a partnership or sub-group. This may include issues such as the role and responsibilities of the partnership or sub-group; frequency of meetings; a statement about use of understandable language in meetings; plans for dealing with persistent absences by members; and the system for reviewing the terms of reference

Source: Some of the definitions above are taken from and/or adapted from Government Office for the South East (GOSE, 2003) *Working Together and Building Links: Partnership Working Toolkit* and HealthKnowledge (2011)

Establishing a partnership in a setting can be thwarted by a number of complexities or obstacles (see the Improvement Network (2010) and Scriven (in press), for a list of the top ten partnership killers and ways of overcoming potential problems). Impediments are to be expected when disparate agencies try to come together with different legislative and/or policy frameworks, competing organizational imperatives and conflicting professional cultures. Under the new organizational measures introduced in the White Paper *Equity and Excellence:*

Table 4.2 Examples of the benefits of working in partnerships across a setting

Benefits and opportunities of partnership working
A forum to share evidence across sectors, build best practice and coordinate service delivery within the setting and between settings where relevant
Pooled resources with the potential to save time, energy and funding, with access to additional networks, support, knowledge, capacity and competences
Wider access to target groups and/or hard-to-reach communities/populations
Increasing commitment of all possible stakeholders and ensuring that others' views are heard and needs are taken into account across sectors
Greater cohesion and the possibility of building long term relationships, with opportunities to develop other collaborative projects
A stronger voice to influence policy agendas both within and outside the setting, maximizing the potential and contribution of each partner
Break down barriers, create dialogue between different agencies within a setting and create mutual understanding and respect between diverse sectors, including community groups
Opens up new funding streams, helps share the risks and widen the benefits of health promotion action, develops potential for long term programmes across settings

Liberating the NHS (Department of Health, 2010), local authorities in England are charged with promoting the joining up of local NHS services, social care and health improvement. These novel arrangements will hopefully enable greater potential and fluidity in terms of both establishing and sustaining partnerships, with the consequent benefits for those working for health gain in settings. As Table 4.2 indicates, partnership working offers a range of opportunities that can enhance health promotion action in and between settings. For these to be fully realized, however, the barriers to partnership working highlighted by the Improvement Network (2010) have to be identified and strategies put in place to overcome these.

Different types of partnerships in settings

There are many examples of partnership arrangements linked to setting. The most common are those that are specific to the setting to ensure effective functioning. Healthy Schools Partnerships, for example, are generally joint initiatives between the public health services (currently being reorganized and moved to local authorities) and the Education Service. These partnerships generally support schools to develop an ethos and environment that enables learning and promotes health and wellbeing through a whole school approach. This might involve curriculum development which covers personal, social and health education (including drugs, and sex and relationship education), physical activity, healthy eating, emotional health and wellbeing, and education for a sustainable environment. For examples see the myriad of Healthy Schools Partnerships that

have their own websites, such as Manchester (see www.manchester.gov.uk/
info/200104/youth_support/1446/health_promotion_with_young_people/2)
(see also Part II, Chapter 9 for details of Healthy Schools programmes).

Other types of partnership might span the spectrum of cooperation, coordination and collaboration (see Table 4.1) to full partnerships that are within or
across settings and might be long term or based on short-lived projects. Some of
these will be similar to those outlined earlier under health alliances. Mohajer
(2011) highlights three examples of some of the partnerships that might be
found in settings when outlining the Royal Society for Public Health (RSPH)
Health Promotion and Community Well-Being Organization and Partnership
Awards. All three winners of the award in 2010 offer positive examples of the
type of linkages that can be established in settings, demonstrating active engagement with partner organizations, charities and local agencies to build strong
relationships.

Some settings are more complicated than others and partnership working will
reflect more intricate arrangements. For a useful compilation of ideas for people
working in partnerships in more unusual settings, see Bartel et al. (2007) who
have written a practical guide to beginning and sustaining interagency partnerships in conflict-affected settings.

Establishing partnerships for health in settings

Whatever the setting, in order for partnerships to be effective they must be
transparent and accountable and be based on agreed ethical principles,
mutual understanding and respect (see Box 4.1 for an ethical behaviour protocol designed to enhance partnerships), with adherence to mutually agreed
guidelines and protocols.

Box 4.1   Partnership behaviour protocol (for use in local authority partnerships)

Achieve intended outcomes

Our priorities are evidence-based and our decision making is transparent.
We will:

- Share resources to achieve joint outcomes
- Monitor how well we have used our resources
- Actively encourage ideas and innovation
- Ensure that decision making is transparent
- Be committed to continuous improvement
- Ensure that claims of improved performance are based on clear evidence
- Establish accountability both across the partnership (horizontally) and within
  each organization (vertically)

Public interest

We act in the interest of the public and demonstrate value.
We will:

- Focus on long term as well as short term issues
- Act in the interests of the public good over individual interests
- Demonstrate to the community how we are achieving publicly valued outcomes
- Agree a protocol for the handling of complaints that relate to our joint work

Building partners' capacity

We build capacity in our partnership.
We will:

- Be committed to developing individual partners' skills to achieve our aims
- Encourage partners to be confident working outside of their organizational culture
- Be open to partners' suggestions and help

Value and respect each other

We respect and value everyone's contribution.
We will:

- Ensure that all partners contribute appropriately and openly
- Acknowledge the capabilities of all members
- Recognize and embrace the role of voluntary and community sector partners
- Avoid dominance by one or two individuals
- Respect each other's roles and needs
- Actively encourage the participation of all partnership members
- Build effective working relationships with each other
- Recognize the value of all partners' contributions

Act ethically

We act ethically. We are open and objective and encourage constructive challenge.
We will:

- Agree a mechanism for whistleblowing and dealing with complaints
- Ensure whistleblowers are supported
- Actively promote a 'no-blame' culture
- Support partners to both understand and constructively challenge any poor behaviour
- Use appropriate, unambiguous and simple language

(Continued)

(Continued)

- Agree how we will achieve democratic accountability
- Ensure that our dialogue is open and transparent
- Declare conflicts of interest and address them
- Make sure that the purpose of all meetings is made clear
- Be honest and objective

Aligning strategies and networks

We harness our collective efforts through joint planning, delivery and governance arrangements.
  We will:

- Ensure that partners can influence the decision making of member organizations
- Allow sufficient time and capacity to be given to understand an issue and to reflect on its impact
- Make sure that actions taken by the partnership are clear, time-limited and task-orientated
- Encourage all partners to actively shape the strategy
- Ensure that agreed actions are carried out

Source: Standards for England (2010).

A large number of partnership development tools have been produced and are available on various national and international websites. For example, the partnership behavioural protocol template in Box 4.1 (Standards for England, 2010) is available online for local authorities (LAs) and others to download wholly or amend it as appropriate (including adding organizational logos) to suit their own requirements. The document is not designed to be prescriptive and the values and behaviours listed are not exhaustive. They are based on a research project undertaken by Standards for England with Manchester City Council and partners in 2009. The recommendation is that the template protocol is personalized with the individual authority's corporate identity and used to aid the establishment and the maintenance of partnerships.

The International Union of Health Promotion and Education (IUHPE) is also producing an online database that supports partnership activities in health promotion. This web portal is being put together to include a set of tools that both assists and evaluates levels and types of health promotion activities undertaken in partnership (see IUHPE, 2011).

An earlier set of tools was published by the Health Development Agency, now no longer in existence, but the tools are available from the National Institute for Health and Clinical Excellence (NICE). This set of guidelines and tools produced by Markwell et al. (2003) provides, amongst other components discussed below, a comprehensive checklist of elements that make up a successful partnership (see Box 4.2). While some of these elements are similar to the behaviour protocol listed in Box 4.1, either or both can be adapted and used as guides to practice when establishing and maintaining partnership.

Box 4.2 Key elements of effective partnership work

Leadership – Effective leadership involves attention to:

- Developing a shared vision
- Embodying and promoting ownership of and *commitment* to the partnership and its goals
- Being alert to factors and *relationships* in the external environment that might affect the partnership

Organization – Clear and effective systems are needed for:

- Public *participation* in partnership processes and decision-making
- *Flexibility* in working arrangements
- Transparent and effective *management* of the partnership
- *Communication* in ways and at times that can be easily understood, interpreted and acted upon

Strategy – The partnership needs to implement its mission and vision via a clear strategy informed by local communities and other stakeholders which focus on:

- Strategic development to agree priorities and define outcome targets
- Sharing *information* and *evaluation* of progress and achievements
- A continuous process of action and review

Learning – Partner organizations need to attract, manage and develop people to release their full knowledge and potential by:

- *Valuing* people as a primary resource
- Development and application of *knowledge and skills*
- Supporting *innovation*

Resources – The contribution and shared utilization of resources, including:

- Building and strengthening *social* capital
- Managing and pooling *financial* resources
- Making *information* work
- Using information and communication *technology* appropriately

Programmes – Partners seek to develop coordinated programmes and integrated services that fit together well. This requires attention to:

- Realizing added value from *joint* planning
- Focused *delivery*
- Regular monitoring and *review*

Source: Markwell et al. (2003), taken from NICE (2011).

A critical goal to note here should be the involvement of the community or community stakeholders in these partnerships. Unfortunately, partnerships are not usually of equals (Coulson, 2005). Unequal power relationships between professionals and representatives and groups from the setting will skew the partnership agenda. Scriven (2007) argues that in order for people to participate fully there has to be a sharing of power. Laverack (2004) identifies characteristics of participation where the power is more equally balanced. These characteristics form a useful checklist for ensuring health promotion partnerships in settings are fully participatory:

- A strong participant base involving all stakeholders, including marginalized groups, but sensitive to the cultural and social context
- Participants involved in defining need, solutions and actions
- Participants involved in decision making mechanisms, including planning, delivery, evaluation of programmes and services, and also in policy development
- Participation goes beyond the benefits and activities of the specific local partnership and extends to broader issues
- Mechanism exists which allows for the free flow of information between the different stakeholders
- Community stakeholders are appointed by its members

In addition to the above, it must be remembered that building capacity and capability for community participation in settings partnerships is crucial. This will include developing personal skills and understanding and enabling participation through the provision of resources and practical support (Scriven, 2007).

Measuring the success of partnerships in settings

It is important that all stakeholders involved in partnerships reflect on their own effectiveness, benchmark the status of their partnership and provide a framework for development. This can be difficult, as the nature of partnerships is such that the inputs, processes and outcomes are not always easy to quantify (Corbin and Mittelmark, 2008). Nonetheless, Watson et al. (2000), following the WHO's Investment for Health Initiative at Verona in 1998 (which discussed the need for a resource to support the development of partnership quality measures), were involved in the design, development and testing of a benchmarking and assessment tool to enable partnerships to determine their progress against evidence-based criteria, and to share good practice. This tool, then known as the Verona Benchmark, was tested in community planning partnerships in Scotland and at 15 pilot sites across Europe. After extensive peer review in the UK involving people with practical research and policy expertise in partnership development, the tool was revised and restructured to support capacity development and to offer greater flexibility in its use. It was then retitled and launched. The Working Partnership (Markwell et al., 2003) is a toolkit for professionals whose job is to support partnership development and improve the quality of partnership working (Box 4.2 is taken from The Working Partnership). While Markwell et al. (2003) argue that there are no unique models for successful partnerships, they point to some common success factors and have drawn upon the available evidence and wide range of the experience in producing the toolkit which comprises an introductory guide, a short assessment manual, an in-depth assessment version, and a collection of photocopiable material, all of which are available on the National Institute for Health and Clinical Excellence web pages (NICE, 2011).

Halliday et al. (2004) have questioned the value of using tools and argue that they are open to misinterpretation and unlikely to foster development other than in those partnerships prepared to invest the necessary resources in broadbased evaluation (see Part I, Chapter 5 for more on evaluation and evaluating settings). Their work drew on the evaluation of two Health Action Zones, which had used a formal assessment tool, adapted from the Nuffield Partnership Assessment Tool and the Verona Benchmark. It is suggested that formal assessment tools can be extremely valuable in terms of the learning that can result both from the process itself and from the outcomes of the assessment.

Corbin and Mittelmark (2008) suggest that partnership working is an act of faith based on the belief of synergistic outcomes, rather than evidence. Dowling et al. (2004) support this claim and argue that the advantages of partnership working are often espoused, but the evidence of success can be limited. Researching how success in partnership working is conceptualized, they found that there were two main elements being measured. The first came under the category of process issues, focusing on how well the partners work together in addressing joint aims and the long term sustainability of the partnership. The second focused on outcome issues, such as changes in service delivery, and subsequent effects on the health or wellbeing of service users. The conclusion drawn was that the research into the effectiveness of partnerships has centred heavily on process issues, while much less emphasis has been given to outcome success. While their findings were specifically focused on partnership relating to service delivery, their findings have relevance to health promotion partnership in settings that span the wide range of public sector agencies and the third sector. Table 4.3 has drawn from the findings of Dowling et al. (2004) and applied these in a generic way to health promotion partnerships designed to deliver services or interventions within settings. The table provides ideas for establishing both process and the outcome measures of success.

An essential premise underpinning partnership working, despite the weak evidence base, is that it is a fundamental principle on which settings work should be established. The opportunities for collaboration, cooperation and

Table 4.3   Process and outcome measures and indicators to use for measuring the success of health promotion partnerships

	Dimension	Indicators of success
Process	Level of engagement and commitment of partners (including community representatives)	Level of enthusiasm of partners for the partnership as reflected in the behaviours and beliefs of the partners
	Agreement of the need and nature of the partnership	Aims and vision are shared and there is interdependency between partners
	High level of trust, reciprocity and respect between partners	The extent to which partners have confidence in each other
	Positive environmental factors, including financial climate, suitable institutional and legal structures and wider interagency activity	Political and social climate conducive to partnership working
	Satisfactory accountability arrangement, plus appropriate audit and monitoring of the partnership	Appropriate lines of responsibility and appraisal arrangements
	Adequate leadership and management of the partnership	Quality of the partnerships executive authority over the strategic direction of the partnership and the management of the activities designed to achieve that broad direction
Outcome	Improvement in the accessibility to the health promotion service or intervention by service users and target groups	Convenience of the service location; service users experience quicker response or earlier intervention
	Distribution of services is more equitable	Distribution of services relating to need, people with the same need receive the same attention and resources, people with different needs receive different attention and resources
	Improvement in efficiency, effectiveness or quality of health promotion services or interventions	Impact and standards of the interventions, taking into account costs and reduction in duplication and overlap between health promotion service providers
	Improvement in the experiences of staff and partners	Changes in the working conditions and/or job satisfaction of staff providing the health promotion service or intervention
	Improvement in the health status, quality of life or wellbeing experienced by individuals, target groups and/or communities	Impact of the intervention on the specific health or wellbeing issue amongst the targeted population group

Source: Based on the finding of the Dowling et al. (2004) literature survey. See the article for full discussion of their methodology and results.

formal partnerships have to be embraced in order to advance settings. A final point to emphasize is that the arguments for a synergistic relationship and a co-dependency between settings and partnerships appear valid. It is easy to make the case for how settings could not function effectively without fully developed participatory approaches and in turn that settings provide the structure and the milieu in which partnerships are formed and maintained. If settings are to continue to thrive, therefore, then the capacity and capability for engaging in partnerships and the nurturing of an environment for such work has to be prioritized.

Summary points

- Developing and sustaining health promotion partnerships is regarded as a fundamental principle of working in settings.

- The increased emphasis on partnership working is deemed to provide a wide range of benefits to those embracing a settings approach.

- The complexity of health promotion partnership working in and across settings is challenging, but necessary to the success of a settings approach.

- Health promoters should enter into health promotion participatory and partnership working with a realistic view of the challenges, vexations and intangible elements to be confronted.

Online Further Reading

Halliday, G., Asthana, S.N.M. and Richardson, S (2004) 'Evaluating partnership: the role of formal assessment tools', *Evaluation*, 10 (3): 285–303.

For those who wish to examine in more detail the evaluation of partnership working, this article assesses the contribution of formal tools to our understanding of partnership. It outlines some key methodological limitations and stresses the continued importance of an understanding of context alongside any measurement of partnership effectiveness.

References

ASH Wales (2011) www.ashwales.co.uk/wtca.php (accessed 16 March 2011).

Bartel, D., Igras, S. and Chamberlain, J. (2007) *Building Partnerships for Health in Conflict Affected Settings: A Practical Guide to Beginning and Sustaining Inter-Agency Partnerships*. London: Care International.

Corbin, J.H and Mittelmark, M.B. (2008) 'Partnership lessons from the Global Programme for Health Promotion Effectiveness: a case study', *Health Promotion International*, 23 (4): 365–71.

Coulson, A.C (2005) 'A plague on all your partnerships: theory and practice in regeneration', *International Journal of Public Sector Management*, 18 (2): 151–63.

Department of the Environment, Transport and the Regions (2001) *Local Strategic Partnerships*. London: DETR.

Department of Health (1994) *The Health of the Nation*. London: The Stationery Office.

Department of Health (2006) *Our Health, Our Care, Our Say*. London: The Stationery Office.

Department of Health (2007) *Partnerships for Better Health: Small Change, Big Difference: Healthier Choices for Life*. London: The Stationery Office.

Department of Health (2010) *Equity and Excellence: Liberating the NHS*. London: The Stationery Office. www.dh.gov.uk/en/Healthcare/LiberatingtheNHS/index.htm (accessed 30 March 2011).

Dooris, M. (2004) 'Joining up settings for health: a valuable investment for strategic partnerships?', *Critical Public Health*, 14 (1): 49–61.

Dowling, B., Powell, M. and Glendinning, C. (2004) 'Conceptualising successful partnerships', *Health and Social Care in the Community*, 12 (4): 309–17.

Halliday, G., Asthana, S.N.M. and Richardson, S. (2004) 'Evaluating partnership: the role of formal assessment tools', *Evaluation*, 10 (3): 285–303.

Health Scotland (2011) www.healthscotland.com/food-and-health.aspx (accessed 16 March 2011).

HealthKnowledge (2011) *Structuring and managing inter-organisational (network) relationships, including intersectoral work, collaborative working practices and partnerships*. Available at: www.healthknowledge.org.uk/public-health-textbook/organisation-management/5b-understanding-ofs/relationships (accessed 30 March 2011).

Improvement Network (2010) *Top 10 Partnership Killers*. Available at: www.improvementnetwork.gov.uk/imp/aio/11465 (accessed on 30 March 2011).

IUHPE (International Union of Heath Promotion and Education) (2011) *Tools for partnership activities in health promotion and evaluating interventions that aim to reduce social inequalities in health*. Available at: www.iuhpe.org/?page=508&lang=en (accessed 18 March 2011).

Jackson, S., Perkins, F., Khandor, E., Cordwell, L., Hamann, S. and Buasai, S. (2006) 'Integrated health promotion strategies: a contribution to tackling current and future health challenges', *Health Promotion International*, 21, Issue supplement 1: 75–83.

Jupp, B. (2000) *Working Together: Creating a Better Environment for Cross-Sector Partnerships*. Demos: London.

Knight, T., Smith, J. and Cropper, S. (2001) 'Developing sustainable collaboration: learning from theory and practice', *Primary Health Care Research and Development*, 2: 139–48.

Laverack, G. (2004) *Health Promotion Practice: Power and Empowerment.* London: Sage.

Local Government Improvement and Development (2011a) *Coalition Government Plans – Implications for Local Partnership Working.* Available at: www.idea.gov. uk/idk/core/page.do?pageId=20784973 (accessed 30 March 2011).

Local Government Improvement and Development (2011b) LSPs – Leadership and governance of an area. www.idea.gov.uk/idk/core/page.do?pageId=15217079 (accessed 30 March 2011).

Markwell, S., Watson, J., Speller, V., Platt, J. and Younger, T. (2003) *The Working Partnership, Book 1.* London: Health Development Agency. Available from NICE: www.nice.org.uk/aboutnice/whoweare/aboutthehda/ hdapublications/working_partnership_book_1__introduction.jsp (accessed 14 March 2011).

Mohajer, G. (2011) 'Health Promotion Awards 2010', *Perspectives in Public Health*, 131 (2): 59–61.

National Institute of Health and Clinical Excellence (NICE) (2011) www.nice.org. uk/aboutnice/whoweare/aboutthehda/hdapublications/working_partnership_ book_1__introduction.jsp (accessed 18 March 2011).

PAHA (2011) www.paha.org.uk/SitePage/about-the-alliance (accessed 16 March 2011).

Scriven, A. (2007) 'Developing local alliance partnerships through community collaboration and participation', in S. Handsley, C.E. Lloyd, J. Douglas, S. Earle and S.M. Spurr (eds), *Policy and Practice in Promoting Public Health.* London: Sage.

Scriven, A. (2010) 'Partnership, collaboration and participatory approaches in health promotion practice', in A. Scriven, C. Kouta and I. Papadopoulos (eds), *Health Promotion for Health Practitioners.* Athens: Paschalides.

Scriven, A. (in press) 'Building partnerships and alliances', in L. Jones and J. Douglas (eds), *Public Health: Building Innovative Practice.* London: Sage.

Standards for England (2010) Partnership Working Protocol Template. www.stand-ardsforengland.gov.uk/Resources/Resourcelibrary/Toolkits/pwptemplate/#d. en.26872 (accessed 09 March 2011).

Tang, K., Beaglehole, R. and O'Byrne, D. (2005) 'Policy and partnership for health promotion action – addressing the determinants of health', *Bulletin of the World Health Organization*, 83 (12), 881–968.

Watson, J., Speller, V., Markwell, S. and Platt, S. (2000) 'The Verona Benchmark – applying evidence to improve the quality of partnership', *Promotion and Education*, VII (2): 16–23.

World Health Organization (1978) *Declaration of Alma Ata International Conference*, 6–12 September 1978. Geneva: WHO.

WHO (World Health Organization) (1986) *Ottawa Charter for Health Promotion.* Geneva: WHO.

WHO (World Health Organization) (1997) *Jakarta Declaration on Leading Health Promotion into the 21st Century.* Geneva: WHO.

WHO (World Health Organization) (1998) *Health Promotion Glossary.* Geneva: WHO.

WHO (World Health Organization) (2002) *Community Participation in Local Health and Sustainable Development: Approaches and Techniques.* European Sustainable Development and Health Series: 4. Geneva: WHO.

WHO (World Health Organization) (2005) *The Bangkok Charter.* Geneva: WHO.

WHO (World Health Organization) (2011) www.who.int/healthy_settings/en/ (accessed 21 March 2011).

5

Planning and Evaluating Health Promotion in Settings

Jane South and James Woodall

Aims

- To examine the principles of health promotion programme planning and evaluation and their application within a settings-based approach
- To highlight the significance of stakeholder involvement in all stages of the planning and evaluation process
- To look at the selection of appropriate indicators for monitoring and evaluation within a settings framework
- To discuss the challenges and opportunities for developing the evidence base for settings-based approaches

Principles of health promotion programme planning and evaluation

Health promotion is a process of enabling individuals and communities to gain greater control over their health and wellbeing and this imperative, whether at individual, organizational or population level, can be contrasted to the maintenance of services based on traditional power structures and practices and an emphasis on systematic programme planning processes in order to be able to effect change (Green and Tones, 2010; Rootman et al., 2001) and on the generation and appraisal of evidence to demonstrate effectiveness (Nutbeam, 1998; Rychetnik et al., 2002; Springett et al., 2007). In settings-based approaches, programme planning and evaluation are informed by an ecological model of health that recognizes that health is determined by various environmental, organizational and personal factors (Dooris, 2009). The focus is on supporting system change through policy development, participation and partnership working. Sharing learning and demonstrating worth is of critical importance in a field of work that seeks to shift policy and practice upstream, and yet settings-based approaches have been critiqued for lacking a strong evidence base (Dooris, 2005) and being legitimized through an act of faith rather than through robust research and evaluation (St Leger, 1997).

Applying the principles of health promotion programme planning and evaluation can help in the identification of priorities for action in settings, in supporting effective implementation and in recognizing achievements. Conversely the lack of rational planning can lead to poorly designed interventions, implementation failure and weak evidence of success. Evaluation of settings-based approaches is informed by wider debates about the development of an evidence base for health promotion and appropriate methodologies for measuring change (Raphael, 2000; Springett, 2001). In practice, health promoters who wish to develop settings-based approaches can be faced with a myriad of choices over targets, indicators and methods. This chapter seeks to provide an overview of the main issues for developing an evidence base and to highlight key decision points.

The purpose of programme planning is to provide a framework for delivering effective health promotion interventions within the setting which will ultimately result in positive health outcomes. In its simplest form, the planning process can be considered as a number of stages (South, 2010) (see Table 5.1).

While it is tempting to view planning as a linear process, cyclic models of programme planning, with the emphasis on processes of change, provide

Table 5.1 Stages of the planning process

Main stages	Key processes
Assessment of the current situation	Problem identification
	Assessment of needs
	Identification of stakeholders
	Interpretation of existing evidence
Planning for change	Goal setting
	Agreeing objectives and targets
	Identification of priorities
	Selection of intervention methods
Delivering change	Allocation of resources
	Capacity building
	Alliance building
	Leadership
	Implementation
	Monitoring and audit
Evaluating change	Developing evaluation frameworks
	Selecting indicators
	Data collection and interpretation
	Feedback and dissemination

Source: South, 2010

a better fit with health promotion than linear models (Whitehead, 2001), and allow for the flexible development of activities in response to both stakeholder involvement and evidence gathered through evaluation. Settings-based approaches may involve multiple planning cycles to develop specific interventions and these cycles will be nested within a wider programme structure.

Many of the principles set out in this chapter have wide application, but the focus will be on planning, delivering and evaluating settings-based approaches. The scale and scope of health promotion activity in settings encompasses large scale regional health programmes, through to small organizations operating with discrete boundaries. The emphasis on horizontal programmes, with programme activities directed at improving general health or determinants of health across a number of areas, can create challenges for planning and evaluation. Therefore the concept of an intervention has to be a broad one, reflecting the diversity of methods and activities that may be adopted as part of a settings approach and the levels of change (individual, organizational, community, policy).

The nature of health promotion requires a shift of emphasis from service delivery *for* people to achieving health outcomes *with* people. Green and Tones (2010: 175) caution that to set systematic planning processes against community participation and flexibility is to impose a false dichotomy, as planning models should be seen as offering valuable frameworks for decision making that can be linked to community development and empowerment goals. Settings-based approaches are characterized by the involvement of multiple stakeholders, not only in consultation and programme design but in goal setting, implementation and monitoring and evaluation. This not only presents practical challenges around coordination and communication, but also there may be conceptual differences in how success is defined (Smith et al., 2008). There needs to be recognition that while frameworks can support planning and evaluation through application of systematic processes, the synergy from effective partnerships in health promoting settings may lead to improvements greater than predicted through the individual parts.

Programme planning and design in a settings-based approach

The development of specialized planning frameworks for health promoting settings has been uneven, although there are examples to be found in settings such as schools (Booth and Samdal, 1997; Deschesnes et al., 2003; for more details on the school setting see Part II, Chapter 9), hospitals (Hancock, 1999; Pelikan et al., 2001; see Part II, Chapter 8) and universities (Tsouros et al., 1998) (see Part II, Chapter 10). The dearth of generic frameworks that support practitioners to plan and design settings work has arguably created a gap between the theory of settings approaches and the implementation in practice (Deschesnes et al., 2003; Nutbeam, 1992; Woodall, 2010). No two settings are alike, which makes the transferability of what works problematic (Dooris, 2005; Poland et al., 2009). Poland et al. (2009) eschew the concept of a prescriptive planning

Table 5.2   An analytical framework for settings

Key aspects of settings		
(1) Understanding settings	(2) Changing settings	(3) Knowledge development and knowledge translation
Diversity across and within categories of settings	Context and history in the setting	Identified knowledge gaps
Received knowledge and underlying assumptions	Capacity – local agencies, government, professionals and communities	Forms of knowledge and information
Localized determinants of health – physical, built and psychosocial environment	Focus	Theory–practice gaps
Stakeholders and interests	Engagement	
Power, influence and drivers for social change	Strategy	
	Evaluation	

Source: Poland et al. (2009)

model and instead propose an analytical framework. This framework recognizes the diversity and uniqueness of settings, and is accompanied by key questions for practitioners to use within the specific contexts with which they are working (Table 5.2). For example, understanding the setting itself and how environmental influences within that setting shape health, is considered the first part of the planning process (Poland et al., 2009).

Health needs assessment remains a cornerstone of health promotion planning within a settings approach. The WHO Health Promotion Glossary (Smith et al., 2006: 343) defines health needs assessment as:

> A systematic procedure for determining the nature and extent of health needs in a population, the causes and contributing factors to those needs and the human, organizational and community resources which are available to respond to these.

Failure to assess health needs is likely to lead to a poor fit between programme elements and the needs of recipients, and therefore misdirected use of resources. Conversely, health needs assessments cannot only provide essential contextual information to aid planning but can also be a mechanism for increasing stakeholder involvement in the programme development. There is a strong case for incorporating lay perspectives on health and health needs to complement evidence of need derived from expert knowledge, such as epidemiological data (Krieger et al., 2002; Popay et al., 1998; Rifkin et al., 2000).

The whole system philosophy of the settings approach (see Part I, Chapter 3 for a detailed overview of whole systems thinking) demands consideration of all those who interact with or are part of the setting (Poland et al., 2009), although this may be built over time (Heritage and Dooris, 2009). For example, involving stakeholders in the needs assessment process in a school setting would constitute the inclusion of the views of teachers, non-teaching staff (including administrators, school cooks, cleaners and caretakers), governors, pupils and parents. The setting itself may hold different meanings to the individuals within it; for example the prison setting is viewed as a workplace for staff, a temporary home for prisoners and a place to visit for families and children (Dixey and Woodall, forthcoming) (see Part II, Chapter 11 for more on prisons as a setting).

An assessment of all aspects of the setting should be considered in this initial stage, including elements of the physical, built and psychosocial environment that may impact upon health as well as a detailed understanding of the existing power relations within the setting that may have an impact on the implementation of a settings approach (Poland et al., 2009). While Barić (1998) advocates that practitioners should work closely with the management and those who hold power within the setting, Poland et al. (2000) discuss the paradox that practitioners aligning themselves too closely with powerful gatekeepers may jeopardize attempts to gain the trust and support of all those within the organization.

Once a detailed assessment of the setting has been undertaken, the next stage is goal setting and identification of clear aims and objectives. Aims are broad statements that describe the overall purpose of the programme, while goals denote the desired outcomes or targets (Spicker, 2006). Objectives are more specific statements that define what programme participants will have achieved or what a programme will deliver. Pragmatically, initial aims and objectives may be considered by a working team of people within an organization or partnership structure who then share their ideas with the setting as a whole (Barić, 1998). The process of setting aims and objectives is not merely a technical exercise, but one where the values and underpinning philosophy of a proposed programme are considered and appropriate approaches agreed. Johnson and Baum (2001), for example, demonstrate a variety of interpretations in the meaning of a health promoting hospital ranging from the provision of health information and education to patients through to the reorientation of services and major organizational reform (see Part II, Chapter 8 for a critical overview of healthy hospitals).

Creating greater ownership of aims and objectives will build commitment to delivery and more likelihood of achieving sustainability. An action planning cycle can mean that communities are involved in a continuous cycle from assessing needs and assets through to monitoring and evaluation (WHO, 2002). There is evidence that participation in health promotion planning can improve project management and sustainability because links between project beneficiaries and planners are strengthened and multidisciplinary working facilitated (Rifkin et al., 2000). For example, Jamison et al. (1998) report that involving pupils in the development of planning within a health promoting school gave them a sense of pride in their school environment. Aims and objectives will undoubtedly be contingent on capacity and feasibility issues as well as senior level commitment from within the organization (Caraher et al., 2002;

Woodall, 2010). The extent to which organizations aspire to, or are able to achieve, the ideal healthy setting may be constrained by the competing forces within the setting acting against the health agenda or limitations in support structures (finance, time, training, expertise) (Green and Tones, 2010; Whitelaw et al., 2001).

Choice of health promotion methods should follow on naturally from the setting of objectives and should be congruent with the overall settings approach. Whitelaw et al. (2001) present a typology of settings-based activity which highlights the spectrum of potential interventions, ranging from a passive model where the setting merely provides access to a population and traditional health education activities are selected, to a comprehensive structural model where system change is achieved through activities such as organizational change and policy development. As part of their analytical framework, Poland et al. (2009: 511) usefully outline four key questions that should be posed by practitioners to guide the development of strategy:

• What emphasis is put on changing individual behaviour as opposed to structural and organizational change?
• How should one work with wider stakeholders outside the setting of focus?
• How much of a participatory approach will be undertaken?
• What type of evidence will be drawn for the intervention design?

A settings-based approach is characterized by a focus on system change and creating more supportive environments, consequently even within a single organization like a school there are likely to be multiple programme strands and different levels of activity as well as specific projects. Ideally these strands will fit within an overarching strategy that links activities in a holistic way. Settings-based approaches are usually seeking change over time; the implications are that planning processes should retain sufficient flexibility to cope with new developments, as, for example, stakeholder involvement is widened in the course of the intervention. Inevitably the planning process will be an iterative one, with stakeholders returning to decisions and refining plans as new information emerges. Theory-Based Evaluation can provide a basis for articulating assumptions at a micro level (de Leeuw, 2009). Developed as an evaluation approach for large, multidimensional programmes (Fulbright-Anderson et al., 1998), Theory of Change (TOC) involves stakeholders working together to identify long term goals, modelling how change is to be achieved and checking assumptions about the programme logic, thereby improving planning processes in the context of the evaluation (Connell and Kubisch, 1988).

Delivering change in settings

There is little guidance given in health promotion planning literature to the implementation stage of programme development. Yet inattention to aspects of delivery can result in an implementation gap, where programme objectives fail to be achieved due to a range of causes, from unrealistic targets to staff resistance.

Implementation is an important subject in policy studies and some of the critiques advanced have relevance to settings-based approaches because of their focus on system and organizational change (Parsons, 1995; Sabatier, 1986). The rationalist top-down model for programme implementation is rarely achieved as there are numerous barriers to perfect implementation, including external constraints, poor links between cause and effect, poor coordination and inadequate resources (Hogwood and Gunn, 1984) but at the same time the role of what Lipsky (1993) refers to as street level bureaucrats, the workers who shape policy through the decisions they make in practice, can have a profound effect on the outcomes. In implementing settings-based approaches, it is useful to consider both the vertical and horizontal dimensions of policy identified by Colebatch (2002). Concern with the vertical dimension in health promoting settings would involve health promoters in setting a clear strategic direction for organizations, ensuring the necessary authority for decisions and allocation of resources was sought, agreeing realistic targets and identifying individuals able to manage programme strands or specific projects. Concern with the horizontal dimension would involve health promoters in working for wider ownership of the programme, facilitating multidisciplinary working, building workforce and community capacity, and collecting feedback from stakeholders.

Many of the pitfalls of implementation can be avoided by robust programme planning processes and by wide stakeholder involvement to ensure that plans are relevant, acceptable and feasible. Some settings, such as health promoting schools (see Part II, Chapter 9), are defined by known boundaries of action and defined populations (Ziglio et al., 1995), which can be considered an advantage in terms of implementation and allocation of resources. Others, such as healthy cities, face the challenges of multisectoral working and programmes operating at many levels with diverse activities. Whatever the setting, the practicalities of delivery are important. This will include aspects like budgeting and financial governance, project management and staff responsibilities, project timelines and milestones and monitoring systems. Pronk (2003) identifies four components that need to be considered in health promotion programmes:

- Size – the extent of the programme in terms of amount of activities (contacts, events, training sessions etc.)
- Scope – the range of activities included
- Scalability – the way a programme will gradually increase its coverage through a series of planned steps
- Sustainability – long term programme support

Settings-based approaches take an ecological approach to health promotion so require the involvement of a range of stakeholders. The implications are that in any one setting a number of professional groups or staff will be involved, as well as community members and/or programme recipients. Developing capacity in the workforce for programme delivery will need to extend beyond those with health roles if settings-based approaches are to be successful. This may require developing knowledge and awareness in the workforce, training and skills development, as well as increasing participation and commitment in other professional groups (Crisp et al., 2000). Indeed, Green and Tones (2010) argue that even in policy-based interventions, change is dependent on a process of learning. Engaging stakeholders can be seen as a critical factor in achieving sustainability. Whitelaw et al. (2001) highlight the challenge of translating isolated and discrete health promotion activities into more penetrative settings-based work. With regard to health promoting universities (see Part II, Chapter 10), Dooris (2001: 58) argues for the need to move beyond projectism, where people see settings work as a discrete and contained project – interesting, important even, but definitely the responsibility of a named coordinator – to mainstreaming of health promotion activity.

Evaluation of healthy settings

Evaluation is a key stage of the planning cycle as it provides an assessment of a programme and its impact. Evaluation is also a mechanism for feedback and improvement and as such should be regarded as an integral component of health promotion programmes (Springett, 1998). Wright (1999) sets out a number of reasons for undertaking evaluation in health promotion practice, all of which have relevance to settings-based approaches, and these include accountability, improving the design or performance of a service, checking progress, informing decision making about which activities should be supported and piloting innovative ideas.

While there is an imperative to evaluate, health promotion evaluation is not unproblematic, both in terms of the practicalities of evaluation in different settings and the existence of profound debates, and indeed methodological divisions, about appropriate approaches to gathering and validating evidence (Fawcett et al., 2001; Green and Tones, 1999; Kelly et al., 2002). Settings literature (see for example (Dooris, 2005; de Leeuw and Skovgaard, 2005) reflects the somewhat troublesome nature of evaluation in terms of attempting to reconcile the need to develop a sound evidence base with an ecological approach based on broad system change. Some of the challenges for creating an evidence base are discussed in the following section, but here the principles of health promotion evaluation and how they might apply to settings-based approaches are discussed.

The focus of a health promotion evaluation should be on evaluating change rather than service delivery. In most evaluations this will involve both assessment of outcomes, that is the changes that result from an intervention (in its broadest sense), and examination of processes, looking at the mechanisms operating within programmes and the influence of contextual factors. There are good reasons to include both process and outcome measures as a fuller, more comprehensive view of a programme will be obtained, and more critically in settings-based approaches, this will help develop understanding of how different programme strands and the contribution of different stakeholders work together within that context to produce positive outcomes. A distinction is often made between formative evaluation, which can usually be conducted during the development of a healthy settings programme for the purpose of providing feedback to refine the activities, and summative evaluation, conducted to provide an assessment of progress at the end of a programme or on reaching milestones. The purpose and resulting focus of an evaluation will be dependent on the stage of development (Nutbeam, 1998) and whether there is existing evidence of effectiveness (Wimbush and Watson, 2000). Curtice et al. (2001: 328) in setting out recommendations on the evaluation of healthy cities, emphasize the collaborative and developmental nature of evaluation in these settings. They argue that evaluation should be justified on the basis that it should contribute to knowledge and policy development in an iterative and continuing way. Even within smaller settings, such as healthy workplaces, evaluation will not be a once-and-for-all event as different programme strands and individual projects will have different measurement priorities. However, an overarching evaluation framework will allow progress towards goals within the healthy setting to be assessed so that results can be fed into programme planning and policy development.

Consideration needs to be given to evaluation design and to underpinning epistemological assumptions about how evidence is to be generated and validated. Methodological debates in health promotion centre on what evaluation means within a social as opposed to biomedical model of health (Green and Tones, 1999; Raphael, 2000). At the heart of many of the debates is the question of what should be measured and how designs can cope with the complexity of health promotion interventions at the same time as valuing the participation and active engagement of stakeholders (Nutbeam, 1998; Springett, 2001). These arguments have particular cogency for settings-based approaches because partnership working and community engagement are core methods and need to be considered within any evaluation.

Experimental design, and specifically randomized controlled trials, which are the gold-standard for evidence-based medicine, are deemed inappropriate for health promotion evaluation as experimental designs fail to take account of the multiple factors affecting health (Green and Tones, 1999). The complexity and diversity of settings precludes the use of experimental design on both pragmatic and methodological grounds (Green et al., 2000). Dooris (2005: 61) argues that theory-based evaluation may offer a way forward in evaluating healthy settings as this involves mapping the links between processes and outcomes at different levels, and could potentially be a means of understanding and capturing added value of whole system working as well as assessing the effectiveness of individual programmes and projects. However, he cautions that a number of issues need to be addressed, including being able to articulate the underpinning theories for settings-based work.

There is wide support in health promotion for use of participatory evaluation approaches that facilitate stakeholder involvement in evaluation design, data collection and dissemination (Feuerstein, 1986; Nguyet Nguyen and Otis, 2003). Seeking stakeholder involvement in evaluation fits with the overall ethos of settings work in terms of developing pluralistic perspectives on the healthy setting, and furthermore there are good pragmatic reasons in terms of research capacity and capturing data across different programme strands and levels. There are strong arguments that collaboration in evaluation will enhance mutual learning and lead to more relevant research that is more likely to be used (Walter et al., 2003; WHO Europe Working Group on Health Promotion Evaluation, 1998).

In considering what aspects to measure in an evaluation of a healthy setting, indicators or measures will need to be chosen that are appropriate to the setting and its context, and will fit with emerging evaluation priorities and information needs. Saunders et al. (2005) suggest seven elements to be included in a process evaluation plan (adapted from Steckler and Linnan, 2002): fidelity (whether the programme was implemented as planned), completeness (whether all elements were delivered to participants), exposure, satisfaction, reach, recruitment and context (whether environmental aspects have influenced the programme). In settings-based approaches evaluation can usefully examine the quality and outcomes from collaborative processes as logically these will deliver more than the sum of the parts of constituent programmes. Dooris (2005: 66) argues that whole systems thinking means evaluation has to capture added value and map interrelationships, interactions and synergies with and between settings.

Outcome evaluation is needed to assess the effectiveness of a healthy settings programme against its goals and objectives; and measures of success or indicators should be selected that are capable of demonstrating the expected outcomes. At the same time, evaluation should be flexible enough to detect unanticipated outcomes, both negative and positive (Rychetnik et al., 2002) and because of concern for equity, examine relative costs and benefits for different stakeholder groups (Poland et al., 2009). Green and South (2006: 164) argue that selection of indicators is key to good evaluation and indicators should be chosen that are valid (measure what they are meant to), meaningful (able to be interpreted by stakeholders) and credible (able to convince stakeholders). Indicators measure different types of health promotion outcomes and can therefore be behavioural, educational, social, policy, environmental or even physiological and will relate to different levels of programme outcomes:

- individual – for example, measuring changes in individuals' attributes, such as knowledge, beliefs or behaviour;
- organizational – for example, measuring changes in staff skills or service improvements;
- community – for example, measuring changes in social capital or increased community mobilization;
- policy – for example, measuring changes in policy to support health or increased participation in policy processes.

Selection of indicators should match the programme plan, objectives and activities, and take account of the predicted time line between programme delivery and any realistic impact. In settings-based approaches most health outcomes will be achieved indirectly through environmental and policy change affecting the determinants of health rather than through any direct impact at an individual level. Blenkinsop et al. (2004), for example, argue that the National Healthy School Standard will not result in a direct impact on health in the short term but suggest instead focusing on health-related behaviours (see Part II, Chapter 9 for more details on National Healthy Schools Standards). Table 5.3 provides examples of criteria on healthy eating from the current Healthy Schools Standard (Healthy Schools, 2009), which reflect the whole systems approach to changing the school environment and the range of types of indicator.

Curtice et al. (2001) argue that indicators for healthy cities (see Part II, Chapter 9) must be developed locally and cannot be developed in isolation from the political context in which the evaluation is taking place. Judge and Bauld (2001: 27) present four key requirements for a change framework:

- Indicators: which indicators will demonstrate that a particular element's outcomes are changing?
- Populations: which target populations should be showing change on these indicators?
- Thresholds: how much change on these indicators is good enough?
- Timelines: how long will it take to achieve these thresholds?

Table 5.3   Examples of Healthy Eating criteria for healthy schools

Criteria	Examples of information collected	Examples of measures/ tools to use
Has a Whole School Food Policy – developed through wide consultation, implemented, monitored and evaluated for impact	Surveys, questionnaires, discussions	Written Whole School Food Policy School Council minutes
Ensures that children and young people have opportunities to learn about different types of food in the context of a balanced diet and how to plan, budget, prepare and cook meals	Outline of the curriculum for Healthy Eating. Balance and breadth of curriculum Children's and young people's knowledge and understanding of healthy eating	Healthy eating/design technology/food technology schemes of work Questionnaires, discussion
Has a welcoming eating environment that encourages the positive social interaction of children/young people	How and when children have been consulted and changes made as a result The attitudes of children and young people to the dining room Number of children and young people who meet in dining room	Questionnaires, discussion Teacher observations Diary of events, minutes of School Council
Ensures provision of training in practical food education	CPD folders	Written Whole School Food Policy

Source: Healthy Schools, 2009 (Crown copyright)

Following selection of indicators, appropriate research methods can then be chosen to gather data, taking into account whether quantitative or qualitative measures are being used. Consideration should be given to ensuring that the methods fit with the setting and the programme ethos and that the different perspectives of stakeholders are included (Green and South, 2006). In many settings, routinely collected data, such as population level indices and monitoring information, can be used in evaluation although there can be disadvantages in terms of lack of specificity and sensitivity and data quality (Kane et al., 2000).

Challenges for developing an evidence-based settings approach

Hancock (1999) suggests that the settings approach is one of the most successful strategies to emerge from the Ottawa Charter, but argues that one major drawback has been a paucity of high quality evaluation leading to an uneven and underdeveloped evidence base (Dooris et al., 2007: 335). There are exceptions to this; for example, the establishment of an evidence base for health promoting schools (Corcoran and Bone, 2007; Dooris, 2007). This has arguably been facilitated by the standards and criteria developed for the health promoting schools and other key texts (see for example Barnekow et al., 2006).

Dooris (2005, 2006) has outlined the main challenges that have inhibited the generation of a convincing evidence base. Firstly, the funding structures for evaluative work are often focused on specific diseases and risk factor interventions and this runs counter to a comprehensive settings-based evaluation. Secondly, the heterogeneity between and across settings, coupled with the diversity and understanding of the approach, creates issues in transferability of research evidence. Indeed, the conceptual variances, pragmatic influences and differences in the size and type of setting makes building a substantive view of what works challenging (Dooris, 2005). Finally, there are problems with evaluating ecological and whole system approaches. If the settings approach is about integration within organizations, it can be argued that the greater the success, the more difficult the evaluation becomes (Dooris, 2005: 59).

Barić and Blinkhorn (2007) see embedded health promotion and health education within organizations as a logical outcome of the settings approach. Sufficient time is needed to consider long term organizational and systems change. Yet, time is often a rare commodity in health promotion programme evaluation (Kickbusch, 1995), where often rapid, measurable success is prioritized over determining longer term achievements. De Leeuw (2009) also notes that the more distal interventions will provide a broad and sustainable impact on health but compared to proximal interventions, require more complex methodology to assess effectiveness.

The evident challenges in constructing a robust evidence base for settings-based approaches leave scope for the further development of practical and analytical frameworks to support the synthesis of evidence and learning. Moreover, de Leeuw's (2009) plea for utility-driven evidence within the policy sphere in the context of healthy cities has wider resonance, as evaluation has the potential to be a mechanism for learning (Springett, 2001). The adoption of systematic programme planning and evaluation processes can assist in developing settings-based approaches and in building an evidence base. This does not mean supporting a narrow reductionist approach that fragments activities and ignores the synergies from collaborative working and capacity-building activities. Planning and evaluation processes can incorporate health promotion values through facilitating cooperation, participation and shared learning. Health promoters will have a key role in arguing for a shift of focus from measuring individual actions in settings to capturing system change in relation to wider determinants.

Summary points

- Systematic programme planning processes can add value to settings-based approaches. Health promoters need to incorporate an analysis of environmental influences and organizational capacity as well as undertaking needs assessment, setting aims and objectives, delivering programme components and undertaking evaluation.
- In line with the whole systems thinking that underpins settings-based approaches, stakeholder engagement should be sought at all stages of the programme planning cycle as this will widen ownership, build capacity for delivery and help to achieve sustainability.
- Evaluation methods and measures can be chosen with the aim of understanding the context, examining the key processes that will deliver change, capturing the synergies that may result, as well as measuring outcomes at individual, organizational, policy and community level.
- There are practical and methodological challenges in constructing an evidence base for settings-based work, however, evaluation can contribute to programme development and learning within and between settings.

Online Further Reading

Poland, B., Krupa, G. and McCall, D. (2009) 'Settings for health promotion: an analytic framework to guide intervention design and implementation', *Health Promotion Practice*, 10: 505–16.

This article provides one of the few templates for developing and evaluating health promoting settings. As well as analysing the challenges of settings-based work, the paper outlines a framework to assist practitioners in the design, implementation and evaluation of activities.

References

Barić, L. (1998) *People in Settings*. Altrincham: Barns Publications.

Baric', L. and Blinkhorn, A. (2007) 'Consumer-driven embedded health promotion and health education', *International Journal of Health Promotion and Education*, 45: 87–92.

Barnekow, V., Buijs, G., Clift, S., Bruun Jensen, B., Paulus, P., Rivett, D. and Young, I. (2006) *Health-Promoting Schools: A Resource for Developing Indicators*. Copenhagen: European Network of Health Promoting Schools.

Blenkinsop, S., Eggers, M., Schagen, I., Schagen, S., Scott, E., Warwick, I., Aggleton, P., Chase, E. and Surmount, M. (2004) Evaluation of the Impact of the National Healthy School Standard. Final Report. London: NFER, Thomas Coram Research Unit.

Booth, M.L. and Samdal, O. (1997) 'Health–promoting schools in Australia: models and measurement', *Australia and New Zealand Journal of Public Health*, 21: 365–70.

Caraher, M., Dixon, P., Hayton, P., Carr-Hill, R., Cough, H. and Bird, L. (2002) 'Are health-promoting prisons an impossibility? Lessons from England and Wales', *Health Education*, 102: 219–29.

Colebatch, H.K. (2002) *Policy*. Buckingham: Open University Press.

Connell, J.P. and Kubisch, A.C. (1988) 'Applying a theory of change approach to the evaluation of Comprehensive Community Initiatives: progress, prospects and problems', in K. Fulbright-Anderson, A. Kubisch and J. Connell (eds), *New Approaches to Evaluating Community Initiatives*. Washington, DC: The Aspen Institute.

Corcoran, N. and Bone, A. (2007) 'Using settings to communicate health promotion', in N Corcoran (ed.), *Communicating Health: Strategies for Health Promotion*. London: Sage.

Crisp, B., Swordsmen, H. and Docket, S. (2000) 'Four approaches to capacity building in health: consequences for measurement and accountability', *Health Promotion International*, 15: 99–107.

Curtice, L., Springett, J. and Kennedy, A. (2001) 'Evaluation in urban settings: the challenge of Healthy Cities', in I. Rootman, M.S. Ronstadt, B. Hyndman, D. McQueen, L. Putin, J. Springett and E. Zillion (eds), *Evaluation in Health Promotion. Principles and Perspectives*. Denmark: WHO Europe.

Deschesnes, M., Martin, C. and Jomphe-Hill, A. (2003) 'Comprehensive approaches to school health promotion: how to achieve broader implementation?', *Health Promotion International*, 18: 387–96.

Dixey, R. and Woodall, J. (forthcoming) 'The significance of "the visit" in an English category-B prison: views from prisoners, prisoners' families and prison staff', *Community, Work and Family*.

Dooris, M. (2001) 'The "Health Promoting University"': a critical exploration of theory and practice', *Health Education*, 101: 51–60.

Dooris, M. (2005) 'Healthy settings: challenges to generating evidence of effectiveness', *Health Promotion International*, 21: 55–65.

Dooris, M. (2006) 'Health promoting settings: future directions', *Promotion and Education*, 13: 4–6.

Dooris, M. (2007) 'Healthy settings: past, present and future'. Unpublished PhD thesis. School of Health and Social Development. Victoria, Deakin University.

Dooris, M. (2009) 'Holistic and sustainable health improvement: the contribution of the settings-based approach to health promotion', *Perspectives in Public Health*, 129: 29–36.

Dooris, M., Poland, B., Kolbe, L., Leeuw, E.D., McCall, D. and Wharf-Higgins, J. (2007) 'Healthy settings. Building evidence for the effectiveness of whole system health promotion – challenges and future directions. In D.V. McQueen and C. Jones (eds), *Global Perspectives on Health Promotion Effectiveness*. New York: Springer.

Fawcett, S.B., Paine-Andrews, A., Francisco, V.T., Schultz, J., Richter, K.P., Berkley-Patton, J., Fisher, J.L., Lewis, R.K., Lopez, C.M., Russos, S., Williams, E.L., Harris, K.J. and Evensong, P. (2001) 'Evaluating community health initiatives for health and development', in I. Rootman, M.S. Goodstadt, B. Hyndman, D. McQueen, L. Putin, J. Springett and E. Zillion (eds), *Evaluation in Health Promotion: Principles and Perspectives*. Denmark: WHO Europe.

Feuerstein, M.T. (1986) *Partners in Evaluation: Evaluating Development and Community Programmes with Participants*. London: TALC, Macmillan.

Fulbright-Anderson, K., Kubisch, A. and Connell, J. (eds) (1998) *New Approaches to Evaluating Community Initiatives. Vol. 2: Theory, Measurement and Analysis*. Washington, DC: The Aspen Institute.

Green, J. and South, J. (2006) *Evaluation*. Maidenhead: Open University Press.

Green, J. and Tones, K. (1999) 'Towards a secure evidence base for health promotion', *Journal of Public Health Medicine*, 21: 133–9.

Green, J. and Tones, K. (2010) *Health Promotion: Planning and Strategies*. London: Sage.

Green, L.W., Poland, B.D. and Rootman, I. (2000) 'The settings approach to health promotion', in B.D. Poland, L.W. Green and I. Rootman (eds), *Settings for Health Promotion. Linking Theory and Practice*. Thousand Oaks, CA: Sage.

Hancock, T. (1999) 'Creating health and health promoting hospitals: a worthy challenge for the twenty-first century', *International Journal of Health Care Quality Assurance*, 12: 8–19.

Healthy Schools (2009) Healthy Eating. National Resources to Help Achieve the Criteria. Available at: www.healthyschools.gov.uk. PowerPoint presentation. http://resources.healthyschools.gov.uk/v/3c2f4382-9221-41a0-a5f7-9cbc00f0463d?c=8d58bfca-39d1-4d7d-927a-9cb501033fb9.

Heritage, Z. and Dooris, M. (2009) 'Community participation and empowerment in Healthy Cities', *Health Promotion International*, 24: 45–55.

Hogwood, B.W. and Gunn, L.A. (1984) *Policy Analysis for the Real World*. Oxford: Oxford University Press.

Jamison, J., Ashby, P., Hamilton, K., Lewis, G., Macdonald, A. and Saunders, L. (1998) *The Health Promoting School: Final Report of the ENHPS Evaluation Project in England*. London: HEA.

Johnson, A. and Baum, F. (2001) 'Health promoting hospitals: a typology of different organizational approaches to health promotion', *Health Promotion International*, 16: 281–7.

Judge, K. and Bauld, L. (2001) 'Strong theory, flexible methods: evaluating complex community-based initiatives', *Critical Public Health*, 11: 19–38.

Kane, R., Welling, K., Free, C. and Goodrich, J. (2000) 'Uses of routine data sets in the evaluation of health promotion interventions: opportunities and limitations', *Health Education*, 100: 33–41.

Kelly, M., Swann, C., Kilogram, A., Naidoo, B., Barnett-Paige, E. and Morgan, A. (2002) *Methodological Problems in Constructing the Evidence Base in Public*

Health. Methodology Reference Group, Public Health Evidence Steering Group, Health Development Agency.

Kickbusch, I. (1995) 'An overview to the settings based approach to health promotion', in T. Teacher and J. Thompson (eds), *The Settings Based Approach to Health Promotion: Conference Report*. Welwyn Garden City: Hertfordshire Health Promotion.

Krieger, J., Allen, C., Chile, A., Ciskei, S., Shier, J.K., Sentara, K. and Sullivan, M. (2002) 'Using community-based participatory research to address social determinants of health: lessons learnt from Seattle Partners for Healthy Communities', *Health Education and Behavior*, 29: 361–82.

de Leeuw, E. (2009) 'Evidence for Healthy Cities: reflections on practice, method and theory', *Health Promotion International*, 24: 19–36.

de Leeuw, E. and Skovgaard, T. (2005) 'Utility-driven evidence for healthy cities: problems with evidence generation and application', *Social Science and Medicine*, 61: 1331–41.

Lipsky, M. (1993) Extract from M. Lipsky, *Street Level Bureaucracy: Dilemmas of the Individual in Public Services* (Russell Sage), in M. Hill (ed.), *The Policy Process. A Reader*. Englewood Cliffs, NJ: Prentice–Hall.

Nguyet Nguyen, M. and Otis, J. (2003) 'Evaluating the Fabreville Heart Health Program in Laval, Canada: a dialogue between the two paradigms, positivism and constructivism', *Health Promotion International*, 18: 127–34.

Nutbeam, D. (1992) 'The health promoting school: closing the gap between theory and practice', *Health Promotion International*, 7: 151–3.

Nutbeam, D. (1998) 'Evaluating health promotion – progress, problems and solutions', *Health Promotion International*, 13, 27–44.

Parsons, W. (1995) *Public Policy: An Introduction to the Theory and Practice of Policy Analysis*. Gloucester: Edward Elgar.

Pelikan, J.M., Krajic, K. and Dietscher, C. (2001) 'The Health Promoting Hospital (HPH): concept and development', *Patient Education and Counselling*, 45: 239–43.

Poland, B., Krupa, G. and McCall, D. (2009) 'Settings for health promotion: an analytic framework to guide intervention design and implementation', *Health Promotion Practice*, 10: 505–16.

Poland, B.D., Green, L.W. and Rootman, I. (2000) 'Reflections on settings for health promotion', in B.D. Poland, L.W. Green, and I. Rootman (eds), *Settings for Health Promotion: Linking Theory and Practice*. Thousand Oaks, CA: Sage.

Popay, J., Williams, G., Thomas, C. and Gatrell, A. (1998) 'Theorising inequalities in health: the place of lay knowledge', *Sociology of Health and Illness*, 20: 619–44.

Pronk, N.P. (2003) 'Designing and evaluating health promotion programs', *Disease Management Health Outcomes*, 11: 149–57.

Raphael, D. (2000) 'The question of evidence in health promotion', *Health Promotion International*, 15: 355–67.

Rifkin, S.B., Lewando-Hundt, G. and Draper, A.K. (2000) *Participatory Approaches in Health Promotion and Health Planning: A Literature Review*. London: Health Development Agency.

Rootman, I., Goodstadt, M.S., Potvin, L. and Springett, J. (2001) 'A framework for health promotion evaluation', in I. Rootman, M.S. Goodstadt, B. Hyndman, D. Mcqueen, L. Potvin, J. Springett and E. Ziglio (eds), *Evaluation in Health Promotion: Principles and Perspectives*. Denmark: WHO Europe.

Rychetnik, L., Frommer, M., Hawe, P. and Shiell, A. (2002) 'Criteria for evaluating evidence on public health interventions', *Journal of Epidemiology and Community Health*, 56: 119–27.

Sabatier, P. (1986) 'Top down and bottom up approaches to implementation research: a critical analysis and suggested synthesis', *Journal of Public Policy*, 16: 21–48.

Saunders, R.P., Evans, M.H. and Joshi, P. (2005) 'Developing a process-evaluation plan for assessing health promotion program implementation: a how-to-guide', *Health Promotion Practice*, 6: 134–47.

Smith, B. J., Cho Tang, K. and Nutbeam, D. (2006) 'WHO health promotion glossary: new terms', *Health Promotion International*, 21: 340–5.

Smith, N., Littlejohns, L.B., Hawe, P. and Sutherland, L. (2008) 'Great expectations and hard times: developing community indicators in a Healthy Communities Initiative in Canada', *Health Promotion International*, 23: 119–26.

South, J. (2010) 'Planning and evaluating health promotion in health practice', in A. Scriven, C. Kouta and I. Papadopoulos (eds), *Health Promotion for Health Practitioners*. Athens, Paschalidis Medical Publications.

Spicker, P. (2006) *Policy Analysis for Practice: Applying Social Policy*. Bristol: The Policy Press.

Springett, J. (1998) *Practical Guidance on Evaluating Health Promotion*. Brighton: WHO Europe.

Springett, J. (2001) 'Appropriate approaches to the evaluation of health promotion', *Critical Public Health*, 11: 139–51.

Springett, J., Owens, C. and Callaghan, J. (2007) 'The challenge of combining "lay" knowledge with "evidenced-based" practice in health promotion: Fag Ends Smoking Cessation Service', *Critical Public Health*, 17: 243–56.

Steckler, A. and Linnan, L. (2002) *Process Evaluation for Public Health Interventions and Research*. New York: Jossey Bass.

St Leger, L. (1997) 'Health promoting settings: from Ottawa to Jakarta', *Health Promotion International*, 12: 99–101.

Tsouros, A., Dowding, G. and Dooris, M. (1998) 'Strategic framework for the Health Promoting Universities project', in A. Tsouros, G. Dowding, J. Thompson and M. Dooris (eds), *Health Promoting Universities: Concept, Experience and Framework for Action*. Copenhagen: WHO Regional Office for Europe.

Walter, I., Davies, H. and Nutley, S. (2003) 'Increasing research impact through partnerships: evidence from outside health care', *Journal of Health Services Research and Policy*, 8: S2: 58–61.

Whitehead, D. (2001) 'A stage planning programme model for health education/health promotion practice', *Journal of Advanced Nursing*, 36: 311–20.

Whitelaw, S., Baxendale, A., Bryce, C., MacHardy, L., Young, I. and Witney, E. (2001) '"Settings" based health promotion: a review', *Health Promotion International*, 16: 339–52.

WHO Europe Working Group on Health Promotion Evaluation (1998) *Health Promotion Evaluation: Recommendations to Policy Makers*. Brighton: WHO Europe.

Wimbush, E. and Watson, J. (2000) 'An evaluation framework for health promotion: theory, quality and effectiveness', *Evaluation*, 6: 301–21.

Woodall, J. (2010) 'Control and choice in three category-C English prisons: implications for the concept and practice of the health promoting prison'. Unpublished PhD thesis, *Faculty of Health*. Leeds: Leeds Metropolitan University.

World Health Organization (2002) *Community Participation in Local Health and Sustainable Development. Approaches and Techniques. European Sustainable Development and Health Series No. 4.* WHO Regional Office for Europe.

Wright, L. (1999) 'Evaluation in health promotion: the proof of the pudding?', in E. Perkins, I. Simnett and L. Wright (eds), *Evidence Based Health Promotion.* Chichester: Wiley.

Ziglio, E., Rivett, D. and Rasmussen, V. B. (1995) *The European Network of Health Promoting Schools: Managing Innovation and Change.* Copenhagen: WHO Regional Office for Europe.

Part 2

Health Promoting Settings

Introduction to Part II

Healthy Settings

Margaret Hodgins and Angela Scriven

The fundamental value that underpins healthy settings relates to the recognition that the physical and social milieu in which population groups live, work and play is both a major determinant of health and the context in which health should be promoted. The chapters in this part of the book draw on this values base and offer a range of critical perspectives on specific settings. What is highlighted is the many and divers factors that influence the ability of health promoters to achieve health gain, providing a critical overview of the array of activities that are delivered in each setting and proffering a detailed assessment of the nature of settings as diverse as schools and prisons. A number of generic issues and themes are raised throughout.

Not all settings are organizations, and those with less well-defined boundaries pose particular challenges. In chapters 6 and 7, two such settings, communities and cities, expose some of these challenges. Both, for example, discuss problems such as alcohol abuse, antisocial behaviour and citizen safety. These are described as 'wicked', a term used in the policy literature, although not generally favoured in health promotion discourse. The term refers to complexity, but also to the fact that such problems have failed policy makers employing traditional linear problem solving models, due to their changing requirements, instability and the interdependency of systems in both creating the problems as well as finding a solution. Healthy Cities and Healthy Community projects have a key contribution to make in addressing these problems, and the settings approach equips them well to do so.

Relatedly, in both communities and cities the scope of the setting gives health promotion a real opportunity to act on health inequalities. While in other settings, for example healthcare or prisons, many of the problems encountered are at the downstream level; in neighbourhoods, communities and cities there is an opportunity to address the upstream interaction of systems and structures that create health inequalities. Both chapters refer to this significant challenge and how the settings approach is being used to address multiple and interacting determinants of health inequity.

In Chapter 6, the potential for working in partnership with local government is explored and some excellent examples of joined up work are given, illustrating the benefits of alliances between public health and local government. The Total Place pilot is given as an example of how this kind of partnership working has highlighted the need for service re-design and for a focus on the context rather the person. The project has exposed the need to design the whole system to improve outcomes for young children, rather than delivering services into which people must fit.

The importance of partnerships is also highlighted in Chapter 7, in which city partnerships with key sectors that influence health across all stages of the lifespan are identified as a critical success factor. The experience of the healthy cities movement is that robust organizational structures for managing change are also critical to making partnerships work on the ground. In this chapter, attention is drawn to the necessity of strategic and operational committees as they bring together the dicision-making authority, processes and resources required to determine goals and facilitate health promotion action in such a fluid and undefined setting.

In Chapter 7 it is observed that the Healthy Cities Programme has stimulated change in the more general governance structures of a city, demonstrating the validity of multisectoral work that underpins the approach. Reference is made to how the mandatory requirements of membership of the WHO European Healthy Cities Network has led to enduring intersectoral partnership structures that have had the capability to drive healthy public policy at the local level, and to the formation of committee structures with diverse membership including, importantly, representatives of the community.

Both chapters 8 and 9 raise the important issue of how placing the term 'healthy' before a given setting is often misleading, as it may suggest that a settings approach is being taken, when in fact this is not the case. In the case of hospitals, for example, a distinction is made between a healthy hospital, which may have specific focused interventions for patients or staff within its campus, and a health promoting hospital which shifts the focus to the role and impact of the hospital beyond its four walls, and into the wider community and environment in which it exists. In Chapter 9, the various ways in which the term 'healthy school' has been employed is explored and, again, the interpretation of healthy schools as places where health education can be extended to a captive audience is contrasted with a healthy school as one which integrates health promotion into every aspect of the school setting, addressing all the people connected with it: pupils, teachers, parents and the wider community. In this, both chapters grapple with the difference between settings as places where health promotion takes place and a setting as a dynamic system, which can both create or compromise health and which must be engaged with at the level of the system.

The growing interest in and commitment to ensuring that business and industry behaves in an environmentally responsible manner is explored in Chapter 8 in the context of health promoting hospitals. This is also explored in Part 3, where examples of good practice in respect of workplace setting include the concept of corporate social responsibility. Respecting the environment, through using resources in a sustainable manner and avoiding harm to ecosystem health as required for a health promoting hospital, is likely to be of increasing importance for all organizational settings. The example given in Chapter 8 of the Health Care Without Harm initiative may also be useful for other settings.

An important point raised forcefully in Chapter 10 when discussing universities as settings within which and through which health can be promoted is the questionable evidence base for justifying a settings approach. The problem relates to not being able to state with certainty that multi-component, whole settings holistic approaches are more successful than one-off health promotion activities. The argument presented is that the evidence points in favour of settings, and supports and reflects more general public health research which has concluded that the complexity and inter-relationships of risk factors and determinants make a compelling case for the futility of isolated initiatives around single factor public health topics or risk factors.

Two other crucial ideas were raised when discussing the university as a setting. The first is the importance to effective health promotion action of fully understanding the overall purpose and nature of each setting and how the groups within it function, adopt roles and interrelate. The second point is to recognize the synergistic relationship between settings, developing a cognisance of the way activities in a specific setting influence the wider community and the society in which it exists, what is referred to as synergistic throughputs. Relating to these ideas is the difficulties caused by health not being seen as the core business or central aim of some of these settings. In this situation there is a real need for health promoters to highlight relevant issues that can impact positively on core business (in the case of the university setting, for example, student recruitment, experience, retention and achievement; widening participation; staff recruitment, retention, performance and productivity).

In some settings there is a significant cultural clash with certain environments by their very nature being hierarchical, disempowering and (in the case of prisons) penalizing structures. What is interesting about Chapter 11 on the prison setting is the evident contradiction in the discourse and ideology of health promotion to a setting that curtails individual freedom and choice. The main argument here, however, is about opportunities that the settings approach offers for health promotion work, with prisons seen as providing an appropriate context to address the health and social circumstances of prisoners who may have been from a hard-to-reach group when living in the wider community. Prisons, therefore, are seen as prime settings to tackle inequalities in health (see Part I, Chapter 2, for further discussion on settings as appropriate forums for tackling inequalities in health amongst hard-to-reach groups). Perhaps more than any other setting, the prisons context also emphasizes the importance of ethical practice and the significance of the Ottawa Charter mediation, enabling and advocacy roles to health promotion work within healthy settings.

Another contradiction that is highlighted in the prison setting and can potentially be seen as a possible conflict in some other settings is the dominance of the biomedical model and the impetus towards prevention, which is inconsistent with the central tenets of health promotion and a settings approach. Arguably, a biomedical view has the danger of obscuring the wider political, psychosocial and environmental determinants that can impinge upon health, such as poverty, education, employment and housing.

Conclusions

There are clear conclusions that can be drawn from the settings discussed in this part of the book. Those professionals with a responsibility to promote health in the different settings are undoubtedly facing challenges that are common in nature. The benefits, the challenges and the potential obstacles to working effectively within and across settings are similar and include the dearth of evidence of effectiveness, the cultural clashes, contradictory perspectives and other barriers which are making the promotion of health a complex process. Confronting these challenges will require a continued and concerted effort and innovatory and outward-looking, rather than insular, ways of working. This must include effective collaborative long term planning and the combining of resources and partnership effort between population groups and different statutory and non-statutory agencies and stakeholders.

Some settings are more advanced in their evolutionary development, with prisons providing the most complex environment for the healthy settings movement. What is also evident, however, is the professional policy and political enthusiasm and momentum for a settings approach. This is not the time for complacency, but the impetus demonstrated in these chapters will hopefully result in a sustained future for the settings approach where means will be found for overcoming some of the identified obstacles.

6

Healthy Neighbourhoods and Communities: Policy and Practice

Susan Biddle and Martin Seymour

Aims

- To develop an understanding of place, neighbourhoods and communities as settings for health improvement and recognize the complexity of this approach and the challenges and opportunities that it presents
- To understand the role that local government in England has and how partners across the statutory and community sectors work together to act on the social determinants of health
- To recognize the influence national policy and local strategic decision making has on place-based settings approaches within the context of the government policy
- To be able to navigate the route from policy into practice and see examples of approaches to improving health through neighbourhood and community settings approaches

---

The health of individuals and populations is determined by factors outside the influence of the health service (Marmot et al., 2010; Orme et al., 2007) and beyond a narrow interpretation of personal choice and lifestyle. In the context of UK government policy, the Local Government Group (2010) asserts that improving health and tackling inequalities is at the heart of what local government is about, while the 2010 public health White Paper (Department of Health, 2010a) acknowledges the influence of local government on many factors that affect health and wellbeing, pointing to the need to tap into this potential and build on its existing important role in public health.

This chapter considers how local authorities in England, as leaders of place and local partnerships, contribute to a neighbourhood and community settings approach to improving health and reducing health inequalities.

The chapter draws on the experience of the Local Government Improvement and Development (LGID) Healthy Communities Programme. The chapter also includes two short case studies that demonstrate the reality of working within community and neighbourhood settings. Many other examples of health improvement work in community and neighbourhood settings are available via the healthy communities website: www.idea.gov.uk/health. The chapter considers how the proposals for the transfer of responsibility for aspects of public health from the NHS to local government, the creation of a national public health service in England and a renewed focus on individual lifestyle and behaviour change (Department of Health, 2010a, 2010b) could manifest in changes to the working lives of public health professionals and different approaches to promoting health in community and neighbourhood settings.

Community and neighbourhoods as settings for health promotion

Barton and Grant's (2006) map of the determinants of health (Figure 6.1) illustrates how the settings into which we are born, where we grow, learn, work and play, impact on our health behaviours, our lifestyles, the choices we make and hence our health and wellbeing. These are social, cultural, economic, political and physical environments that are our neighbourhoods and communities (Mackinnon et al., 2006) and it is these neighbourhood and community settings that have the capacity to be both health promoting and health damaging.

Neighbourhoods and communities are less well defined as health promoting settings than are schools, workplaces, hospitals or universities. These latter examples generally have defined boundaries with known populations and a common association that formally binds the participants in that setting. Many also have defined organizational structures and buildings around which whole place policies and interventions can be designed and delivered.

Neighbourhoods and communities share some of these characteristics but are less formal, more fluid and more difficult to define. Jewkes and Murcott (1996) conclude there is no common, agreed definition of community, that there are a variety of meanings found and that each is generally constructed by people who regard themselves as non-members of those communities. Freeman et al. (1997) define community as a group of people who share an interest or a common set of circumstances. A community setting approach, subtly different from a community development approach, requires a place to bring people together, which may be the neighbourhood. Hence a community or neighbourhood setting may be locality bound by geographical limits and be defined by people or organizations external to that community with deficit connotations of shared problems and needs. Hawtin et al. (1994) discuss the idea of a common bond existing between members of a community and Sulliman (1983) identifies a common perception of collective needs and priorities, and an ability to assume a collective responsibility for

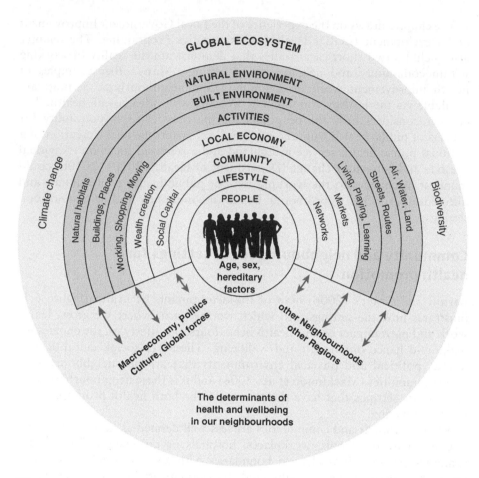

Figure 6.1 Map of health determinants (Barton and Grant, 2006)

community decisions, when defining a community. It may be unwise to assume such a notion of collective responsibility in a geographic community defined by professionals or organizations external to that community. Yet the succession of government-driven, area-based initiatives for regeneration and addressing inequalities within England, such as Health Action Zones, implies such an assumption within a definition of community by place.

A more recent example of the area-based approach is the Communities for Health programme (Department of Health, 2009; IDeA 2009a). Eighty-three local authorities were funded directly by the Department of Health to engage the most disadvantaged communities to involve them in adopting healthier lifestyles and empowering them to take more responsibility for improving their own health. The programme built upon the community engagement role of local government to build capacity within communities and the wider public health workforce. Barnsley's community parents' programme, for example, has trained 33 volunteer parents to provide peer support to new parents and other families in need. Using a semi-structured support package the intervention has been shown to build confidence, reduce social isolation, anxiety and depression and contributes to giving children a better start in life.

It is important to distinguish between interventions delivered within a community or neighbourhood setting and a settings approach which takes a whole systems approach to address the social, cultural, economic, political and physical environments illustrated in Barton and Grant's (2006) model. Using the example of physical activity, the former might include a programme of led health walks while the latter would look to address the social norms that influence walking and travel choices, increase the walkability of a neighbourhood, provide environmental improvements, promote policy to reduce car travel and so on. (For a more detailed discussion of a whole systems approach see Chapter 3.)

Harris et al. (2009) considers how improving health and reducing health inequalities within a community or neighbourhood setting requires a whole systems approach with multifaceted solutions and interagency collaboration to take account of the broader social, cultural, economic, political and physical environments that shape people's experience of health and wellbeing. Taking a settings approach to promoting health in neighbourhoods and communities is enshrined within the five action areas of the WHO (1986) Ottawa Charter for Health Promotion. Health promoting communities and neighbourhoods require the creation of a supportive environment that includes both the social and physical aspects of people's surroundings.

The Marmot Review (Marmot et al., 2010) also notes the importance of places and communities on health and wellbeing, referring to the physical and social characteristics of places and communities and the degree to which they promote and enable healthy behaviours. While highlighting the contribution these have to the social gradient of health inequalities the authors point to the need to address the psychosocial effects of neighbourhood deprivation and suggest that increasing social networks, reducing social isolation and increasing individual and community empowerment will all have a positive impact on improving health and reducing inequalities. Friedli (2009) suggests that higher levels of social capital, health assets and resilience, and salutogenic factors may explain why one poor neighbourhood can have lower mortality rates than an equally poor neighbourhood. She goes on to suggest that such resilience and collective efficacy, the very characteristics that communities need to survive adversity, may be eroded away by the injustice of the differences in life chances and opportunities in Britain today.

Gilchrist (2003) discusses the concept of social capital and its positive impact on wellbeing and refers to the formal and informal networks that exist within community and neighbourhood settings. Such networks might be defined as communities of interests and add to the sense of place, the association that community members have with the locality. In this respect communities of interest within a locality can be regarded as contributing to the make-up of that community of place. This is recognized in neighbourhood settings approaches which might focus on a defined area but which would recognize the various communities of place and interest that are layered upon each other and which contribute to the broader sense of community.

Community involvement: a feature of a health promotion approach

A neighbourhood or community setting approach may follow some of the principles and practice common with other settings and described within other chapters in this book but promoting health in these settings is more rooted in community development approaches. In advocating a community development approach, Seabrooke in SOLACE (2010) notes the requirement for collaboration amongst local people themselves and between local people and government together with innovative approaches to funding and service provision. Emmel and Conn (2004: 8), for example, in describing the benefits of successful community involvement note that:

> Communities can identify the wider determinants of health and develop plans and frequently implement strategies to address inequalities in health ... and that ... communities can be empowered and their capacity released to promote self-control and self-confidence to address their health needs.

The Marmot Review (Marmot et al., 2010) in setting out priorities for addressing health inequalities through action on the social determinants of health also calls for an approach in which organizations and people work together with activity at national, regional and local level. At a local level the review identifies three strands on which to focus:

- Creating opportunities for individuals and communities to set the agenda for change to define local problems and search out local solutions.
- Developing, commissioning and improving good quality, integrated local services co-produced with the public to achieve better outcomes for communities and individuals.
- Appropriate links between these levels and organizations ... to create partnerships to address health inequalities ... to shift in power and resources towards local communities. (Marmot et al., 2010: 151)

Marmot et al. (2010) refer to the crucial role that councils play in the lives of citizens and in the prospects for the area through the services they provide or commission and in their role as place shaper (Lyons, 2007). Box 6.1 illustrates the way councils may seek to renew their relationship with their local communities. In this example from South Ribble in England, local councillors in collaborating with the community, discovered the strength and assets within their community and redefined what it is to be a local leader.

Box 6.1 Improving health equity through collaboration and partnership

South Ribble Council wanted to undertake a scrutiny review to improve health equity, recognizing the socio-economic diversity of their population and the potential impact that a sense of community can have on health and wellbeing. Starting with a small but ambitious aim to improve health equity for the people of Broadfield by building community capacity and resilience, a broad partnership of organizations and community representatives worked and dreamed together using appreciative inquiry techniques to revive the sense of community in the area:

> Before we used to think about what we can do in communities to identify problems and deliver services. This way we ask the community what they want. What has come out of the inquiry is very different – how do we build on the assets such as the green space? The young people came out with achievable ideas. We would not have thought of the benches as the community did. (Senior Officer – South Ribble Council – March 2010)

Key to the approach was the active involvement of elected members. This enabled councillors to rethink their leadership role and relationship with the community:

> The inquiry influenced the next scrutiny review subject and orientation. It has been a vehicle for the community leadership role of the council. In the past we have been inward looking, see officers making things happen, looking at problems, not what we can do. It made us look at our role re community engagement. (Councillor – South Ribble Council – March 2010)

For more information please see www.nwtwc.org.uk/uploads/South_Ribble_case_study.pdf.

Local government as place shaper

Campbell (2010) acknowledges the broad role played by local government in England in shaping neighbourhoods and communities and in promoting health, illustrated through her adaptation of the health map (see Figure 6.2).

Councils have been working for many years to improve the health of their local populations. The Local Government Improvement and Development (LGID) Healthy Communities Programme recognizes and elaborates on this. The LGID (formerly the IDeA) is part of the Local Government Group. Its purpose is to support improvement and innovation in local government. The Healthy Communities Programme was established in 2006, with funding from the Department of Health, with a remit to improve the capacity, capability and confidence of local government throughout England to improve health and tackle health inequalities. It brings together a wide range of programmes and activities with one clear aim, to help local government improve the health of their local communities and particularly to help them narrow the gap between those that have the best health and those that have the poorest health. The programme has offered a wide range of support to local authorities and ensures good and innovative practice is recognized and learning is shared. This work includes delivering support that raises the profile of health inequalities and health improvement within the sector and of local government as a key player in addressing health inequalities. Additionally it is intended that local government contributes to policy development. The programme has a particular focus on the key role that local elected councillors play in the leadership of health in

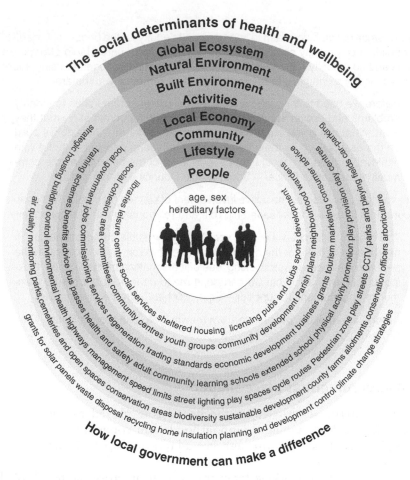

Figure 6.2   How local government can make a difference to community health (Campbell, 2010)

the locality setting and places an emphasis on developing self improvement capacity within the sector via extensive use of peer support. It works from a core model, or benchmark, of what a health promoting local authority looks like and seeks to promote a whole council approach that acknowledges the contribution of all services.

Part of the remit of the Healthy Communities Programme has been to capture examples to make it available to others as case study material. This not only charts the development of the sector's approach over the period of the programme but also enables councils, and their partners, to learn from each other, critical in an area where little useful evidence exists of what works in reducing health inequalities. For councils, who often work in the arena of emerging practice, this is essential and learning from the success and failure of others will be increasingly important in times of reduced resources when a business case will be needed.

The New Economics Foundation (2010) considers the role of local government in promoting wellbeing and points to five key areas of activity, each of which contributes to a whole systems approach. These are outlined in Box 6.2.

The Marmot Review (Marmot et al., 2010) identifies a real challenge for local government and partners to increase political and workforce capacity and confidence in addressing the social determinants, and points to the need to disseminate successful initiatives while also understanding the limitations of lifestyle interventions. The LGID Healthy Communities Programme has sought to assist councils with this by developing a benchmark of what a health promoting council looks like. This forms the basis of many improvement activities within the Healthy Communities Programme, including LGIDs flagship peer review process. The peer review process illustrates the Local Government Group's core belief that the sector has the knowledge and capacity for self-improvement. Drawing together the knowledge within the sector and its close partners the benchmark is created around four key areas: leadership, empowering communities, making it happen and improving performance. Teams of peers are brought together to provide the review challenge to individual councils. The healthy communities peer review advocates an integrated approach and makes explicit the health promoting benefits of many everyday council activities: for example, showing the strong links and potential health outcomes between the actions councils may take to regenerate an area and the development of open spaces and built environments, and the creation of meaningful employment opportunities.

Box 6.2   Key areas of local government activity contributing to a whole systems approach to wellbeing

1. Strategic leadership	2. Services and commissioning
• vision for local wellbeing • designated senior officer and strategic oversight • wellbeing in resource allocation • promoting use of local government powers	• commissioning for wellbeing outcomes • using wellbeing proofing methods • building wellbeing into service design • co-producing services • wellbeing promotion activities within a range of local provision

(Continued)

(Continued)

3. Strengthening communities	4. Using organizational levers
• develop asset-based approaches to draw on residents' capabilities • foster social connections and networks • devolve genuine power and control to communities	• support psychosocial wellbeing of council staff and help local businesses do same for their employees • use procurement and recruitment policies to strengthen local economy and wellbeing of local residents
5. Measuring outcomes	
• measurement at the universal level, the population as a whole • measurement at the targeted level, specific communities or service users • mental wellbeing impact assessment	

Source: New Economics Foundation (2010)

The role of local government needs to be seen in the context of a policy shift within the UK not just in the proposed transfer of responsibility for public health improvement from primary care trusts to local government (Department of Health, 2010a) but also in the move away from a model that relies upon defined public bodies as the primary vehicles for public health improvement to the more complex mix of providers in the private, public, voluntary and social enterprise sector. In engaging with this mixed provider economy councils become a critical vehicle for improved community engagement, providing a channel for bottom-up approaches while at the same time being provider, enabler, market maker and advocate for the community. This is a dynamic environment in which to work, involving juggling of priorities and a commitment to localism that it expected to increase as this policy plays out (Secretary of State for Communities and Local Government, 2010). The introduction of public health professionals, used as they are to working to nationally determined targets and an upward-facing performance regime, into this local authority context is likely to result in some tension between the role of the professional expert and the leadership role of the locally elected councillor. Developing the skills necessary to navigate this complex local environment will be key to the success of the public health workforce; knowing when to challenge and when to persuade and how to align action to improve the health of the public with other local strategies and priorities. Elson (2009: 22) writes:

> Those who hold these [Director of Public Health] posts need to establish exceptional personal credibility to be successful. The personal skill set that each DPH holds must be matched to the capacity that the local authority has to manage change and deliver real outcomes for citizens.

He goes on to describe six models of practice for Directors of Public Health: the expert, the critical friend, the adviser, the provider, the catalyst and the community advocate and leader, and the interplay between these roles in various local authority settings. Some of these areas were explored by the IDeA et al. (2010), who examined the experience and challenges involved in the tri-partite working arrangements between the Director of Public Health, the Director of Adult Services (DAS) and Director of Children's Services (DCS), particularly on the Joint Strategic Needs Assessments (JSNA).

A critical role for partnerships

The concept of partnership is fundamental to public health policy and action (Peckham, 2007) and multisectoral collaborative working or the joining up of agencies is now embedded in national UK policy and local delivery mechanisms (MacPherson, 2006). (See Chapter 4 for a more detailed discussion on partnerships.) In respect to addressing health inequalities Local Strategic Partnerships (LSP) are, or ought to be, well placed to deliver the whole systems approach recognized as essential by Marmot (Marmot et al., 2010). Interagency collaboration through LSPs can take account of the broader social, cultural, economic, political and physical environments that shape people's experience of health and wellbeing. Just how the role of LSPs will develop, and the way they will work in relation to the proposed Health and Wellbeing Boards (Department of Health, 2010b) is yet to be understood but it is clear that, whatever the structures locally, there is recognition that the complex and intractable public health problems we face will not be tackled successfully by working in silos.

Partnership working is seen as inherently good. A lot of time and effort has been invested in developing and maintaining partnerships both at a practitioner level and at a local strategic level in the UK, where past government policy has advanced the development of multiagency strategic working. The UK government's Total Place pilot programme (HM Treasury, 2010a) aimed to increase efficiency and effectiveness through taking an area-based partnership approach, aligning budgets across public sector agencies to address specific 'wicked' issues, defined by the Audit Commission (1998) as complex problems that cross organizational boundaries and which include tackling alcohol abuse, minimizing reoffending and creating safer, stronger and healthier neighbourhoods. An example can be seen in Box 6.3. This approach is set to continue through a programme of Community Budgets, seen as both a mechanism for reducing costs, duplication and bureaucracy and a means for a more focused community and neighbourhoods approach.

Box 6.3 *Total Place*: problem- and population-based approaches

Ten partner organizations in the Leicestershire and Leicester City area used *Total Place* to understand how public money can be better spent on reducing

(Continued)

(Continued)

levels of alcohol and drug abuse. Binge drinking, antisocial behaviour and violent crime associated with alcohol and drug use were identified as key issues, impacting as they do on the budgets and policy objectives of a range of organizations, not just health. The partners mapped £6 billion of public sector spend and identified considerable savings and benefits from increasing investment in preventative services on alcohol abuse. Addressing this required a change of focus from the service to the person and the place in which they live and a move from organizational silos to partnership working.

A whole systems approach was adopted with steps that included piloting a normative marketing campaign in selected universities and educational establishments; robust approaches to policing the night time economy and strengthening the approach to licensing across the place and a new alcohol care pathway that recognized the significant opportunity to improve engagement from agencies whose services are integral to the recovery of misusers within a whole system approach including, for example, housing, education, training and employment and between community and custody for offenders (Leicester and Leicestershire Public Service Board, 2010).

Jointly led by Croydon Council and NHS Croydon, and drawing in all LSP partners, Croydon adopted Early Years as its Total Place theme and set out to map the costs involved in reactive response to children from birth to seven years and reconfigure the system to facilitate greater emphasis on early intervention. Following the child through the system the pilot learned of fragmented solutions that failed families at key points, the dangers of failing to pick up early warning signs, and of poor response times and the costs on services of decisions made elsewhere in the system. The pilot recognized that concentrating on the child misses the importance of dealing with the context that they live in, their families, that often need significant support too if the resources invested on their children are not to be wasted. The *Total Place* pilot has highlighted the need for service redesign to solution-focused, rather than delivering services into which people must fit, ensuring children and families themselves are recognized as a resource and, crucially, designing the whole system to improve outcomes for young children, to ensure all the parts fit and work together well for the family. The experience and lessons learned are informing Croydon's progress as a Community Budget pilot area and early intervention city (NHS Croydon and Croydon Council, 2010).

A key driver for local strategic partnership working is the requirement since 2008 for primary care trusts and upper tier local authorities to produce a Joint Strategic Needs Assessment (JSNA) to fulfil the vital need for public sector and other local organizations to have a comprehensive understanding of the factors that influence the health and wellbeing of their populations and to shape commissioning priorities. The JSNA process is intended to provide a considerable opportunity to strengthen partnership working and address key strategic challenges. JSNA is about people and the places they live in, about their health needs but also increasingly about their assets and their potential to contribute improving health. The JSNA process is enhanced through the engagement of local communities and some areas have demonstrated innovative ways of involving the voluntary and community sector and local people in identifying needs and assets and establishing health priorities. The IDeA (2009b) recognizes how the JSNA process has been both a litmus test for the state of local health partnerships and a catalyst for change.

The current emphasis on localism within UK policy (Boyle, 2009) together with the advancement of total place methodology through community budgets (HM Treasury, 2010b) and the imperative of financial constraints provides a strong indication that area-based partnership working both at a strategic and operational level is set to continue. Marks (2007), however, notes how the Audit Commission raised doubts over the effectiveness, accountability, leadership and purpose of local partnerships and the extent to which they add value. Hamer and Smithies (2002) identified the difficulty in demonstrating the added value of partnership working for different partners. More recently, the National Support Team for Health Inequalities (Bentley, 2008), while acknowledging examples of seamless partnership working between local authorities and primary care trusts, reported that partners continue to work in isolation, suggesting that no advantage is being gained.

There is little research into the effectiveness of partnership working on improving health, something recognized by Perkins et al. (2009) in their systematic review, which set out to thematically explore the theories on partnership working. Their findings point to process issues that can support or restrict partnership working but found more limited evidence on the health outcomes. The authors conclude that this does not mean that partnership working for health improvement is not a good thing, just that the evidence to support the continued belief in this approach is not available.

Seymour (2010) explored practitioner perspectives on how effective LSPs are at promoting health through the concept of collaborative advantage, defined by Huxham (2003) as delivering outcomes that organizations working alone would not achieve. Participants in the study recognized that while operational partnerships frequently brought together organizations and communities to deliver successful outcomes, strategic partnerships needed to progress to a state of maturity in order to deliver the whole system, socioecological approach to addressing the social determinants of health (see Figure 6.3). The study identified process and external contextual factors that constrain strategic partnership working and progress towards a mature partnership where health is seen as everybody's business and there is recognition of and a commitment to structuralist approaches to health improvement with a focus on healthy public policy, social, ecological and environmental measures (Douglas, 2007).

The LGID Healthy Communities Programme has developed a partnership compendium and is working with LSPs across the country highlighting how effective health partnerships are operating, how they are assessing their own

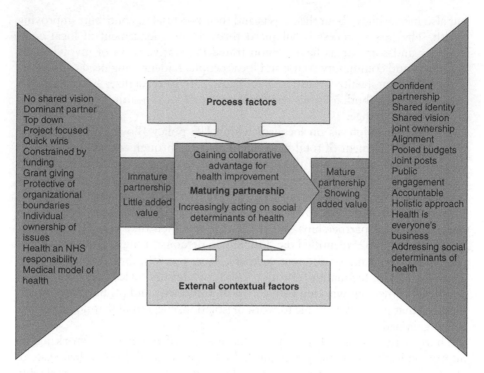

Figure 6.3 Theory of maturing partnerships for health improvement (Seymour, 2010)

impact on the health of the public, and how they are evolving to respond to the changing health policy landscape, including the abolition of Primary Care Trusts and Strategic Health Authorities, and the creation of Health and Wellbeing Boards.

From community assets to localism

The Marmot Review (Marmot et al., 2010), in relation to partnership working, calls for a shift in power and resources towards local communities, a concept wholly in keeping with the commitment to localism. It talks about creating opportunities for individuals and communities to set the agenda for change, to define local problems and search out local solutions. It puts the empowerment of individuals and communities at the heart of action to reduce health inequalities and recognizes that achieving this requires social action to create the conditions in which people are able to take control of their own lives.

This is in keeping with an approach that moves away from the dominant deficit model with its tendency to define a community through connotations of deprivation, poor health, low standards of education and other aspects of poverty and need towards an approach that recognizes the value that people, organizations, buildings and so on contribute to a community. *A Glass Half-full* (Foot with Hopkins, 2010), produced by LGID Healthy Communities Programme, discusses asset-based community development and advocates a positive approach to capturing the profile of a community through assets mapping, that captures the building blocks of every community. Kretzmann (1995) identifies three types of assets: the gift of individuals; the community, including building assets; and the groups and organizations within a community and the institutions – the schools, libraries, parks and the resources that they bring. Working closer with and within community and neighbourhood settings delivers another key message for public health professionals: people's lives are complex and approaching health improvement via a conditions-focused approach fails to acknowledge this. Seeing people and communities in the round and recognizing the active role they can play in their own health improvement may lay better foundations for success. Semenza and Krishnasamy (2007) provide an analysis of positive health and lifestyle benefits that can result from community engagement in neighbourhood design and urban landscape improvements. They point to multiple benefits beyond the landscape improvements, including strengthened social networks and social capital.

The drive for localism in many ways builds upon the notion of community participation and engagement inherent in the healthy setting concept. The transfer of power from government to communities and individuals that is inherent in the policy objectives of localism is in keeping with the health promotion objectives of strengthening community action and creating supportive environments. While we must heed concerns over austerity measures that will constrain local authority spending and put at risk many community and voluntary sector organizations there may yet be opportunity provided by the localism agenda to develop community action for improving health based not on prescribed localities but on communities and neighbourhoods defined by community members.

Health: everyone's business

Local government in England, as it absorbs its new public health responsibilities and takes up a lead role in improving health within its locality, must ensure that improving health is seen to be everyone's business both within and without the authority. This means developing more effective, mature partnerships with other agencies and transferring the power to improve health to communities and neighbourhoods. Those within the council with responsibility for planning and transport, environmental health, housing and neighbourhoods, culture and sport, open spaces, waste management and so on need also to be confident in their role as health promoters and able to work with communities to address the social determinants of health. Many local authorities are on this path. The London Borough of Greenwich pioneered a *Health is Everyone's Business* (IDeA, 2007) programme that sought to do just this: to focus all services on the contribution they could make to better community health and reducing health inequalities.

There is a challenge in the need for local government to improve the wellbeing and resilience of local populations, to continue to create the conditions for material wellbeing and to nurture psychosocial wellbeing in local populations (New Economics Foundation, 2010). Working through a community and neighbourhood setting framework local government can contribute to reducing social isolation, increasing social networks, helping people to feel in control of their lives and creating the conditions in which people and communities are able to flourish.

In times of change there is a natural inclination to look inwards and focus on organizational structures and processes. As leaders of place and local partnerships, local government and others must look outward and focus on the pursuit of better health for local people. At the time of writing this chapter it is too early to say how things will play out but the transfer of health improvement functions to local government and the arrival of GP consortia onto the new health and wellbeing boards could enable a more localist, community approach to improving health and addressing inequalities. We may be on the brink of a renaissance in community settings-based health improvement.

Summary points

- Communities and neighbourhoods are a powerful setting for health improvement work but also represent a dynamic environment in which to operate, requiring flexibility, variation and inclusive approaches.

- Communities are not passive entities. Their involvement in the definition of the issues of concern and the planning and delivery of action is critical to success.

- Problem-focused initiatives not only fail to acknowledge the assets within a community that can aid traction but can also be over-simplistic, failing to acknowledge the complexity of people's lives. Approaches based on understanding a whole system are more likely to succeed in complex environments.

- With a democratic mandate to lead in localities, local government and particularly elected members are key to success and their role in coordinating multisectoral partnerships is of increasing importance in the new health environment.

Online Further Reading

Semenza, J. and Krishnasamy, V. (2007) 'Design of a health promoting neighbourhood intervention', *Health Promotion Practice*, 8: 243–56.

This article considers the positive health and lifestyle benefits that can result from community engagement in neighbourhood design. It details an initiative in Portland, Oregon, to develop an urban gathering space for local people. It highlights the challenge and complexity of such programmes, particularly when involving re-design of urban space environments but acknowledges the powerful effect environment has on community wellbeing and the social capital advantages of designing community meeting and conversation spaces. It is of particular interest to this chapter in that it advocates the full involvement of the community in such projects, mentioning asset mapping amongst other approaches to community engagement.

References

Antonovsky, A. (1993) 'The structure and properties of the sense of coherence scale', *Social Science and Medicine*, 36 (6): 725–33.

Audit Commission (1998) *A Fruitful Partnership, Effective Partnership Working*. Abingdon: Audit Commission Publications.

Barton, H. and Grant, M. (2006) 'A health map for the local human habitat', *Journal for the Royal Society for the Promotion of Health*, 126 (6): 252–61. Available at: http://dx.doi.org/10.1177/1466424006070466 (accessed 9 September 2010).

Bentley, C. (2008) *Systematically Addressing Health Inequalities*. London: Department of Health.

Boyle, D. (2009) *Localism: Unravelling the Supplicant State*. London: New Economics Foundation. Available at www.neweconomics.org/publications/localism (accessed 23 November 2010).

Campbell, F. (ed.) for the IDeA (2010) *The Social Determinants of Health and the Role of Local Government*. London: IDeA.

Department of Health (2009) *Communities for Health: Unlocking the Energy within Communities to Improve Health*. London: Department of Health.

Department of Health (2010a) *Healthy Lives, Healthy People: Our Strategy for Public Health in England*. London: Department of Health.

Department of Health (2010b) *Equity and Excellence: Liberating the NHS*. London: Department of Health.

Douglas, J. (2007) 'Promoting the public health: continuity and change over two centuries', in J. Douglas, S. Earle, S. Handsley, C.E. Lloyd and S. Spur (eds), *A Reader in Promoting Public Health: Challenge and Controversy*. London: Sage.

Elson, T. (2009) 'Joint Director of Public Health appointments – six models of practice', in D. Hunter (ed.) for the IDeA and Durham University (2009), *Perspectives on Joint Director of Public Health Appointments*. Durham: Durham University.

Emmel, N. and Conn, C. (2004) *Towards community involvement: Strategies for health and social care providers. Guide 21: Identifying the goal and objectives of community involvement*. The Department of Health Portfolio Programme. London: Department of Health.

Freeman, R., Gillam, S., Shearin, C. and Pratt, J. (1997) *Community Development in Primary Care: A Guide to Involving the Community in COPC*. London: The King's Fund.

Friedli, L. (2009) *Mental Health, Resilience and Inequalities – A Report for WHO Europe and the Mental Health Foundation*. London/Copenhagen: Mental Health

Foundation and WHO Europe. Available at: www.euro.who.int/document/e92227.
pdf (accessed 23 November 2010).

Foot, J. with Hopkins, T. (2010) *A Glass Half-full: How an Asset Approach Can
Improve Community Health and Wellbeing.* London: Local Government
Improvement and Development.

Gilchrist, A. (2003) 'Community development and networking for Health', in
J. Orme, J. Powell, P. Taylor, T. Harrison and M. Grey (eds), *Public Health for
the 21st Century: New Perspectives on Policy, Participation and Practice.*
Maidenhead: Open University Press.

HM Treasury (2010a) *Total Place: A Whole Area Approach to Public Services.*
London: HM Treasury www.hm-treasury.gov.uk/psr_total_place.htm (accessed
30 December 2010).

HM Treasury (2010b) *The Spending Review 2010.* London: The Stationery Office.

Hamer, L. and Smithies, J. (2002) *Planning Across the Local Strategic Partnership
(LSP). Case Studies of Integrating Community Strategies and Health Improvement.*
London: Health Development Agency.

Harris, A., Hastings, N. and McCormick, J. (2009) 'Scotland's future wellbeing', in
J. Murray (ed.), *Perspectives on Health Improvement: A Contribution to the
Consultation on the Scottish Government's Action Plan on Health and Wellbeing.*
Edinburgh: Health Scotland.

Hawtin, M., Hughes, G., Percy-Smith, J. and Foreman, A. (1994) *Community
Profiling: Auditing Social Needs.* Buckingham: Open University Press.

Huxham, C. (2003) 'Theorising collaborative practice', *Public Management
Review*, 5 (3): 401–23.

IDeA (2009a) *Communities for Health: The Story So Far ...* London: Improvement
and Development Agency.

IDeA (2009b) *Joint Strategic Needs Assessment: Progress So Far.* London:
Improvement and Development Agency.

IDeA, ADASS, and ADCS (2010) *Leading Together Better.* London: Improvement
and Development Agency.

IDeA (2007) *Greenwich Tackles Health Inequalities.* Available at: www.idea.gov.
uk/idk/core/page.do?pageId=6288177 (accessed 30 December 2010).

Jewkes, R. and Murcott, A. (1996) 'The meaning of community', *Social Science and
Medicine*, 43 (4): 555–63.

Kretzmann, J.P. (1995) 'Building communities from the inside out', *Shelterforce
online* National Housing Institute. Available at: www.nhi.org/online/issues/83/
buildcomm.html (accessed 9 January 2011).

Leicester and Leicestershire Public Service Board (2010) *Leicester and Leicestershire
Total Place Final Report.* Available at: www.oneleicester.com/leicester-partnership/
total-place/ (accessed 23 November 2010).

Local Government Group (2010) *The Health of the Public: Local Government
Group Discussion Paper.* London: The Local Government Group.

Lyons, M. (2007) *The Lyons Inquiry into Local Government. Place Shaping: A
Shared Ambition for the Future of Local Government.* London: HMSO.

Mackinnon, J., Reid, M. and Kearns, A. (2006) *Communities and Health Improvement:
A Review of Evidence and Approaches.* Glasgow: NHS Health Scotland.

MacPherson, S. (2006) 'Promoting "strategic" working within area based and the-
matic social inclusion partnerships in Scotland', *Local Economy*, 21 (2): 180–96.

Marks, L. (2007) 'Fault lines between policy and practice in local partnerships', *Journal of Health Organization and Management*, 21 (2): 136–48.

Marmot, M., Allen, J., Goldblatt, P., Boyce, T., McNeish, D., Grady, M. and Geddes, I. (2010) *Fair Society, Healthy Lives: A Strategic Review of Health Inequalities in England post-2010* (The Marmot Review). London: The Marmot Review.

New Economics Foundation (2010) *The Role of Local Government in Promoting Wellbeing*. London: Local Government Improvement and Development.

NHS Croydon and Croydon Council (2010) Child: Family: Place. Radical efficiency to improve outcomes for young children. Available at: www.croydon.gov.uk/democracy/dande/policies/cypl/totalplace/ (accessed 30 December 2010).

Orme, J., Powell, J., Taylor, P. and Grey, M. (2007) 'Mapping public health', in J. Orme, J. Powell, P. Taylor and M. Grey (eds), *Public Health for the 21st Century: New Perspectives on Policy, Participation and Practice*, 2nd edn. Maidenhead: Open University Press.

Peckham, S. (2007) 'Partnership working for public health', in J. Orme, J. Powell, P. Taylor and M. Grey (eds), *Public Health for the 21st Century: New Perspectives on Policy, Participation and Practice*, 2nd edn. Maidenhead: Open University Press.

Perkins, N., Smith, K., Hunter, D.J., Bambra, C. and Joyce, K. (2009) 'What counts is what works? New Labour and partnerships in public health', *Policy and Politics*, 38 (1): 101–17.

Secretary of State for Communities and Local Government (2010) *The Localism Bill*. London: The Stationery Office.

Semenza, J. and Krishnasamy, V. (2007) 'Design of a Health Promoting Neighbourhood intervention', *Health Promotion Practice*, 8: 243–56.

Seymour, M. (2010) Do Local Strategic Partnerships Provide Collaborative Advantage for Health Improvement? A Practitioner's Perspective Using Grounded Theory. Unpublished student dissertation.

SOLACE Foundation Imprint (2010) *Health, Wealth and Wellbeing*. London: SFI.

Sulliman, A. (1983) 'Effective refugee health depends on community participation', *Carnets de l'enfant* 2, 2, cited in Jewkes, R. and Murcott, A. (1996) 'The meaning of community', *Social Science and Medicine*, 43 (4): 555–63.

WHO (World Health Organization) (1986) *Ottawa Charter for Health Promotion*. Geneva: WHO.

7

Healthy Cities: Comprehensive Solutions to Urban Health Improvement

Sally Fawkes, Colin Fudge and Katrin Engelhardt

Aims

- To outline the challenges of increasing urbanization
- To review the origins, development and structures of the WHO European Healthy Cities Project and the scope of the Healthy Cities movement
- To describe healthy cities' work in relation to a key issue: health inequalities
- To discuss the implications of the urban age and other social movements on future developments of the Healthy Cities approach

---

By mid-2009, the number of people living in urban areas (3.42 billion) had surpassed the number living in rural areas (3.41 billion) (UN Population Division, 2010a). By 2050, the percentage of the world's population living in cities is expected to rise from the current figure of 50.5% to about 70% in 2050. We have entered an urban age. Designing and instituting actions that improve and sustain the health and equity of people living and working in urban settings are outstanding social challenges with major co-benefits for the environment and economy. Over the past 25 years, the Healthy Cities approach, described in this chapter, has been used by the World Health Organization (WHO) and others to support cities in placing health and the process of health promotion at the centre of public and organizational policies, programmes, decision making and resource allocation in order to bring about better health and equity in cities. The key issue explored in this chapter is whether, even though health can be an outcome of urban regeneration and development (Fudge, 2003), the Healthy Cities approach is still relevant for driving comprehensive solutions to improving population health and equity in the urban age.

The urban age: figures, facts and consequences

The urban age has its roots in the industrial revolution of the nineteenth century. Emerging industries generated an immense need for labour and facilitated the creation of large population clusters. Cities grew to be dynamic centres of activity, offering jobs, opportunities for cultural expression, social interaction, learning and education and access to health and social services. Cities are the hub of technological advancements in information and communication, medicine, food, environment and transportation and other areas. A sharp rise in urbanization between 1950 and 1990 around the world has been followed by a steady rise, which is predicted to continue through to 2050 and see almost 90% of the European population living in cities. Predictions are that urbanized populations will be older, comprise people from different countries and tend to live in smaller urban centres. The number of older persons worldwide has more than tripled since 1950 and will almost triple again by 2050 (UN Population Division, 2010b). More developed regions have older and more urbanized populations, but the number of older persons is growing most rapidly in urban areas of less developed regions. Between 2009 and 2025, small urban centres with fewer than half a million inhabitants are predicted to account for 45% of the expected increase in the world's urban population (UN Population Division, 2010a).

Innovations in various fields of technology, such as information and communication, healthcare and medicine, food production, environmental management and transportation, have revolutionized many aspects of life in cities. They have also created new risks and impacts, including contributing to the widening of social inequalities in cities (UN-HABITAT, 2010). A highly visible side effect of technological innovation has been an increasing volume of various types of waste in cities and an increase in energy consumption. The demand in urban settings for non-renewable and renewable (but scarce) resources is immense. Indeed, the urban spatial footprint is expanding due to increasing resource consumption and waste production arising from major activities in cities related to the supply of, for example, food, transport, housing, and consumer goods and services. This is making resource management a pressing agenda for urban governance.

Cities are especially vulnerable to the impacts of changing environmental conditions (IPCC, 2009; World Bank, 2010). The nature of the built environment makes urban settings prone to higher temperatures due to heat generation from buildings and paved structures, which negatively affects the health of populations, especially more vulnerable groups (such as the very young and very old), workers' productivity and residents' daily living activities. Risks of flooding are increased as buildings, roads, and infrastructure alter the water cycle by preventing rainfall from infiltrating into the soil, causing contamination of freshwater supplies and creating new breeding grounds for disease-carrying insects (Satterthwaite, 2007). Generally speaking, the fundamental prerequisites for achieving and maintaining health, such as clean air and water, sufficient food and shelter, will be affected by the changing climate (WHO, 2009) and pose particular problems for large metropolises.

A key factor shaping urban life is transport, which concerns both the movement of people and freight. Road-based forms of transport and lack of attention to broader options for whole-of-population mobility in cities create unsustainable transport systems and can produce numerous and severe problems for the environment and people: air and noise pollution, global climate change, waste disposal, visual intrusion, mental stress, congestion, energy security and accidents (UNCRD, 2010; WHO, 2010a).

An important demographic change, and a positive outcome of improved public health, education and healthcare over the past century (Fried and Paccaud, 2010), is that in many countries people are living longer. While representing an immense opportunity for societies, there will be increased demand for chronic disease healthcare, long term care and social services, posing a burden on already troubled service systems and the reduced numbers of people in the productive age group able to provide support and protection for older people (OECD, 2010). Individuals living alone (estimated at 100 million, globally) are more likely to be poor and socially isolated and often dependent on various types of support if they have to manage chronic illness and/or disabilities (UN Population Division, 2010b). When their levels of self-sufficiency decline, individuals have to decide whether they are able to stay in their home or within their communities, termed 'ageing in place', or require housing with care services. Public policy goals include the provision of affordable housing options that cater to differing levels of independence and are accessible, and designing support services that both meet the daily needs of older people and are financially and geographically accessible (OECD, 2003).

This initial review of urban age challenges related to demography, technology, transport and housing highlights the interconnectedness between issues and underscores the 'wicked' nature of challenges facing cities in the twenty-first century. The complexity of issues facing cities, though daunting, does not justify inaction. There is no one-size-fits all approach to resolving complex, urban issues (The Global Compact, 2010). This is in part because each city is unique in terms of its socio-political dynamics, its governance arrangements and priorities, its capability to mobilize community support and effort or resources, the complexion of issues competing for attention and other characteristics. There are, however, processes that can be considered fundamental to sustainable and healthy urbanization. These are geared towards the principles of health promotion and are central to the Healthy Cities approach.

Cities as a setting for health promotion: transition from a WHO project to a worldwide movement

Linking health and cities is an idea that has a long history with important works including *The Urban Condition* (Duhl, 1963) setting out its rationale and parameters. Together with public health physician Trevor Hancock, WHO executive Ilona Kickbusch and others, Duhl activated the idea of urban settings as a focus for policy work within the WHO European region. In 1986, a Healthy Cities Project Planning Group meeting, involving 21 European cities, was held in Lisbon, Portugal. It set the scene for the instigation of a demonstration project in which cities would work together on better approaches to urban health development. The project was launched by WHO as a platform for translating the *Health for All* strategy to the local level of government in European member states (see for example Hancock and Duhl, 1986; Hancock, 1993).

Embodied in the project were three key ideas. Firstly, local governments are well placed to pursue strategies based on the holistic ideas of health that underpin WHO work because their functions closely connect them to the lives of individuals, families and communities. Secondly, local governments can facilitate the new public health (Ashton et al., 1986) by requiring all policy areas to make evident their contribution to, and impacts on, population health such as housing, transport, local health services, early childhood services, neighbourhood/city infrastructure development and cultural development. (The role of local government is considered in more detail in Chapter 4.) Thirdly, cities need to be planned, governed and organized in fundamentally different ways if health is to be high on the political, social and economic agendas of cities. The project was founded on the idea that any city can be a healthy city, regardless of the current health status of its population, as long as there is a commitment to health and a process and structure for:

> Continually creating and improving those physical and social environments and expanding those community resources which enable people to mutually support each other in performing all the functions of life and in developing to their maximum potential. (WHO, 1998: 13)

A checklist was devised to communicate key ideas and a vision for cities participating in the WHO project (see Box 7.1). Healthy Cities expanded beyond a project into a growing movement (Kickbusch, 1989), even at a relatively early stage of the project. Healthy Cities has grown from a WHO demonstration project in 35 European cities, to national networks seeded by these project cities, to international networks, and what some call a movement, of over 2,000 cities. Healthy cities in Europe and Canada were followed by healthy cities, towns, communities, municipalities and villages in Australia, the United States and countries in South America and Asia, tailored to the settlements, ideas and symbols of the countries and regions concerned. Through a series of five-year phases (see, for example, Tsouros, 1990, 2009), the WHO European Healthy Cities Network has sought growth, institutional and programmatic innovation, measurable impacts and contemporary relevance, maintaining wide appeal despite the changing political, social, economic and administrative landscape in which it grew (Lawrence and Fudge, 2003, 2009). The various changes in strategic emphasis through the phases are reflected in a series of declarations. For example the Belfast Declaration (WHO 2003) highlights the power of local action and the Zagreb Declaration (2009), which informs the latest phase, emphasizes the need for health equity in all policies.

Experience and evaluations over 25 years of Healthy Cities initiatives in Europe (see for example, Ritsatakis, 2009) and elsewhere point to a cluster of key success factors in the Healthy Cities approach: municipal leadership reflecting political commitment to Healthy Cities principles and strategies; capacity for action, new, robust organizational structures for managing change; city partnerships with key sectors with an influence on health across all stages of the lifespan, business, industry, transport, education, economic sector and environment sector.

Box 7.1   Qualities of a healthy city

A healthy city aims to provide:

- a clean, safe physical environment of high quality, including housing quality
- an ecosystem that is stable now and sustainable in the long term
- a strong, mutually supportive and non-exploitative community
- a high degree of participation in and control by the citizens over the decisions affecting their lives, health and wellbeing
- the meeting of basic needs (for example, food, water, shelter, income, safety and work) for all the city's people
- access by the people to a wide variety of experiences and resources, with the chance for a wide variety of contact, interaction and communication
- a diverse, vital and innovative economy
- connectedness with the past, with the cultural and biological heritage of city dwellers and with other groups and individuals
- an optimum level of appropriate public health and sickness care services, accessible to all
- high health status (for example, high levels of positive health and low levels of disease)

A healthy city is characterized by:

- explicit political commitment
- leadership
- institutional change
- intersectoral partnerships

(WHO Europe, 1997)

Now, the urban age brings with it unprecedented urgency for cities to mobilize action across these sectors to prevent or redress very complex issues. However, since many of these issues may be strongly driven by forces located well outside of cities and even countries, such as multinational corporate interests in food and beverage products, entertainment or consumer goods (Freudenberg and Galea, 2008), the influence of city-level decision making authority may sometimes be weaker than necessary to leverage change. In the face of these globalized forces shaping lifestyles and environments, it is important to question whether the Healthy Cities settings model and tools have the relevance and power needed to make a difference to population health and inequalities through policy, planning and health promotion solutions. To explore this question, three aspects are briefly considered: the principles and values of Healthy Cities; the organizational model underpinning Healthy Cities; and approaches taken to promoting health.

The principles and values of Healthy Cities

Healthy Cities' principles and values (see Box 7.2) have been tested in different countries, political systems and economic circumstances and underpinned initiatives across diverse health issues for many years. They have remained relatively robust despite the diverse contexts in which they have been applied. Indeed, they have become increasingly pertinent for tackling the types of health problems seen in urban settings, such as epidemics of chronic diseases. In the Zagreb Declaration, the principles and values of the Healthy Cities Project were presented as a basis for action by countries in the WHO European Region (WHO Europe, 2009).

Box 7.2 Principles and values of the Healthy Cities Project

Equity: addressing inequality in health, and paying attention to the needs of those who are vulnerable and socially disadvantaged; inequity is inequality in health that is unfair and unjust and avoidable causes of ill health.

Participation and empowerment: ensuring the individual and collective rights of people to participate in decision making that affects their health, healthcare and wellbeing.

Working in partnership: building effective multi-sectoral strategic partnerships to implement integrated approaches and achieve sustainable improvement in health.

Solidarity and friendship: working in the spirit of peace, friendship and solidarity through networking and respect and appreciation of the social and cultural diversity of the cities of the Healthy Cities movement.

Sustainable development: the necessity of working to ensure that economic development is environmentally and socially sustainable; meeting the needs of the present in ways that do not compromise the ability of future generations to meet their own needs.

(WHO Europe, 2009)

Healthy cities' organizational structures

Strategic and operational committees are fundamental to the work of healthy cities, bringing together the decision making authority, processes and resources required to determine goals and facilitate health promotion action in urban settings. As healthy cities lead local level action on many issues that have little to do with healthcare services and much more to do with the mandate and concerns of other sectors (WHO Europe, 1997), membership of committees is multisectoral and multidisciplinary. Healthy cities projects operate as mediating structures, viewing city life through the dual lenses of health and equity and linking diverse stakeholders around these two broad social goals. An example of the organizational arrangements in Belfast is provided in Box 7.3. Belfast was among the first group of cities designated to the European Healthy Cities Network in 1987, and hosted the 2003 conference at which the Belfast Declaration, focusing on the power of local action, was adopted.

Box 7.3   Organizational arrangements: Belfast Healthy Cities

Belfast Healthy Cities, in Northern Ireland, is an **independent, partnership-based organization** within the city with a mandate to act on the priority themes of the WHO European Healthy Cities Network within the local context. It is a limited company with charitable status, governed by an **elected Board of Directors** that represents the public, university, voluntary and community sectors. A **small professional team** is responsible for action and includes a director, a health development manager, a support manager and a support officer, a senior health development officer and an inequalities officer. It works with relevant organizations to bring about change and develop tools, strategies and ways of working that can be applied by other organizations.

In 2002 Belfast Healthy Cities produced *Planning for a Healthy City*. This set out jointly agreed action plans on four themes identified as priorities through consultation. A new strategic planning group method was used to develop the plan, which involved intersectoral groups being set up around each theme. To bring the plan to life, actions were implemented as part of the corporate plans of partner agencies.

(Visit their website at http://www.belfasthealthycities.com/about-us.html for more details)

As well as operating to deliver programmes in some cities, one of the most important roles of healthy cities may be as a driver of new governance structures for public health and health promotion at the city level (Green et al., 2009). In their review of healthy cities' partnership structures, Green et al. (2009) observed that the mandatory requirements of membership of the WHO European Healthy Cities Network led to intersectoral partnership structures forming that were enduring, largely successful and that had the capability to drive healthy public policy at the local level and, in turn, deliver better health outcomes. Committee structures enabling partnerships were found to have diverse membership including, importantly, representatives of the community.

Healthy cities' organizational structures have developed at local, national and regional levels since the late 1980s to support growth, innovation and organizational sustainability. At the national and international levels, networks are the main mechanisms that have evolved for supporting and promoting the work of healthy cities and sharing experiences and lessons learnt. Networks have sought institutional partners to assist in elevating the profile of health and cities such as the European Union, Local Governments for Sustainability and other organs of the United Nations (for example, UN Development Program or UN-HABITAT). Networks have been important for intersectoral collaboration and also the mainstreaming of ideas, policy innovations and effective programs.

Approaches taken to promoting health

A rich and diverse range of health promotion work has been undertaken by healthy cities in the European region, as well as cities not formally involved in the Healthy Cities Network, reflecting the relevance and adaptability of cities as a setting for health promotion. The issues address local priorities across a wide range of areas: increasing physical activity, preventing crime, promoting social connectedness and mental wellbeing, chronic disease prevention, supporting vulnerable population groups (young children, older adults, newly arrived migrants) and many others. To shed light on practical efforts, healthy cities' approaches to addressing a complex but increasingly important issue, health equalities, are explored below.

Health equity has been a longstanding priority of healthy cities. As well as part of the original set of commitments, the need to take action on equity was reinforced in the mayoral declaration Action for Equity in Europe (WHO Europe, 2000) which called on healthy cities to develop a vision and strategy locating equity as a core value and key component of the city health development plan. It also called for cities to produce policies and programmes for reducing health inequalities in areas such as poverty, vulnerable social groups, access to health, education and social care, and people living in poor neighbourhoods of the city. While operationalizing the principle of equity has proven to been a significant challenge, the emphasis given to action on equity by the European Healthy Cities Network has led to a shift from rhetoric to action in cities (Ritsatakis, 2009). An evaluation of initiatives promoting health equity in healthy cities (Ritsatakis, 2009) showed that the main areas of action, initiated by the Healthy Cities project or others, concerned the provision of support to vulnerable groups, although the effectiveness of these interventions is not clear. Examples of projects discussed in this evaluation are summarized in Table 7.1.

At the heart of the efforts identified are some common requirements for effective action on health inequalities. These include political commitment and

Table 7.1   Summary of actions on health equity taken in Healthy Cities projects

Target population	Areas of action on equity
Children (18 cities)	Free fruit and breakfast (UK cities); dairy products (Zagreb); student meals (Maribor); summer camps, foster homes, youth hostels, support for abused children (Athens); support for children of alcoholic parents (Gyor); lower fees in kindergartens for disadvantaged children (Dresden); reading recovery programme (Belfast)
Elderly and/or disabled (18 cities)	Improving access to buildings and public transport (range of cities); summer camps (Athens, Padua); tele-alarm (Maribor); nursing care (Jerusalem); strategic plan for mentally and physically disabled people (Helsingborg)
Immigrants, ethnic minorities and travellers (15 cities)	Representation of immigrants on City Council (Padua); intercultural coexistence (San Fernando de Henares); banking system for poor migrants (Milan); race equality schemes (Camden)
Lifestyles (several cities)	Swimming classes for disadvantaged young people and ethnic minority women (Gothenburg); free access to swimming pools for young people (Glasgow); bicycle paths (Sandnes); cycling and walking projects, including safer routes to school (Camden); volunteer adults who patrol streets in the evening to keep young people safe (Sandnes)
Healthcare (10 cities)	Main focus: free check-ups, other preventive services for disadvantaged groups (number of cities); ensuring transparency in waiting lists (Arezzo); lending medical equipment (Jerusalem)
Unemployment (14 cities)	Main focus: re-training (number of cities); developing infrastructure to attract new enterprises and jobs (Kuressaare); efforts to reduce unemployment among women, ex-prisoners and disabled people (Izhevsk)
Housing and the homeless (13 cities)	Ensuring high-quality drinking water by providing new pipes (Izhevsk); stock transfer of social housing (Liverpool)
Overall development	Regeneration of disadvantaged areas, community strategies, health action zones, education action zones, New Deal programmes, neighbourhood renewal and crime reduction programs (UK); equity linked to development (Athens, Bologna, Gyor, Horsens, Jerusalem, Seixal, Turku); policies to promote equity in health in support of the city's development plan (Maribor)
Other	Outreach programme to help the poor apply for benefits to which they are entitled (Rotterdam); government reporting on cross-cutting spending (Liverpool); equity experts on call (Liverpool); focus of city contracts and local education contracts on disadvantaged areas (Rennes); neighbourhood councils to improve participation in decision making (Rennes)

partnerships so that support, resources and action can be mobilized, institutional changes so that the issues are understood as integral to the work of local governments and others at the local level, and capacity for action, for example planning, implementation, evaluation and reporting.

While the examples of action indicate the diversity of entry points to reducing health inequalities in urban settings, the potential for the Healthy Cities approach to be used to address health inequalities is largely unfulfilled and represents a core agenda for the next 25 years. Although Ritsatakis (2009) found there had been a demonstrable improvement in measuring, monitoring and acting on health inequalities in healthy cities, there remain considerable opportunities to boost the commitment and ongoing participation of all sectors operating at city level in the pursuit of health equity. Involving the business sector in a Healthy Cities project is a particular challenge, given its fundamental orientation to profit and shareholders. Trends in relation to corporate social responsibility suggest growing opportunities exist for dialogue and engagement. Organizations that successfully partner with businesses on sustainability and health initiatives may have valuable lessons for healthy cities around finding shared goals and leveraging private sector investment for the public good.

Healthy Cities has produced many tested tools and approaches and as a result, considerable international networking. Important know-how has been generated by cities across Europe and other parts of the world concerning a number of key structures, processes and actions for promoting health in urban settings, and as a WHO initiative, Healthy Cities in Europe has given a profile to the legitimacy and potential of urban settings as a place for health promotion. The context for urban settings is changing dramatically and there is an urgency to pre-empt imminent and longer term risks to urban populations such as climate change and address obstinate problems such as health inequalities.

The city as a setting for health promotion: future challenges

The pace of growth of cities, their increasing complexity on many fronts, and their vulnerability to external economic, environmental and other forces suggest that the next 25 years will be a major test for those leading health promotion efforts. While cities have been an important setting for promoting health and have achieved many successes, their potential has not yet been fully exploited. Healthy Cities faces the challenge of remaining relevant and 'fit for purpose' as a force for health promotion innovation in an increasingly risky and complex environment. The Kobe Call to Action (WHO and UN Human Settlements Programme 2010: 4) formulated at the Global Forum on Urbanization and Health in November 2010, articulated the broad set of challenges for cities:

> While cities strive to build their resilience to the impacts of climate change and other troubling environmental changes (for example, air pollution), and to

strengthen their health systems, they also face a triple health threat: infectious diseases which thrive when people are crowded together under inadequate living conditions; violence and injuries (including road traffic accidents) which further burden urban health; and non-communicable diseases and conditions (including mental health) which are in part a result of the globalization of unhealthy lifestyles (for example, tobacco use, unhealthy diets, physical inactivity and harmful use of alcohol) fuelled by urban life. However, one of the most prominent threats of all remains urban health inequities, which are largely hidden by the misleading use of averages.

The task of responding to this call to action has a number of dimensions. Reflecting on the key ideas that led to the creation of the first Healthy Cities project, cities must continue to innovate around public health and urban governance structures and processes to enable cities to deal with complex, interrelated and intractable health-related issues (described earlier as 'wicked issues'). Analysis of the capabilities and responsiveness of existing governance structures in urban settings is fundamental to such innovation. Urban governance refers to the systems, institutions and processes through which policies and decisions concerning public life, economic and social development are influenced and enacted. Governance structures in a city must be capable of convening key actors, formal institutions and civil society, if they are to support action on the urban setting as a whole or address an issue using a comprehensive approach based on systems thinking (whole systems approaches are discussed in more detail in Chapter 3). Thus, developing know-how related to negotiating relationships with private and not-for-profit sectors, including by tapping into corporate social responsibility must receive more focus in healthy cities. Future efforts in healthy cities must mainstream accomplishments so that what was once innovation now becomes the new way of doing business.

It seems likely that a step change will be required in the mindset of key city actors, politicians, decision makers, communities, business leaders and others, concerning Healthy Cities initiatives and health promotion. The determinants of many health issues facing urban populations need to be understood as not easily defined and new forms of partnerships, investments and actions need to be sustained over the longer term. There has always been a delay in finding and implementing fundamental solutions to issues affecting our health and the environment. We must start shifting from solutions that offer short term fixes to finding regenerative solutions (see for example Senge et al., 2008). This is becoming more and more urgent considering the impacts of climate change.

Practical implications of this changed mindset, at the city level, relate particularly to healthy cities' governance, infrastructure and the types of programmes designed to address problems. Urban governance needs to have health and equity positioned as driving forces for decision making and accountability. The composition of the Healthy City steering committee and sub-committees, the nature of partners, the competencies of coordinators and the scale of programmes and the nature of their partners may benefit from review to enable the required authority, policy instruments, processes and resources to be brought together to effect action. Work at the global network level may become even more important, as cities collaborate on research, programmes and advocacy to address determinants of health that lie outside the influence of individual cities.

In addition to the urgent need for regenerative solutions, another implication of the urban age for the Healthy Cities movement (arising from changes in social values, demographic changes and increasing inequalities) is that municipal authorities must foster inclusiveness in their cities (UN-HABITAT, 2009). According to the most recent UN-HABITAT State of the World's Cities report:

> Inclusive policies for cities should ... focus more particularly on any positive components that could be integrated to formal municipal norms and practices, such as the informal economy, social capital and informal institutional arrangements, including affordable land delivery and housing systems etc. (UN-HABITAT, 2010: 56)

While many examples can be found of very fruitful uses of the Healthy Cities approach, it is not the only approach to bringing about the type of comprehensive solutions to public health issues needed in the urban age. The early framing of Healthy Cities ideas drew on social movements such as women's, social justice, ecology and community development movements (Baum, 1993). Other movements with a concern for how the life of cities is changing and how to make cities better have emerged over the past two decades to sit alongside healthy cities as engines for change. These include sustainable cities, resilient cities, compassionate cities, age-friendly cities and child-friendly cities. In addition, numerous non-government and other types of organizations have developed to tackle contemporary agendas that are directly or indirectly related to health. For example, Groundwork UK is a group of charities working across England, Wales and Northern Ireland that supports people and organizations to make changes that lead to better neighbourhoods, enhanced skills and job prospects, and 'green' ways to live and work. The organization emphasizes a flexible, interconnected agenda around environmental, urban regeneration, health, safety, employment and other issues and engages business and the third sector.

A challenge lies ahead for cities to benefit from the leadership, knowledge, tools and resources produced by diverse urban initiatives such as those noted above and create synergy between them and impacts on health and equity. In addition, the achievements of Healthy Cities and other initiatives that strive to achieve sustainable improvements in urban health and the environment (Dooris, 1999) need to be mainstreamed. That is, they need to shift from being special, time-limited projects working in parallel to shaping new norms for how cities function and do business (Plümer et al., 2010). A number of core components identified by WHO for mainstreaming health promotion could be applied to ensure Healthy Cities makes an ongoing impact on the way health is understood and enhanced in cities.

Gaps in existing knowledge about how best to strengthen cities as a setting for health promotion point to a broad research agenda. While often neglected and underfunded, evaluation of existing actions and programmes and dissemination of these findings is fundamental to improving knowledge.

Particular forms of research, such as action research, may promote participation in research activities, and interest in health promotion, by a range of stakeholders. The nature of problems and opportunities facing cities underscores the need for transdisciplinary research. The use of futures studies (Fawkes, 2009) may help to engage diverse groups in exploring trends, scenarios and optional courses of action to promote health at the local level.

Summary points

- Changes are occurring rapidly in the populations and environments of urban areas to create problems that have no easy solutions. However, there is inadequate understanding among decision makers of the urgency of acting given the nature, pace and impacts of changes.

- In light of emerging challenges for people's health in cities, the 'wicked' problems and the rapid rate of urbanization, the Healthy Cities movement needs to be proactive in adapting its principles, values and approaches to the urban age context. Action that is geared to sustainable development needs to be fast tracked.

- National and international partnerships and networks involving public, private and other sectors are essential for expanding learning and mentoring activities for developing cities as healthy settings.

- Research into and debate about how to build capacity for resilience to change needs to be prioritized alongside how to achieve population health goals.

Online Further Reading

Kjellstrom, T. and Mercado, S. (2008) 'Towards action on social determinants for health equity in urban settings', *Environment and Urbanization*, 20: 551–75.

This paper draws attention to the need to address social determinants of health, in meeting the challenge of urbanization. Strong urban governance can address social determinants of health such as housing and living conditions, access to safe water and good sanitation, efficient waste management systems, safer working environments and neighbourhoods, food security and access to services such as education, health, welfare, public transportation and childcare. The paper explores how urban development and town planning are key to creating supportive social and physical environments for health and health equity.

Portney, K.E. and Berry, J.M. (2010) 'Participation and the pursuit of sustainability in US cities', *Urban Affairs Review*, 46: 119–40.

In this paper the relationship between political and civic participation and the pursuit of sustainability is explored, in the context of American cities. The paper compares cities that have sustainability programmes with those that have modest programmes and those that have no sustainability programmes at all, in terms of participation, finding that cities that are most committed to pursuing sustainability policies do tend to be more participatory places with respect to signing petitions, participating in demonstrations, belonging to local reform groups and joining neighbourhood associations.

References

Ashton, J., Grey, P. and Barnard, K. (1986) 'WHO's new public health initiative', *Health Promotion International*, 1: 319–24.

Baum, F. (1993) 'Healthy Cities and change: social movement or bureaucratic tool?', *Health Promotion International*, 8 (1): 31–40.

Dooris, M. (1999) 'Healthy Cities and Local Agenda 21: the UK experience – challenges for the new millennium', *Health Promotion International*, 14: 365–75.

Duhl, L. (1963) *The Urban Condition: People and Policy in the Metropolis.* New York: Basic Books.

Fawkes, S. (2009) 'Taking the long view in health policy making: the use of futures studies'. Unpublished PhD thesis. La Trobe University, Melbourne.

Freudenberg, N. and Galea, S. (2008) 'Cities of consumption: the impact of corporate practices on the health of urban populations'. *Journal of Urban Health*, 85 (4): 462–71.

Fried, L. and Paccaud, F. (2010) 'Editorial', *Public Health Reviews, Ageing Societies*, 32 (2): 2–5.

Fudge, C. (2003) 'Health and sustainability gains from urban regeneration and development', in T. Takano (ed.), *Healthy Cities and Urban Policy Research*. London: Spon Press.

Green, G., Price, C., Lipp, A. and Priestly, R. (2009) 'Partnership structures in the WHO European Healthy Cities project', *Health Promotion International*, 24 (S1): i37–i44.

Hancock, T. and Duhl, L. (1986) *Promoting Health in the Urban Context.* Copenhagen: World Health Organization Regional Office for Europe.

Hancock, T. (1993) 'The evolution, impact and significance of the Healthy Cities movement', *Journal of Public Health Policy*, 14: 5–18.

IPCC (2009) Scoping for the IPCC 5th Assessment Report. Concept paper for an IPCC expert meeting on human settlement, water, energy and transport infrastructure – mitigation and adaptation strategies (submitted by Working Group III Co-Chairs). Thirteenth Session, Antalya, 21–23 April 2009. Geneva: Intergovernmental Panel on Climate Change.

Kickbusch, I. (1989) 'Healthy Cities: a working project and a growing movement', *Health Promotion International*, 4: 77–82.

Lawrence, R. and Fudge, C. (2003) 'Urban health and healthy cities: context and relevance', in A.D. Tsouros and J.L. Farrington (eds), *WHO Healthy Cities in Europe: A Compilation of Papers on Progress and Achievements*. Copenhagen: World Health Organization Regional Office for Europe.

Lawrence, R. and Fudge, C. (2009) 'Healthy Cities in a global and regional context', *Health Promotion International*, 24 (51), November (Special issue on European Healthy Cities).

OECD (2003) *Ageing, Housing and Urban Development*. Paris: OECD.

OECD (2010) *Pensions at a Glance 2009: Retirement-Income Systems in OECD Countries* Paris: OECD. www.oecd.org/dataoecd/10/26/43060101.pdf (accessed 1 February 2011).

Plümer, K.D., Kennedy, L. and Trojan, A. (2010) 'Evaluating the implementation of the WHO Healthy Cities Programme across Germany (1999–2002)', *Health Promotion International*, 25(3): 342–54.

Ritsatakis, A. (2009) 'Equity and social determinants of health at a city level', *Health Promotion International*, 24 (Suppl 1): i81–i90.

Satterthwaite, D. (2007) *Climate Change and Urbanization: Effects and Implications for Urban Governance*. United National Expert Group Meeting on Population Distribution, Urbanization, Internal Migration and Development. Population Division, Department of Economic and Social Affairs, United Nations Secretariat, New York, 21–23 January 2008.

Senge, P., Smith, B., Kruschwitz, N., Laur, J. and Schley, S. (2008) *The Necessary Revolution. How Individuals and Organizations Are Working Together to Create a Sustainable World*. London: Nicholas Brealey.

The Global Compact (2010) 'The Global Compact Cities Programme', *Sustainable Cities*, Volume 1. Melbourne: Global Contact Cities Programme.

Tsouros, A.D. (1990) *World Health Organization Healthy Cities Project: A Project Becomes a Movement*. Copenhagen: World Health Organization Regional Office for Europe.

Tsouros. A. (2009) 'City leadership for health and sustainable development: The World Health Organization European Healthy Cities Network', *Health Promotion International*, 24 (Suppl 1): i4–i10

UN-HABITAT (2009) Planning sustainable cities: Global report on Human Settlements 2009. Available at: www.unhabitat.org/content.asp?typeid=19&catid=555&cid=5607 (accessed 20 November 2010).

UN-HABITAT (2010) *State of the World's Cities 2010/11: Bridging the Urban Divide*. Press kit: Bridging the Urban Divide. Inclusive Cities, page 2. Kenya: United Nations Human Settlements Programme. Available at: www.unhabitat.org/documents/SOWC10/R11.pdf (accessed 24 March 2011).

UN Population Division (2010a) *World Urbanization Prospects. The 2009 Revision. Highlights*. New York: United Nations.

UN Population Division (2010b) *World Population Ageing 2009*. New York: United Nations.

UNCRD (2010) *Environmentally Sustainable Transport for Asian Cities: A Sourcebook*. Nagoya: United National Centre for Regional Development.

WHO (World Health Organization) (1998) *Health Promotion Glossary*. Geneva: WHO. Available at: www.who.int/hpr/NPH/docs/hp_glossary_en.pdf (accessed 1 February 2011).

WHO (World Health Organization) (2003) The Belfast Declaration for Healthy Cities: The Power of Local Action. Available at: www.euro.who.int/en/what-we-do/health-topics/environmental-health/urban-health/publications/2003/belfast-declaration-for-healthy-cities (accessed 27 March 2011).

WHO (World Health Organization) (2009) *Protecting Health from Climate Change. Connecting Science, Policy and People.* Geneva: WHO.

WHO (2010a) *Environmentally Sustainable and Healthy Urban Transport: A Strategic Focus on Urbanization and Health.* Draft working document, updated 17 March 2010. Manila: World Health Organization Regional Office for the Western Pacific. Available at: www.wpro.who.int/NR/rdonlyres/73A7E616-0CEF-4CE9-87CC-232CE2A958EC/0/ESHUTPrimer.pdf (accessed 7 February 2011).

WHO (2010b) The Global Forum on Urbanization and Health. Kobe Call to Action. Available at: www.who.or.jp/index_files/Kobe%20Call%20to%20Action%20FINAL_4p.pdf (accessed 6 February 2011).

WHO Europe (1997) *20 Steps for Developing a Healthy Cities Project.* Copenhagen: World Health Organization Regional Office for Europe.

WHO Europe (2000). Action for Equity in Europe. Mayors' statement of the WHO Healthy Cities Network in Phase III. Available at: www.euro.who.int/__data/assets/pdf_file/0012/101172/Horsens_Stat_E.pdf (accessed 4 January 2011).

WHO Europe (2009) *Zagreb Declaration for Healthy Cities. Health and Health Equity in All Local Policies.* Copenhagen: World Health Organization Europe Regional Office for Europe.

WHO and United Nations Human Settlements Programme (2010) *Hidden Cities: Unmasking and Overcoming Health Inequities in Urban Settings.* World Health Organization, The WHO Centre for Health Development, Kobe, and United Nations Human Settlements Programme (UN-HABITAT).

World Bank (2010) *Cities and Climate Change: An Urgent Agenda.* Washington, DC: World Bank.

8

The Healthy Hospital: A Contradiction in Terms?

Trevor Hancock

Aims

- To present and distinguish between the concepts of a healthy and a health promoting hospital
- To describe a healthy hospital, as one that creates a healing environment for patients and a healthy workplace for staff
- To describe a health promoting hospital, as one that is an environmentally responsible organization and that contributes to the process of creating a healthier community
- To provide examples of health promoting hospitals and the networks and international organizations which support them

---

When conducting healthy hospital workshops with hospital staff, the following few simple questions almost always trigger uncomfortable and somewhat embarrassed responses:

- Can someone get a good night's sleep in this hospital?
- Does this hospital have the healthiest food in the community?
- Is this hospital the healthiest workplace in the community?
- Is this hospital the greenest facility in the community?

The answer to these questions, unfortunately, is usually negative. So what is wrong with this picture? Shouldn't hospitals, these hugely expensive temples of healing, be able to answer yes to these and similar questions? Shouldn't these places where people heal be the very model of healthy places? Yet we all know that only too often that is not the case. This chapter sets out to explore what is a healthy hospital and a health promoting hospital, and following from this, how can a hospital become one? The answers to these questions, which apply not just to hospitals but to all healthcare facilities, and indeed to the healthcare system as a whole, will be illustrated by examples throughout the chapter.

Historical overview

The concept of health promoting hospitals, like other settings-based approaches, owes its origins to the Ottawa Charter for Health Promotion (WHO, 1986). As part of the follow-up work to the Charter, WHO Europe launched the Health Promoting Hospital Network in 1988, in partnership with Ludwig Boltzmann Institute in Vienna. Over time the network has grown to the point that it now has more than 750 hospitals and national and regional networks in 23 countries in Europe and North America as well as Taiwan, and an international secretariat in Copenhagen.

However, while the work of creating healthier and more health promoting hospitals has been under way in many countries for a number of years, two recent reviews of the evidence have both concluded that, although there is a significant amount of information available in internal reports, databases and progress reports (Groene, 2005) there is a lack of documentation of the experience in the academic literature and a lack of good research, resulting in a dearth of evidence on how best to intervene.

Whitehead finds this disconcerting, and furthermore notes that much of what is described as health promoting work:

> would be more appropriately defined within the context of Health Educating Hospitals ... with ... pockets of health programme activities ... primarily based on disease management/avoidance issues. (Whitehead, 2004: 262)

A more recent review (McHugh et al., 2010) came to similar conclusions, finding a dearth of published English language systematic reviews or randomized controlled studies, and no high level research having been conducted. Not surprisingly, they concluded that more rigorous research on Health Promoting Hospitals and dissemination of results is needed.

Healthy, or health promoting?

It is useful to distinguish between, but link, two different concepts: the healthy hospital and the health promoting hospital (Hancock, 1999).

- A healthy hospital puts the focus on the hospital itself, and what goes on within its four walls. There are two very different broad populations within those walls; patients and their families, on the one hand, and staff, from the cleaner to the CEO, on the other. Clearly the latter exist to serve the former, but in order for this to happen, staff themselves need to have a healthy workplace.

- A health promoting hospital, on the other hand, shifts the focus to the role and impact of the hospital beyond its four walls, in the wider community and environment in which it exists. A hospital, after all, does not exist in isolation, and is often a prominent organization in its community. So two broad questions arise: first, is the hospital being an environmentally responsible organization and second, is the hospital playing its part in creating the conditions for health in the community?

Thus there are four broad areas of activity involved in creating a healthy and health promoting hospital (Hancock, 1999):

- Creating a healing environment for patients.
- Being a healthy workplace for staff.
- Being an environmentally responsible organization.
- Contributing with other partners to the creation of a healthy community.

These four areas of activity are similar to the five foci of activity and four types of health promoting hospitals identified by Johnson and Baum (2001). Fundamental to this work is the need for leadership at the highest level and a shift in organizational culture that embeds these issues in the way of working by all staff at all levels. This shift in organizational culture is addressed in the final section of this chapter.

However, before getting to these more sophisticated concepts of a healthy and health promoting hospital, the more basic principle of *primum noc nocere* should be addressed. It is, or should be, a golden rule of the settings approach that it begins with safety. Before moving on to the more sophisticated aspects of health promotion in a home, school, workplace or community, it is essential to ensure that the building or the community environment is safe, that it won't fall down, or catch fire, or leak, that it meets all applicable building codes, that the community is not built in a floodplain or a landslide zone, and that the activities within it won't kill people or make them sick. So in the case of workplaces, for example, all relevant occupational health and safety legislation, regulations and codes should be followed, machinery should be guarded, toxic substances controlled, appropriate safety equipment used and so on (this is discussed in more detail in Chapter 12). And so it is with hospitals, with the added distinction that there is a very clear ethical directive in the Hippocratic Oath, *primum non nocere* – first, do no harm. Hospitals, perhaps above all other workplaces, have a clear obligation to do no harm to either their patients or their staff. Yet the shocking reality is that hospitals, and the healthcare system more broadly, do a great deal of harm to patients. Hospitals can also be among the least safe and healthy workplaces in their communities.

Medical error is a major cause of death, injury and disability for patients. For example, in Canada, it was estimated that in 2000 between 9,000 and 23,000 deaths resulting from adverse events were preventable (Baker et al.,

2004), making this among the largest causes of death in the country! These medical errors are not only harmful for patients, they are also expensive for the system in economic terms, requiring longer stays, readmissions and additional interventions to fix the errors. Happily, given that the issue of patient safety constitutes a *sine qua non* for the creation of a healing environment for patients, improving both patient safety and the quality of care has become a much more important focus of concern for healthcare in the past decade.

Creating a healing environment for patients

While a safe environment and high quality care is fundamental to the creation of a healing environment for patients, it is not enough. The concept of a healing environment is a broader one than just providing safe care of good quality; it includes providing a truly caring, compassionate, even loving environment for patients, with staff that are committed to caring, a beautiful physical environment that incorporates art and nature, healthy food, and a commitment to the engagement and empowerment of the patient and their family in the process of caring and healing. If this sounds utopian, and expensive, it is not. It is being done in many hospitals, it is affordable and it brings many benefits, not only in terms of improved patient satisfaction and better quality care but also in a much-improved working environment for staff.

The example par excellence of creating a healing environment for patients is Planetree, a US-based Alliance that has been leading this work for more than 20 years. A brief description can be found in Box 8.1. The approach of the hospitals within the Alliance is broad, seeking to address the physical, mental, social and spiritual needs of their patients through what the Alliance calls patient-centred care. In practice, this means creating physical, social and organizational environments that support patients, which ultimately means a change in the organizational culture of the hospital or the health system of which it is a part. Thus the second edition of their book on patient-centred care (Frampton et al., 2008) includes the following topics:

- relationship-centred caring
- access to information to inform and empower diverse populations
- involving patients, families and volunteers in healing partnerships
- the nurturing and healing aspects of food
- spiritual and cultural diversity as inner resources for healing
- the integration of complementary and alternative practices
- the effects of viewing art on health outcomes
- design aspects of creating a healing environment
- expanding the boundaries of health care to create healthier communities

> ## Box 8.1 Planetree and Griffin Hospital: a health promoting hospital
>
> The strongly humanistic and compassionate core values that underpin the work of Planetree are reflected in their statement of beliefs, which can be found on their website, www.planetree.org/about.html.
>
> How this is put into practice is perhaps best exemplified by the Griffin Hospital in Derby, CT, where Planetree is now based. Griffin Hospital adopted the Planetree philosophy in 1992 and its North Wing is the first facility and remains the largest fully Planetree facility in the United States. Griffin is recognized for having industry-leading patient satisfaction ratings and has received a number of quality and clinical excellence awards. For example, Griffin was awarded the Health-Grades *Distinguished Hospital for Clinical Excellence Award* in both 2009 and 2010, putting it in the top 5% of hospitals nationally, significant given that patients receiving care at a hospital rated in the top 5% in the country have, on average, a 71% lower chance of mortality and a 14% lower risk of complications. It is the only hospital to be named on FORTUNE Magazine's '100 Best Companies to Work For' list for ten consecutive years, ranking fourth in 2006, the highest ranking ever achieved by a hospital.
>
> To measure the satisfaction of its inpatients, Griffin Hospital contracts with an independent, private market research company to conduct a telephone survey of 100 discharged patients (about 15% of discharges) each month. In 2009, patient satisfaction with inpatient care was 96%, with the emergency department 92% and with ambulatory care 97%. Griffin was one of the first hospitals in the state and only a small percentage of hospitals nationwide to make a number of quality reports and other performance indicators available to those they serve.
>
> (Visit their website at www.griffinhealth.org/AboutUs.aspx for more details)

A healthy workplace for staff

It should be noted that, in this chapter, only staff health and safety matters that are unique to healthcare are addressed. The healthcare setting is also a workplace setting like many others, and many of the issues that are applicable to other workplaces in creating a healthy workplace apply to healthcare settings as well. They are addressed in the section and in the chapters on healthy workplaces (Chapters 12–15). Moreover, many of the issues relating to a healthy workplace for staff have already been addressed in dealing with issues of patient and staff safety and a healing environment.

In a review of the health of healthcare workers in the Canadian province of British Columbia (BC) the Auditor General for BC stated that three main factors contribute to the health of a workplace:

- The physical safety of the workers, involving such issues as prevention of injury and protection from violence
- The psychological and social environment of the workplace, with an emphasis on the need for respectful working relationships

- The promotion of a healthy lifestyle, involving such issues as the nutrition easily available to workers, and recognition of the need for a life–work balance. (Office of the Auditor General for BC, 2004a)

One would like to think that a hospital would see that its staff are the most important asset it possesses, and thus strive to meet these conditions. Yet Lowe (2002) reports that in Canada in 2000, nursing, technical and support staff in healthcare had the highest number of days lost due to personal illness or injury of any occupation, double or more than the national average. The main risks they faced were from infectious diseases, violence from patients/residents with dementia, allergic reactions from chemical agents, and ergonomic issues associated with patient handling (OHSAH, 2004).

The psychosocial demands of the hospital as a workplace are also considerable. Shift work, work-related exhaustion and burnout are common among healthcare professionals (Leach, 1995), particularly as the intensity of care increases. These strains can be heightened in a time of cutbacks and rapid change (Ryndes, 1997) and by the interaction between workplace and home stressors. Leach suggests that job sharing, flexible work hours, on-site daycare, parenting seminars and arrangements that enable staff to care for sick children or older relatives can help to reduce workplace stress (Leach, 1995). Perhaps not surprisingly, given the difficult physical and psychological conditions of the healthcare workplace, Lowe (2002: 51) notes that:

> Health professionals have the weakest employment relationships on all four dimensions [of employee relationships], trust, commitment, communication and influence, of any occupation in Canada, including unskilled manual and service workers.

The costs to the healthcare system of these unsafe and stressful working conditions are very high, according to the Office of the Auditor General for British Columbia (2004b). He estimated that for this Canadian province of only 4 million people, for five of the six health authorities in BC (data was not available for the smallest health authority in the north) the direct costs of absenteeism and injury to the health authorities in 2002/03 was $247.1 million. Add to that the indirect costs of absences, such as the cost of relief staff to replace absent workers or of overtime, that are estimated to be 2–10 times the direct cost ($103.2 million) and the total cost is anywhere from $309 million to $1.135 billion out of a total budget that year for the five health authorities of $5.639 billion (Health Authority Performance Agreements, 2002/03), amounting to between 5.5 and 20% of their entire budgets. The Auditor General added that:

> Also not included is the cost of decreased productivity when staff attend work but are not feeling well. This is sometimes referred to as presenteeism. The cost of presenteeism is unknown, but some reports have estimated it to be two to four times the direct cost of illness and injury. (Health Authority Performance Agreements, 2002/03: 19)

In addition to the costs of absenteeism and presenteeism, there is the cost of replacing staff that leave. Jones and Gates (2007) state that the cost of a nurse turnover has been estimated to be 1.3 times the annual salary of the departing nurse, with recent estimates ranging from $22,000 to $64,000 (USD). An international study, with data from hospitals in Australia, Canada, New Zealand, Scotland and the United States found that the average cost of a new nursing hire was $22,000 (2002 USD), with the main costs coming from decreased productivity, followed by orientation and training (Stone et al., 2003).

Thus it is important to understand and address the factors that affect staff health and retention; many of these also relate to the health of the workplace and the overall organizational culture and leadership styles within the organization. These issues are discussed later in the section on organizational culture.

An environmentally responsible organization

In recent years, there has been a growing interest in and commitment to ensuring that business and industry behaves in an environmentally responsible manner. This includes not polluting the environment, using resources in a sustainable manner and avoiding harm to ecosystem health and biodiversity. Given that our health and continued economic and social development is ultimately dependent upon the health of the planet and our local environment, it is only logical that a healthy hospital will be exemplary in its environmental practices and its use of resources; doing no harm extends to not harming the environment, so a health promoting hospital is necessarily a 'green' hospital.

Yet there are many ways in which hospitals may contribute to environmental damage. Among the more obvious ones are their use of energy and other resources, especially plastics, paper and other disposables, their emissions of carbon dioxide and toxic chemicals, including incinerator emissions, and their production of solid and liquid wastes and other environmentally harmful practices (Hancock, 2001). In response to these challenges, the healthcare sector has seen a dramatic growth in the movement towards environmentally responsible healthcare in the past 10–15 years. At a global level, this is epitomized by Health Care Without Harm, and many individual hospitals or health systems have inspiring stories to tell (see Box 8.2). On the design side, the Green Building Council in the United States has recently approved a Leadership in Energy and Environmental Design (LEED) standard for healthcare facilities. LEED certification indicates that a building is addressing a number of environmental concerns, including energy savings, water efficiency, CO_2 emissions reduction, improved indoor environmental quality, and stewardship of resources and sensitivity to their impacts.

The bottom line is that there is a great deal of energy and enthusiasm among health professionals for this issue, and a great deal of knowledge and expertise has been developed, along with many resources. No hospital in the twenty-first century should have any excuse for not being more environmentally responsible, especially when it is understood that these initiatives can readily be linked to efforts to improve patient and staff health and safety, as well as saving costs and reducing healthy and environmental impacts.

Box 8.2   Helping hospitals become environmentally friendly

Health Care Without Harm (HCWH) began in the United States in 1996 after the US Environmental Protection Agency identified medical waste incineration as the leading source of dioxin, one of the most potent carcinogens. Today it is a broad-based international coalition of almost 500 organizations in 52 countries. It works on a wide range of issues providing information and resources, organizing campaigns and working with many NGO partners and government and international agencies (Health Care Without Harm, 2011).

The Interior Health Authority (IHA) serves a population of 750,000 people in southeastern British Columbia, Canada. IHA recognizes that minimizing its ecological footprint is of key importance to staff, residents and other stakeholders. In the process it has been able to show that green initiatives are good for the environment and our communities, but they also make financial sense. Among its many initiatives, it has:

- established a Department of Environmental Sustainability
- implemented a policy to build new facilities to meet LEED Gold standards
- undertaken other energy conservation measures such as implementing more energy-efficient lighting and adding solar power to some of its buildings
- implemented a policy to make all new vehicle purchases hybrid and encouraging and supporting active transportation among staff members
- instituted a number of measures to reduce paper use
- developed a mercury thermometer exchange programme in the community
- increased its recycling programmes and purchasing of more recycled products
- implemented a policy to reduce cosmetic pesticide use in grounds-keeping

IHA's leadership has been recognized, among other awards, by being awarded a *Champions for Change Award* from the US-based Hospitals for a Healthy Environment in 2007 (IHA 2011).

A partner in creating a healthier community

This is perhaps the most challenging aspect of being a health promoting hospital, because it takes hospitals well beyond their usual comfort zone of providing health care. It requires that the hospital be one part of the process of creating healthier communities, which is the application at the local level of the strategies of health promotion outlined in the Ottawa Charter. However, the hospital needs to recognize that the major determinants of health lie beyond the healthcare sector in the broad environmental, social, political, economic and cultural conditions of the community. Since many of these factors lie beyond their realm of expertise and jurisdiction, hospitals should not own or manage the project as a healthcare project. However, because of their status within the community hospitals can and should be important partners in the process of creating a healthier community.

Based on the Ottawa Charter for Health Promotion, among the actions a hospital can take are the following (see Hancock (1999) for a fuller discussion):

- Assess the health of the community in partnership with the community
- Identify and address inequalities in health
- Become an advocate for healthy public policies within the community
- Partner with those in the community who are working to create environments supportive of health
- Strengthen community action by actively supporting community groups and organizations that are working to build personal and community capacity
- Help people develop personal skills for health, including such basic skills as literacy

Designing safe, healthy and healing environments

The physical design of the hospital is an important part of creating a healthy hospital. A recent review by a team led by one of the leading experts in this area (Ulrich et al., 2008) found a growing number of rigorous studies that help establish the relationship between the physical design of hospitals and key outcomes. The outcomes they considered included patient safety issues, such as infections, medical errors and falls; other patient outcomes, such as pain, sleep, stress, depression, length of stay, spatial orientation, privacy, communication, social support and overall patient satisfaction; and staff outcomes, such as injuries, stress, work effectiveness and satisfaction.

A review by Joseph and Rashid (2007) notes that design can contribute to or help prevent adverse events through its effect on staff working conditions. They suggest that the evidence is sufficient to influence hospital design now, while Henriksen et al. (2007: 68) report that a business case analysis of evidence-based design for quality and safety in the United States suggests that:

> a slight, one time incremental cost for ensuring safety and quality would be paid back in two to three years in the form of operational savings and increased revenues.

Guidelines have now been proposed and/or put in place in a number of areas with respect to improved design for healthcare facilities. For example, the 2006 version of the *Guidelines for Design and Construction of Health Care Facilities* (American Institute of Architecture, 2006) includes the designation of single-bed rooms as the minimum standard for medical/surgical and postpartum nursing units in general hospitals, an expansion of the environment of care chapter and an appendix on green design. There is also a proposed guideline from the US Pharmacopeia (2008) that would ensure safe medication administration as well as guidelines for environmentally responsible or green design for health care facilities (described later).

Finally, the California-based Center for Health Design (2011) has a number of initiatives that support evidence-based design for health, including a training and accreditation program for practitioners, a newly launched open source, searchable database (RIPPLE) containing information about evidence-based design, and the Pebble Project, which promotes and supports research on the health impacts of facility design in collaboration with scholars, design professionals and industry partners.

Tying it all together: a shift in organizational culture

A healthy and health promoting hospital, which corresponds to the fourth level of Johnson and Baum's (2001) typology, is one that brings together all four of the components identified at the outset; it is one that is dedicated to being a healing environment for patients, a healthy workplace for staff, an environmentally responsible organization and one that partners with others to create a healthier community beyond its four walls and beyond the bounds of healthcare. This requires an integration of several streams of action that are, or should be, complementary and mutually supportive. Interestingly, that integration is beginning to happen. An example is outlined in Box 8.3.

Box 8.3   The Healthier Hospitals initiative

In 2010 six leading healthcare systems in the United States, in partnership with three leading NGOs announced the formation of the Healthier Hospitals Initiative (HHI). The Initiative aims to develop a coordinated sector-wide approach to the design, building and operation of hospitals, to improve patient outcomes and workplace safety, prevent illnesses, create extraordinary environmental benefits, in addition to cost savings. HHI has a the following agenda:

- Improve environmental health and patient safety

  - Design and operate healthier and safer facilities for patients and employees
  - Purchase safer and more sustainable products and materials
  - Support the use of safer chemicals and green chemistry
  - Promote nutritious, sustainable food choices

- Reduce healthcare's use of natural resources and generation of waste

  - Reduce the consumption of energy
  - Support the transition to renewable energy sources
  - Conserve water
  - Minimize waste and emissions; decrease/eliminate incineration
  - Address pharmaceutical waste
  - Improve transportation strategies for patients and staff

(Continued)

(Continued)

- Institutionalize sustainability and safety

  - Make sustainability and safety a strategic imperative
  - Promote environmental health literacy internally and through community programmes
  - Invest in sustainability research and innovation
  - Engage in public policy to promote sustainability and safety

(Healthier Hospitals Initiative, 2011)

Fawkes (1997: 394) argues that there are organizational preconditions if hospitals and other healthcare facilities and services are to become more health promoting. These include:

A supportive philosophy and policy framework; an organizational infrastructure and culture that values and facilitates health promotion; adequately trained staff; clear delineation of responsibilities among staff for various roles ... (and) ... budgetary management that contributes to sustainable health promotion activities.

Shirey and Fisher (2008), writing in the context of the work of the American Association of Critical Care Nurses to create healthier work environments, point to a critical distinction between management and leadership. Management, they note, addresses operational efficiency and work unit management and deals with problems that need managing; we might say that it accepts the givens of the situation and asks the question how do we do this better. Leadership, on the other hand, is focused on the future, on a vision of what we should be doing and why. It is, they say, about transformation and innovation, about people and relationships. They agree that organizations in the United States have been for too long over-managed and under-led.

Hospitals cannot manage their way to being healthy and health promoting. The successful integration of the separate streams of healing environments, healthy workplaces, environmental responsibility and community partnership, and the execution of the needed actions, requires something more than a token gesture or the sort of partial approaches characterized by Johnson and Baum (2001) as Type 1 or 2. It requires a complete commitment of the organization starting at the top, and the creation of an organizational structure and culture that fits this new model. That is very much the key lesson from the work of the Planetree Alliance, and from other hospitals that have shown leadership in any or all of the four components identified. It takes leadership to transform hospitals into the safest, greenest and healthiest organizations in their communities, partners and leaders in creating a healthier community. But why would any hospital aspire to being anything less?

Summary points

- Creating a healthy and health promoting hospital requires a significant shift in organizational culture, which has to be led from the top and must be organization-wide and long term. It requires inspirational and transformational leadership, a participatory culture, involving patients and their families as well as staff at all levels, and the commitment of all members of the organization.

- The first priority for a hospital in its healing and caring role is to do no harm to patients and their families, staff, the community and the global commons. At the same time, the creation of a healthy workplace for staff at every level in the organization is a prerequisite for the safety and health of patients.

- Creating a truly healing environment for patients requires an examination of all aspects of the hospital's physical, social and organizational environments, its food services, the inclusion of nature, the arts and spiritual aspects of caring and anything else that can contribute to healing and caring.

- The hospital should be a model environmentally responsible corporate citizen and a leader, partner and catalyst in the community-wide process of creating a healthier community, using its credibility and status in the community to secure community-wide benefits.

Online Further Reading

Delobelle, P., Onya, H., Langa, C., Mashamba J. and Depoorter, A. (2010) 'Advances in health promotion in Africa: promoting health through hospitals', *Global Health Promotion*, 17: 33–6.

This paper describes a project that aims to adapt the Health Promoting Hospital concept to the context of rural South Africa. The project involves a partnership between the health authority and local stakeholders and is described as an advance in health promotion in the region. It is informed by the principles of health promotion and takes a settings-based approach to promoting the health and wellbeing of hospital staff, patients and relatives.

References

American Institute of Architecture (2006) *Guidelines for Design and Construction of Health Care Facilities.* Available at: http://info.aia.org/nwsltr_aah.cfm?page name=aah_gd_hospcons (accessed 30 January 2011).

Baker, G.R., Norton, P.G., Flintoft, V., Blais, R., Brown, A., Cox, J., Etchells, E., Ghali, W. A., Hebert, P., Majumdar, S. R., O'Beirne, M., Palacios-Derflingher, L., Reid, R.J., Sheps, S. and Tamblyn, R. (2004) 'The Canadian Adverse Events Study: the incidence of adverse events among hospital patients in Canada', *Canadian Medical Association Journal*, 170: 1678–86.

Center for Health Design (2011) www.healthdesign.org/chd (accessed 30 January 2011).

Fawkes, S. (1997) 'Aren't health services already promoting health?', *Australia and New Zealand Journal of Public Health*, 21: 391–7.

Frampton, S., Charmel, P. and Planetree (2008) *Putting Patients First*, 2nd edn. San Francisco: Jossey–Bass.

Groene, O. (2005) 'Evaluating the progress of the Health Promoting Hospitals Initiative? A WHO perspective', commentary on: Whitehead, D. (2004) The European Health promoting Hospitals (HPH) project: how far on?', *Health Promotion International*, 20: 205–7.

Hancock, T. (1999) 'Healthy and health promoting hospitals', *Leadership in Health Services/International Journal of Health Care Quality Assurance*, 12 (3): viii-xix.

Hancock, T. (2001) *Doing Less Harm: Assessing and Reducing the Environmental and Health Impact of Canada's Health Care System*. Toronto: Canadian Coalition for Green Health Care.

Health Authority Performance Agreements (2002/03) www.health.gov.bc.ca/socsec/performance.html (accessed 30 January 2011).

Health Care Without Harm (2011) www.noharm.org/all_regions/about/history.php (accessed 30 January 2011).

Healthier Hospitals Initiative (2011) http://healthierhospitals.org/ (accessed 30 January 2011).

Henriksen, K., Isaacson, S., Sadler, B. and Zimring, C. (2007) 'The role of the physical environment in crossing the quality chasm', *Joint Commission Journal on Quality and Patient Safety*, 33 (11 Suppl): 68–80.

Interior Health Authority (2011) www.interiorhealth.ca/information.aspx?id=10724 (accessed 30 January 2011).

Johnson, A. and Baum, F. (2001) 'Health promoting hospitals: a typology of different organizational approaches to health promotion', *Health Promotion International*, 16: 281–7.

Jones, C. and Gates, M. (2007) 'The costs and benefits of nurse turnover: a business case for nurse retention', *OJIN: The Online Journal of Issues in Nursing*, 12 (3): Manuscript 4. Available at: www.nursingworld.org/MainMenuCategories/ANA Marketplace/ANAPeriodicals/OJIN/TableofContents/Volume122007/No3 Sept07/NurseRetention.aspx (accessed 29 January 2011).

Joseph, A. and Rashid, M. (2007) 'The architecture of safety: hospital design', *Current Opinion Critical Care*, 13: 714–19.

Leach, E. (1995) 'The Canadian health care facility as a model environment', *Canadian Health Care Management*, July: 88–90.

Lowe, G.S. (2002) 'High-quality healthcare workplaces: a vision and action plan', *Hospital Quarterly*, 5 (4): 49–56.

McHugh, C., Robinson, A. and Chesters J. (2010) 'Health promoting health services: a review of the evidence', *Health Promotion International*, 25: 230–7.

Office of the Auditor General for BC (2004a) 'Auditor General says health authorities need to improve the work environment', Press Release, 22 June 2004. Available at: www.llbc.leg.bc.ca/public/pubdocs/bcdocs/370018/bcoag_nr_jun_22_04.pdf (accessed 30 January 2011).

Office of the Auditor General for BC (2004b) *In Sickness and in Health: Healthy Workplaces for British Columbia's Health Care Workers.* Victoria, BC: Auditor General for BC. Available at: www.llbc.leg.bc.ca/public/pubdocs/bcdocs/370018/report2_in-sickness-and-health.pdf (accessed 30 January 2011).

OHSAH (Occupational Health and Safety Agency for Health Care in British Columbia) (2004) *Trends in Workplace Injuries, Illnesses, and Policies in Healthcare across Canada.* Vancouver: OHSAH.

Ryndes, T. (1997) 'Creating an environment to prevent burnout', *Healthcare Forum Journal*, 40 (July/August): 54–7.

Shirey, M. and Fisher, M. (2008) 'Leadership agenda for change towards healthy work environments in acute and critical care', *Critical Care Nursing*, 28 (5): 66–78.

Stone, P., Buchan, J., Duffield, C., Hughes, F., O'Brien-Pallass, L. and Shamian, J. (2003) 'An international examination of the cost of nurse turnover', *Abstracts of Academy of Health Meeting*, (20), abstract no. 328.

Ulrich, R.S., Zimring, C.M., Zhu, X., DuBose, J. Seo, H., Choi, Y., et al. (2008) 'A review of the research literature on evidence-based healthcare design', *Health Environments Research & Design*, 1: 61–125.

US Pharmacopeia (2008) 'Physical environments that promote safe medication use (In-process revision)', *Pharmacopeial Forum*, 34: 1549–58.

Whitehead, D. (2004) 'The European Health Promoting Hospitals HPH project: how far on?', *Health Promotion International*, 19: 259–67.

World Health Organization (1986) *The Ottawa Charter for Health Promotion.* Geneva: WHO.

9

How Effective are Schools as a Setting for Health Promotion?

Colin Noble and Marilyn Toft

Aims

- To discuss a range of interpretations of the term healthy school and the implications for successfully realizing health promotion goals and school improvement
- To discuss the possibilities for, and challenges associated with, achieving effective healthy schools practice
- To explore evidence of impact and outcomes for healthy schools
- To consider future possibilities and the potential of the school setting in the context of promoting health and improving schools

---

What do we mean by a healthy school?

Promoting the health of children through schools has been an important global goal of the World Health Organization (WHO) for many years (Moon et al., 1999). In 1992 the European Network of Health Promoting Schools started with pilot schools in four countries. Some 12 years later more than 40 countries are members of this network (Clift and Bruun Jensen, 2005). Although some articles presume that healthy schools projects in the UK have been homogenous, in reality there have been, and still are, a range of models, their common link being that they perceive the school as an ideal setting in which to educate and/ or influence children and young people.

In England a number of local healthy school programmes started during the 1990s, for example the Kirklees Healthy School Programme and the Wessex Health Promoting Schools Programme, and by the time the National Healthy School Programme was launched in October 1999 well over a third of the country had their own local scheme. From the outset, the local programmes displayed a variety of goals and philosophies regarding the concept of the healthy school, which often reflected their origins. Those that were more based within the local education authority tended to be more interested in how a healthy school could help the process of school improvement (measured primarily by success in external examinations, but also by standards of behaviour, levels of attendance and numbers of exclusions). Those programmes that were based within Health (more often than not, health promotion departments or units) tended to see schools either as places where young people could be encouraged to be healthy, as a goal in itself, largely divorced from educational matters, or as places where health education should be taught. Indeed, health promotion units within primary care units (PCTs) were still known as health education units in some parts of the country. So, there were at least three schools of thought regarding healthy schools:

1. healthy schools as places to inculcate healthy behaviours such as physical exercise, healthy eating, safer sex, safer drug use and anti-bullying
2. healthy schools as places where health education could take place universally to a captive audience through the teaching of skills and knowledge
3. healthy schools as a means, or an aid, to school improvement. This was an argument rarely recognized by school improvement officers themselves and tended to be championed by Personal and Social Education (PSE) advisers and the more education-minded health promotion officers. Healthy schools see the school as a dynamic setting in which the school is constantly questioning and reviewing its practice, responding successfully to change and empowering children and young people, staff and parents/carers to have leadership roles in the school and influence its strategic and operational direction.

There also emerged an argument as to whether schools should be healthy by input (for example, healthy meals offered, several hours of PE and sport, anti-bullying measures, drinking water easily available, a good PSE curriculum) or by outcomes (for example, lower levels of bullying incidents, fewer teenage pregnancies, lower levels of obesity, higher levels of attendance). The former might be called the health promoting school, that is, the school is promoting health actively and comprehensively, but with less emphasis on outcomes. The argument for this is that it recognizes the limitations of what schools can do, for example on average a school pupil gets only 18 per cent of his/her diet from school (breakfast clubs, lunch, tuck shop, vending machines) so account should be taken of the school's context. The latter, measured by outcomes, is much more of a healthy school. The argument for this is that, at the end of the day, it is outcomes that matter and the route to them is, and should be, varied and flexible, responding to specific needs and priorities. The arguments against are twofold:

1. such measurements are often not an indication of a school's healthiness but a reflection of the intake to the school; and
2. a school never reaches a state of perfect health, but can always improve, so the title healthy school can be misleading and becomes a trap for complacency

The European Network of Health Promoting Schools (see Box 9.1) recognized the legitimate existence of different models from an early stage. For example, at the first workshop on Practice of Evaluation of the Health Promoting School, held in Thun, Switzerland (WHO, 1998: 3) the first conclusion was that:

> There is a continuing need to debate what the health promoting school is and to allow that it will take different forms in different countries. Useful debates occurred about the biomedical model and the eco holistic approach. Most felt that both had a necessary place in evaluation thinking about health promotion.

Box 9.1   European network of health promoting schools

Health education has a long tradition in schools, but has usually been only a part of the curriculum and focused on single causes of ill health in individuals, such as smoking and alcohol and drug abuse. Starting with this link between education and health, the three leading organizations, the European Commission (EC), the WHO Regional Office for Europe and the Council of Europe (CE), developed the idea of integrating health promotion into every aspect of the school setting, addressing all the people connected with it: pupils, their teachers, all other school staff, parents and eventually the wider community. In enabling schools to become healthier places, the European Network of Health Promoting Schools aims to integrate health promotion into every aspect of the curriculum, introduce healthy programmes and practices into schools' daily routines, improve working conditions and foster better relations both within the schools and between them and their local communities. The first phase of the project focused on developing activities suited to the needs and circumstances of each participating school, and sharing the results with others. These pilot or demonstration projects generated a vast body of experience that formed the basis for the project's second phase, whose aim is to create a vehicle to influence education policy and practice throughout Europe. (Burgher et al., 2005)

The advent in England of the National Healthy School Standard in October 1999 to some extent settled this debate, at least in England. The adoption and promotion of the whole school approach was based on classic school improvement thinking. Ten aspects were recommended:

1. Leadership and management
2. Policy and policy development
3. Curriculum planning and resources, including working with outside agencies
4. Learning and teaching
5. School culture and environment
6. Pupil voice
7. Provision of support services for schools and young people
8. Staff professional development needs, health and welfare
9. Partnership with parents/carers and local communities
10. Assessing, recording and reporting children's and young people's achievement

In its original manifestation, the National Healthy School Standard in England included eight key areas of activity:

1. Personal, Social and Health Education (PSHE)
2. Citizenship
3. Drug education (including tobacco and alcohol)
4. Emotional health and wellbeing
5. Healthy eating
6. Physical activity
7. Safety
8. Sex and relationship education

However in 2005, after the programme had become hosted by, and located within, the Department of Health (although still with Department for Education and Skills civil servants serving on its Board), it became more heavily concerned with health issues. The eight key areas were reduced to four (PSHE, including drug and sex education; healthy eating; physical activity; and emotional health and wellbeing). The whole school approach, although still informing the way in which schools addressed these four areas, was less evident. The changes also coincided with increasing anxiety, at government level, with the rise of childhood obesity and the programme was seen as a ready-made mechanism to help address that issue. Thus, the move to the Department of Health tended to emphasize the contribution the programme could make to health promotion, a trend that was probably accelerated by the National Institute for Health and Clinical Excellence (NICE) (2008) recommending the use of the programme in its guidance, which had significant impact on health authorities and primary care trusts which were accustomed to respecting and using NICE guidance, but negligible effect on local education authorities and schools which, generally, did not view NICE guidelines as relevant to their work. In the meantime Cathie Hammond and colleagues published work that illustrates the symbiotic relationship between education and health (Feinstein et al., 2006), but the tension between whether healthy schools are about promoting health, or have a wider agenda that includes attainment, remains.

An aim of the National Healthy Schools Programme (NHSP) was to improve pupils' attainment levels. However, there was a difference in the emphasis between schools and local coordinators. Schools felt that raising attainment was a secondary aim of the programme, while some local coordinators stressed the importance of the link between the NHSP and improving results as a primary aim, partly depending on which local authority department they were associated with:

> We do link it very strongly to the raising attainment agenda, and make that link very firmly with schools. Because we sit within the school effectiveness service that has to be our No. 1, so it has to link with raising attainment. (Local coordinator) (Barnard et al., 2009: 19)

The possibilities and challenges associated with achieving effective healthy schools practice

One of the challenges facing healthy schools is that there is no clear agreement about what schools are for. The English education White Paper *The Importance of Teaching* (Department for Education, 2010) seemed to assume that their main purpose was to enable pupils to gain as much learning as possible about English, mathematics and science as well as a strengthening of the knowledge base, such as history. The first part of the foreword by the Prime Minister and Deputy Prime Minister states:

> So much of the education debate in this country is backward looking: have standards fallen? Have exams got easier? These debates will continue, but what really matters is how we're doing compared with our international competitors. That is what will define our economic growth and our country's future. The truth is, at the moment we are standing still while others race past. (Department for Education, 2010: 3)

It then goes on to bemoan the apparent fall of England in some of the international education league tables. In other words, nothing much matters in education apart from how much it is playing its part in building a prosperous economy. The rest of the White Paper is very much about how the quality of teaching needs to improve in order to meet this end. This is a far cry from the concepts of Every Child Matters (HM Treasury, 2003) that clearly spelled out five aims for schools along with all children's services:

> The Government's aim is for every child, whatever their background or their circumstances, to have the support they need to:
> - be healthy
> - stay safe
> - enjoy and achieve
> - make a positive contribution
> - achieve economic wellbeing.
>
> (Every Child Matters, 2003: 6)

This takes a much broader view of the purpose of schools, recognizes the holistic nature of children's experience of life at school and outside, and views schools as having key parts to play in promoting health, safety, happiness, the democratic process and civic involvement, as well as in learning. Many practitioners recognized the complex interdependence between these five aims, which in turn helped to gain more support for healthy schools. It seemed clear to many teachers and parents that a happy, healthy child who lived and learned in a safe environment would be more likely to participate in community activities and also learn better. It confirmed the life experiences of many adults and seemed to view the child more holistically, not just as a pupil. This view is reflected in the WHO criteria for health promoting schools (see Box 9.2).

Box 9.2 WHO criteria for a health promoting school

- Fosters health and learning with all the measures at its disposal.
- Engages health and education officials, teachers, teachers' unions, students, parents, health providers and community leaders in efforts to make the school a healthy place.
- Strives to provide a healthy environment, school health education, and school health services along with school/community projects and outreach, health promotion programmes for staff, nutrition and food safety programmes, opportunities for physical education and recreation, and programmes for counselling, social support and mental health promotion.
- Implements policies and practices that respect an individual's wellbeing and dignity, provide multiple opportunities for success, and acknowledge good efforts and intentions as well as personal achievements.
- Strives to improve the health of school personnel, families and community members as well as pupils; and works with community leaders to help them understand how the community contributes to, or undermines, health and education.

WHO (2011)

The more recent, narrower view of schools as described in *The Importance of Teaching* (Department for Education, 2010) is probably as much due to a less comfortable and less confident analysis of the country's economic future as to any particular ideology. It can be likened to a school which, confronted by lower than expected SAT or GCSE results, decides to remove the non-academic experiences and investment from its offer. So, out goes the annual school trip, PSHE, circle time and the history trip to the Somme battlefield, in favour of extra time for maths, English and science, more revision time, and a focus and pressure on those on the margins of passing/failing. There is no analysis of the impact of any of these things on learning or the wider development of the child. The days of hand wringing and anxiety over such reports as the Innocenti (UNICEF) Social Monitor in October 2006, which showed UK children as some of the least happy in Europe, are seemingly over.

In England, the 2010 Education White Paper has to be read in the context of announced health reforms which envisage the abolition of the local primary care trusts (PCTs) by 2013 with most of their functions and budgets going to general practitioners (GPs) or groups of GPs. Given that the PCTs have been a backbone of local healthy school programmes this may well have serious implications as local GPs are unlikely to see the need to use their budgets in such a way. At the same time, however, local authorities will be obliged to employ Directors of Public Health (DPH) who may, depending on their background and the political leadership of the local authority, want to invest in healthy school programmes as an expression of their commitment to lifelong public health. The extent to which such programmes will be able to capture the more dynamic and successful models of healthy schools will, to a large degree, depend upon the ability of the local DPH and the Head of School Improvement (employed by the same council) to understand its potential in terms of nurturing pupil wellbeing and achieving confident and effective learners, connecting health and learning, as well as each other's needs.

One of the unknown variables in the situation will be the media. Governments, both local and national, appear to make or adjust policy as a response to media pressure or interest. Hence, in England, some of the consequences of the Jamie Oliver school lunch programmes in 2005 were the changing of the regulations regarding school food, the establishment of the School Food Trust and an escalation of the importance of healthy eating within the National Healthy Schools Programme. Thus, in a free society powerful media interest or campaigns about young people and alcohol and drug misuse, eating disorders, mental health, sexual health, obesity, sloth, behaviour or any number of issues could easily lead any government to re-examine how it might best get universal or targeted education or campaigns to young people. In such cases, schools are often considered because they have a captive audience of the vast majority of young people and they are a ready-made conduit. Whether such concern or desire to do something is conducive to constructing the most effective and appropriate healthy school programmes or rather creating flavour-of-the-month isolated project activities is open to debate. However, it does suggest that until young people cease causing anxiety to adults the case for healthy schools will be revisited again and again. Government guidance on such things as sex and relationship education (Department for Education and Skills, 2004a) and drug education (Department for Education and Skills, 2004b) are regularly reviewed and tend to reflect contemporary concerns as well as a developing understanding of good practice. If significant and sustainable progress is to be made with a positive effect on children and young people's wellbeing and achievements, it appears that healthy schools continue to be well placed to respond to this need.

Demonstrating evidence of impact and outcomes for healthy schools

There are a number of challenges that have emerged regarding demonstrating evidence of impact and outcomes for healthy schools, not least confusion about what the terms 'impact' and 'outcomes' actually mean in the context of healthy schools. For the sake of argument we have decided to view **impact** as usually being about process, for example, School X has introduced a healthy eating policy as a consequence of being a healthy school, or School Y now has a very strong peer mentor and circle time programme; while **outcomes** are more about the answering the 'So what?' question, for example, 30% of Year 7 pupils now feel completely safe from bullying at, or on, the journey to and from school compared to only 10% before a, b and c measures were introduced. In other words, outcomes are about the actual experience of children and young people as opposed to their education or the schemes and policies introduced by the school.

The English National Healthy Schools Programme (NHSP) was evaluated first jointly by the National Foundation for Education Research and the Thomas Coram Research Unit, Institute of Education, University of London (Warwick et al., 2004) and again in 2009 by the National Centre for Social Research (Barnard et al., 2009) (see Box 9.3). The latter showed that the programme was making a significant contribution to participating schools. The research revealed significant links between achieving and working towards National Healthy School Status (NHSS), and better Ofsted ratings of school effectiveness, lower total and unauthorized pupil absence, higher contextual value added scores, and higher levels of pupil participation in high quality PE. Under the terms of this chapter, these would be called outcomes.

The report concludes that whole school approaches to promoting health can impact on health and education outcomes, and that NHSP is widely perceived as having an impact on schools. In particular, it has been perceived to bring about changes associated with improved learning among pupils, such as improved concentration, greater participation in physical activity and increased confidence as learners (Barnard et al., 2009).

Box 9.3   The design of the National Centre for Social Research study of the National Healthy Schools Programme

Measuring impact [note that this is the term used by the researchers and is not consistent with the use made in this chapter]

The main challenge for the study in terms of measuring impact is to be able to tell whether improvements are due to the NHSP rather than other factors. This will be done by conducting surveys among pupils and selected school staff within a large sample of schools. At the beginning of the research period, a survey of pupils will be conducted in order to provide a baseline measure of pupil outcomes. The survey will measure attitudes and knowledge of health issues along with healthy behaviour. At this point a survey of appropriate school staff will also

(Continued)

(Continued)

be conducted to establish how many of the NHSP's policies and procedures schools have in place. After two years, the surveys will be repeated, again measuring pupil outcomes and how close to validation schools are.

The impact of NHSP will be assessed by comparing the degree to which pupil outcomes have improved with the degree to which schools have adopted the NHSP's polices and procedures. If pupil outcomes have improved more in schools that have gone further in adopting NHSP's polices and procedures, then the study will conclude that there is good evidence that the programme has had an impact. (Barnard et al., 2009)

It can be seen from the above design that a longitudinal study was used. Other studies, for example the Welsh Network of Healthy School Schemes (Rothwell et al., 2010) and the Scottish Health Promoting School Programme (this programme takes on a healthy school model described in the first part of this chapter) (see for example, Young and Lee, 2009) suggest both significant impact of the healthy school schemes and different approaches from the usual random controlled approach which was used in the first English healthy schools research in 2004 and, for example, the 2010 study of Social and Emotional Aspects of Learning (SEAL) by the University of Manchester. The main problem found with this approach is that the control schools are not isolated from the prevailing educational and health pressures and, despite not formally taking part in the programme under scrutiny, are likely to have introduced some measures to address the issues. For example, the comparatively few schools in England that had not joined the Healthy Schools Programme by 2008 were still compelled by statute to address healthy eating in school, were likely to have been part of a school sports partnership and may well have introduced SEAL.

The Welsh study used a single-case study using data from documentary analysis, interviews with Healthy Schools Coordinators and stakeholder discussion of interim findings at three regional workshops. The study found almost universal adherence to a national framework based on Ottawa Charter principles, with substantial progress on advocacy and mediation, although the framework provided less specific guidance regarding enablement. All-Wales training for coordinators, the commitment of coordinators to working across administrative and professional boundaries, and support from local education and health partnerships, were important determinants of healthy school schemes' growth and efficiency (Rothwell et al., 2010). The Scottish research used data from the 2006 Health Behaviour in School-aged Children (HBSC, 2008) survey which was analysed using multi-level linear progression analyses for outcome measures: happiness, confidence, life satisfaction, feeling left out, helplessness, multiple health complaints and self-rated health.

It is important that any research of healthy school programmes ensures that it has clarified and communicated its meaning of impact and outcomes and that they are not used interchangeably; secondly that the researchers have made every effort to understand the complexity of the research when a number of contributory factors may be at play; and thirdly that it takes account of the context of the school and the population it serves.

Future possibilities and the potential of the school setting in the context of promoting health and improving schools

So, what of the future of healthy schools? We have already made the point that one of the appeals of healthy schools to governments is the near-universal access to all children and young people. However, this has to be tempered by the current desire of governments to cede as much authority to schools' own management to develop their own future and create their own strategies to meet their goals. In this light it is unlikely that governments will be inclined to insist upon, or even encourage, a national healthy schools programme. However, governments have a habit of getting what they want when they sense a need. They could, for example, incentivize local authorities to establish health education or health promotion experiences for young people without actually specifying how that might be done. Local Directors of Public Health (in England) or their equivalents elsewhere may feel that a healthy schools programme would answer many local and national needs, and they would need to work with local politicians, educationalists and school leaders to construct a scheme that was designed to appeal to both schools and to educational and public health priorities.

However, this is to view healthy schools as the creature of national government, created and dismissed by political whims that owe more to the transient needs of ministers than to a national consensus about what schools might achieve in public health. In reality, many healthy schools and many healthy schools schemes will continue to flourish irrespective of government views, as a large number of school leaders and local health and education officers have been convinced that the healthy schools initiative supplies both a structure and process to optimize the school environment in order effectively to promote health and learning. Indeed, educationalists and health officers may pay increasing heed to work such as Hammond (2004), which explores the connection between health and education, the Marmot Review (2010) and the English Public Health White Paper (Department of Health, 2010). The Marmot Review was requested in 2008 by Secretary of State for Health Alan Johnson with the aim of developing the most effective strategies for reducing health inequalities in England from 2010. The Review follows a report by the Global Commission on Social Determinants of Health (CSDH), entitled *Closing the Gap in a Generation*, which was published by the World Health Organization in 2008, and which indicated a need for nation-specific strategies in combating health inequalities in the quest for good health. The review found that reducing health inequalities will require action on six policy objectives:

- Give every child the best start in life
- Enable all children young people and adults to maximise their capabilities and have control over their lives
- Create fair employment and good work for all
- Ensure healthy standard of living for all
- Create and develop healthy and sustainable places and communities
- Strengthen the role and impact of ill health prevention

Marmot Review, Executive Summary (2010: 9)

The opportunities outlined in the English Public Health White Paper of 2010 are of particular relevance:

> Directors of Public Health (DsPH) will be able to work with their local authority children's services colleagues, schools and other partners to determine local strategies for improving child health and wellbeing. They will be supported by consolidation of existing guidance into best practice resources for schools, further education and training providers. The Healthy Schools, Healthy Further Education and Healthy Universities programmes will continue to be developed by their respective sectors, as voluntary programmes, collaborating where appropriate and exploring partnership working with business and voluntary bodies. (Department of Health, 2010: 34)

One area where healthy schools, in its widest sense, could play more of a role is in Initial Teacher Training. According to the White Paper *The Importance of Teaching* (Department for Education, 2010), pupil behaviour is a key issue for new teachers and those contemplating a career in the profession:

> The greatest concern voiced by new teachers and a very common reason experienced teachers cite for leaving the profession is poor pupil behaviour. We know that a minority of pupils can cause serious disruption in the classroom. The number of serious physical assaults on teachers has risen. And poorly disciplined children cause misery for other pupils by bullying them and disrupting learning. It is vital that we restore the authority of teachers and head teachers. And it is crucial that we protect them from false allegations of excessive use of force or inappropriate contact. Unless we act more good people will leave the profession – without good discipline teachers cannot teach and pupils cannot learn. (Department for Education, 2010: 9)

The emerging evidence from studies of healthy school programmes suggests that the type of healthy school programme adopted will be a significant factor in determining the impact and outcomes for young people and institutions.

Summary points

- A healthy school is a driver for school improvement as it is dynamic, where staff and pupils alike welcome and are responsive to change and willing to take risks to secure improvement and a rich learning experience for the whole school community.

- The most successful healthy schools are those that are able to explicitly demonstrate a meaningful relationship between education and health priorities, with a strong focus on pupil wellbeing and the joint ambition of providing accessible learning opportunities for all pupils to raise achievement.

- The healthy school provides opportunities for both universal and targeted education and health activity and in so doing can champion the most vulnerable and those at risk of exclusion by providing excellent provision.

- The healthy school is well positioned to respond to the demands of the current (at time of writing, June 2011) White Paper in that its strong ethos, supportive climate for learning, positive relationships and culture and safe and secure environment will enable all teachers to teach and all pupils to learn.

Online Further Reading

Barnekow Rasmussen, V (2005) 'The European Network of Health Promoting schools – from Iceland to Kyrgyzstan', *Promotion and Education*, XII: 169–72.

In this paper the criteria and principles of the European Network of Health promoting Schools (ENHPS) are outlined. The network is a practical example of a health promotion activity that has successfully incorporated the energies of three major European agencies in the joint pursuit of their goals in school health promotion. The article finds that coordinators of programmes agree that a key element of success is to work together with the school community, parents and young people themselves as well as with health and education ministries.

References

Barnard, M., Becker, E., Creegan, C., Day, N., Devitt, K., Fuller, E., Lee. L., Hayley, N., Purdon, S. and Ranns, H. (2009) *Evaluation of the National Healthy Schools Programme. Interim Report.* London: National Centre for Social Research.

Burgher, M.S., Barnekow, V. and Rivett, D. (2005) *The European Network of Health Promoting Schools: The Alliance of Education and Health.* Geneva: WHO Europe.

Clift, S. and Bruun Jensen, B. (2005) *The Health Promoting School: International Advances in Theory, Evaluation and Practice.* Copenhagen: Danish University of Education Press.

Commission on Social Determinants of Health (2008) *Closing the Gap in a Generation: Health Equity through Action on the Social Determinants of Health.* Final Report of the Commission on Social Determinants of Health. Geneva: World Health Organization.

Department for Education (2010) *The Importance of Teaching.* London: Department for Education

Department for Education and Skills (2004a) Sex and Relationship Education – Schools' Responsibilities. Available at: http://publications.education.gov.uk/

default.aspx?PageFunction=productdetails&PageMode=publications&ProductId=SEX-EDUCATION (accessed 22 March 2011).

Department for Education and Skills (2004b) Drugs: Guidance for Schools. Available at: http://publications.education.gov.uk/default.aspx?PageFunction=productdetails&PageMode=publications&ProductId=DfES+0092+2004 (accessed 22 March 2011).

Department of Health (2010) White Paper: *Healthy Lives, Healthy People: Our Strategy for Public Health in England.* London: Department of Health.

Feinstein, L., Sabates, R., Anderson, T.A., Sorhaindo, A. and Hammond, C. (2006) *What Are the Effects of Education on Health? Measuring the Effects of Education on Health and Civic Engagement.* Copenhagen: OECD.

Hammond, C. (2004). 'Impacts of lifelong learning upon emotional resilience, psychological and mental health: fieldwork evidence', *Oxford Review of Education,* 30: 551–68.

HM Treasury (2003) *Every Child Matters.* London: The Stationery Office.

HBSC Scotland National Report (2008) Health Behaviour in School-Aged Children: WHO collaborative cross-national study. University of Edinburgh, Child and Adolescent Health Research Unit.

Marmot, M., Allen, J., Goldblatt, P., Boyce, T., McNeish, D., Grady, M. and Geddes, I. (2010) *Fair Society, Healthy Lives: A Strategic Review of Health Inequalities in England post-2010* (The Marmot Review). London: The Marmot Review. Executive Summary, p. 9. Available at: www.marmotreview.org/AssetLibrary/pdfs/Reports/FairSocietyHealthyLivesExecSummary.pdf (accessed 22 March 2011).

Moon, A., Mullee, M., Rogers, L., Thompson, R., Speller, V. and Roderick, P. (1999) 'Helping schools become health promoting: an evaluation of the Wessex Healthy Schools Award', *Health Promotion International,* 14: 111–22.

NICE (2008) *Promoting Children's Emotional and Social Wellbeing in Primary Education.* NICE Public Health Guidance 12. Available at: http://guidance.nice.org.uk/PH12 (accessed 14 September 2011).

Rothwell, H., Shepard, M., Murphy, S., Burgess, S., Townsend, N. and Pimm, C. (2010) 'Implementing a social-ecological model of health in Wales', *Health Education,* 110: 471–89.

UNICEF (2006) *Innocenti Social Monitor: Understanding Child Poverty in South-Eastern Europe and the Commonwealth of Independent States.* Florence: UNICEF Innocenti Research Centre.

Warwick, I., Aggleton, P., Chase, E., Blenkinsop, S., Egger, M., Schagen, I., Schagen, S., Scott, E. and Zuurmond, M. (2004) *Evaluation of the Impact of the National Healthy School Standard. Project Report.* London: Thomas Coram Research Unit, Institute of Education, University of London/National Foundation for Educational Research.

WHO (World Health Organization) (1998) *Practice of Evaluation of the Health Promoting School.* Available at: www.schoolsforhealth.eu/.../FirstWorkshoponpracticeofevaluationoftheHPS.pdf (accessed 22 March 2011).

WHO (World Health Organization) (2011) *What Is a Health Promoting School?* Available at: www.who.int/school_youth_health/gshi/hps/en/index.html (accessed 25 March 2010).

Young, I. and Lee, A. (2009) 'Sustaining the development of health-promoting schools: the experience of Scotland in the European context', in Case Studies in C.E. Aldinger and C.V. Whitman (eds), *Global School Health Promotion: From Research to Practice.* New York: Springer.

10

The Healthy Universities Approach: Adding Value to the Higher Education Sector

Mark Dooris, Sharon Doherty, Jennie Cawood and Sue Powell

Aims

- To provide a background and context to Healthy Universities
- To outline the history and development of the Healthy Universities approach
- To discuss how healthy settings theory has been applied to higher education and influenced practice
- To explore challenges and opportunities for progressing Healthy Universities

---

The crucial importance of shifting the focus and resources from treating sickness to improving health has been highlighted consistently over recent years in both national and international health policies (Department of Health, 2004, 2008, 2009; HM Government, 2010; Wanless, 2002, 2004; WHO, 1998). Within this policy context, there has been growing appreciation of the need for effective multidisciplinary and multisectoral partnership working in order to build and release capacity and capability for public health and, specifically, for investment for health within and through educational settings. It follows that higher education has an important role to play as a partner in health improvement, as a setting in and through which to promote health, as a key contributor to citizenship development and as a driver for societal change.

While the healthy settings approach provides an overarching conceptual framework that can be applied to a range of contexts, it is also important to understand the particularities of specific settings. Within the UK alone, there are 169 higher education institutions (HEIs) with more than 2.3 million students and 370,000 staff (HESA, 2009; Universities UK, 2008), pointing to the enormous potential offered by universities worldwide as settings in which and through which to promote public health. The term university is being used here as an umbrella term for higher education institutions (HEIs), although it is important to note that a number of these do not have university status. While universities have for many years been branded as settings characterized by privilege and elitism, the UK government's focus on widening access and participation has resulted in an increasingly diverse student body. Recent research indicates that during the past 10 years young people from disadvantaged areas have been substantially more likely to enter higher education and that differences in participation rates between advantaged and disadvantaged neighbourhoods have reduced (HEFCE, 2010).

As explored by Dooris and Doherty (2009), universities have long served as settings for the delivery of specific projects on various priority issues, resulting in student focused guidance on drugs, alcohol, mental health and other key themes (see, for example, Crouch et al., 2006; Grant, 2002; Polymerou, 2007; Universities UK, 2000). Alongside this, there has been a growing focus on staff wellbeing, reflecting the strengthened national policy focus on workplace health (Black, 2008; Department for Work and Pensions, Department of Health, and Health and Safety Executive, 2005; Health and Safety Executive, 2006; HM Government, 2010; and the chapters in Part III of this book). However, it is only relatively recently that there has been increasing interest in moving beyond a focus on single topics and population sub-groups to develop a more holistic and strategic whole university approach (Dooris and Doherty, 2009), reflecting the success of other educational settings initiatives such as those for healthy schools (see Part II, Chapter 9) and healthy further education.

A review of evidence relating to schools supports a whole school approach, suggesting that effective programmes are likely to be complex, multifactorial and involve activity in more than one domain (St Leger et al., 2010; Stewart-Brown, 2006; see also Part II, Chapter 9 for a more detailed examination of healthy schools), while a review focused on further education has concluded that while it is not possible to state with certainty that multicomponent, whole settings approaches are more successful in college and university settings than one-off activities, the evidence points in this direction (Warwick et al., 2008: 27). This thinking supports and reflects more general public health research such as the Foresight Report on Obesity, which concluded that the complexity and interrelationships of risk factors and determinants make a compelling case for the futility of isolated initiatives (Butland et al., 2007: 10).

For the higher education sector, this means adopting a whole system perspective that takes account of the role of universities as:

- centres of learning and development, with roles in education, research, capacity and capability building, and knowledge exchange
- foci for creativity and innovation, developing knowledge and understanding within and across disciplines, and applying them to the benefit of society

- places within which students undergo life transition, exploring and experimenting, developing independence and lifeskills, and facing particular health challenges
- workplaces and businesses, concerned with performance and productivity within a competitive marketplace
- contexts that future-shape students and staff as they clarify values, grow intellectually and develop capabilities that can enhance current and future citizenship within families, communities, workplaces and society as a whole
- resources for, and influential partners and corporate citizens within, local, regional, national and global communities.

The history and development of Healthy Universities

Over the past 15 years or so, there has been growing interest in applying the settings approach within the context of higher education (Doherty and Dooris, 2006; Dooris, 2001; Dooris and Doherty, 2010a). In the mid-1990s, following the first international conference on settings-based health promotion (Theaker and Thompson, 1995), Lancaster University and the University of Central Lancashire (UCLan) established Health Promoting University initiatives; and the Faculty of Public Health Medicine (1995) published an issue of its newsletter that took Health Promoting Universities as its focus theme. In the editorial, Beattie (1995: 2) noted that while initiatives in universities have emerged more or less in parallel with projects on the health promoting workplace, school and hospital, they lack any national or international infrastructure, and so are only just beginning to generate a momentum of research and development.

A conference organized in 1996 by Lancaster University in collaboration with the World Health Organization (WHO) served as the catalyst for a WHO Round Table meeting and the publication of the seminal book *Health Promoting Universities: Concept, Experience and Framework for Action* (Tsouros et al., 1998). This included conceptual and contextual chapters, case studies of practice in English universities and strategic frameworks for future development at university and European levels (the latter within the framework of the WHO Healthy Cities Project). Although the book proved significant in raising the profile of the Healthy Universities concept and in providing European-level endorsement, its potential influence was weakened by the lack of any subsequent international or national programme to facilitate the translation of rhetoric into policy or practice.

Nationally, having championed the National Healthy Schools Programme since 1999, the Department of Health for England responded to a groundswell of interest and activity in healthy colleges and healthy universities by including reference to further education and higher education sectors in its 2004 White Paper *Choosing Health*. The White Paper expressed commitment to support the initiatives being taken by some colleges and universities to: develop a strategy for health that integrates health into the organization's structure to create healthy working, learning and living environments; increase the profile of health in teaching and research; and develop healthy alliances in the community(Department of Health, 2004: 72). In the absence of any follow-up development or resources, UCLan responded to an increasing demand for information and advice by establishing the English National Healthy Universities Network as a means of facilitating the sharing of experience and practice and providing peer support (Doherty and Dooris, 2006). The following year, partly in response to the pioneering work of the rapidly expanding Healthy Colleges Network, the Department of Health appointed a Further Education Adviser within its National Healthy Schools Team and subsequently commissioned an evidence review (Warwick et al., 2008) and launched a Healthy Further Education Programme (www.excellencegateway. org.uk/hfep). Concurrently, it established regional Teaching Public Health Networks. While the primary focus of these networks was to strengthen public health curricula in higher education, their secondary aim was to create health promoting universities and colleges.

In 2008, UCLan received funding from both the Higher Education Academy Health Sciences and Practice Subject Centre and the Department of Health to conduct a National Research and Development Project on Healthy Universities (Dooris and Doherty, 2009, 2010a, 2010b). Building on this, it secured further funding from the Higher Education Funding Council for England for Developing Leadership and Governance for Healthy Universities, a project that it has jointly led with Manchester Metropolitan University (MMU). This aims to strengthen the National Network, develop and disseminate web-based guidance packages and case studies, and support national developments (see Box 10.1 for an overview of the project). In parallel, the Royal Society for Public Health received funding from the Department of Health and commissioned UCLan and Manchester Metropolitan University to coordinate the development of a model and framework for healthy universities.

Box 10.1   Developing Leadership and Governance for Healthy Universities

Developing Leadership and Governance for Healthy Universities is a two-year project funded by the Higher Education Funding Council for England (HEFCE) Leadership, Governance and Management Fund.

The project is led jointly by the University of Central Lancashire (UCLan) and Manchester Metropolitan University (MMU), working in partnership with Leeds Trinity University College, Nottingham Trent University, Teesside University, the University of the West of England, the Royal Society for Public Health and the Leadership Foundation for Higher Education.

The project receives strategic guidance from a high level Leadership Advisory Group comprising senior representatives from partner HEIs and national stakeholder organizations, and is operationally managed by a project board made up of representatives from the six partner HEIs. Alongside this, the National Network membership provides an important wider reference group.

The project has three key aims:

1. Strengthen, formalize and expand the English National Healthy Universities Network.

The National Network was established in 2006 by UCLan in response to growing demand from the sector. Since then its membership has grown and at the end of 2010 included over 55 HEIs from across England along with a number of partner organizations (such as local National Health Service (NHS) Trusts, National Union of Students (NUS) and other national bodies).
The aims of the network are to:

- Facilitate the exchange of information, research, practice and experience related to the implementation of Healthy Universities.
- Develop and promote models of good practice.
- Advocate and advise on the Healthy Universities approach at regional and national levels.
- Encourage collaborative development and research.

Network members meet twice a year, with meetings comprising a national progress report, local updates, networking and exchange; and a guest speaker and facilitated interactive workshop session.

2. Generate and disseminate web-based guidance tools and case studies that enable HEIs to develop as Healthy Universities

A national website, www.healthyuniversities.ac.uk, has been developed and features the Healthy Universities Toolkit, a set of Guidance Packages and Case Studies designed to support Higher Education Institutions (HEIs) that wish to adopt a whole system university approach.
The toolkit includes a set of Guidance Packages that have been designed to provide guidance to HEIs at all stages in developing and implementing Healthy University initiatives. Each Guidance Package explores a different theme and includes a Resources section which incorporates features such as 'talking head' video clips, 'top tip' checklists and template PowerPoint presentations. The toolkit also includes a growing number of institutional case studies which offer actual examples of Healthy University-related initiatives which have been implemented in institutions across England. The case studies can be accessed using a searchable database, categorized according to topic, method and population group.

3. Support further national developments, building on the findings of the National Research and Development Project.

Alongside this project, UCLan and MMU were commissioned by the Royal Society for Public Health (RSPH) to work on a Department of Health funded project which involved the development of a model for Healthy Universities and the production of recommendations for the development of a National Healthy Universities Framework. The project aimed to articulate a model for Healthy Universities and to produce recommendations for the development and operationalization of a National Healthy Universities Framework.

Healthy Universities theory and practice

Tsouros et al. (1998) advocated a settings approach tailored to take account of the higher education context, acknowledging that as a setting, a university is influenced by its own history and infused with its own distinctive culture and ethos. Drawing on these perspectives and integrating them with reflections on the experience of UCLan in developing and implementing its own Health Promoting University initiative, Dooris (2001) set out a conceptual framework and proposed a social ecosystem model. The model articulates the potential value of the Healthy Universities approach as an investment in the health and wellbeing of students and staff within, outside and beyond their university lives, a systems approach that has been explored further in more recent work (Dooris, 2005). Representing a commitment to the future shaping role of higher education referred to above, this highlights the potential for universities to increase understanding of health, wellbeing and sustainable development (and of their underpinning social, political, economic, cultural and environmental determinants) and encourage the development of value-based perspectives that students and staff will take into their future lives (see Figure 10.1). Other papers similarly draw on UCLan's experience, applying the conceptual framework to mental health promotion (Dooris, 1999) and exploring opportunities and challenges and offering reflections on the processes involved in moving from idea to implementation (Dooris, 2002). Box 10.2 offers an up-to-date case study of practice.

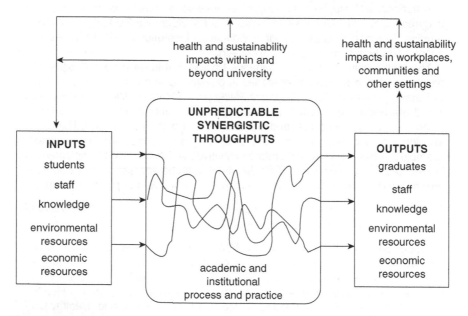

Figure 10.1 Settings as systems – the example of a university (Dooris, 2005; reproduced with permission from Oxford University Press http://heapro.oxford journals.org)

Box 10.2　A healthy university: University of Central Lancashire, England

Building on its involvement with other programmes such as Health Promoting Hospitals, UCLan decided to explore what it might mean to apply the settings approach to itself as an organization. In 1995, its Faculty of Health funded a two-year Health Promoting University pilot that was subsequently made permanent. Fifteen years later, the initiative (now called Healthy University, www.uclan.ac.uk/hu) is going from strength to strength and the university has embedded a commitment to health, wellbeing, sustainability and sustainable development within the core values of its Medium Term Strategy.

Coordinated from the Healthy Settings Development Unit within the School of Public Health and Clinical Sciences, the Healthy University aims to:

- integrate within the university structures, process and culture a commitment to health and to developing its health promoting potential
- promote the health and wellbeing of staff, students and the wider community

It works to a three-year planning cycle overseen by the Healthy University Steering Group and reporting to the University's Safety, Health and Environment Committee and Senior Management Team. The work programme, which is delivered by a number of multiservice, multidisciplinary (and where appropriate, multiagency) working groups, is structured to ensure that it supports the university's core business and contributes to the implementation of key strategies such as Learning and Teaching, Student Retention, Human Resources and Sustainability. Current working groups include Staff Wellbeing, Rethinking Student Mental Health, Healthy and Sustainable Food, and Alcohol and Drugs.

The Healthy University seeks to apply a whole system perspective to all of its work, involving all relevant stakeholders and adopting a range of approaches and mechanisms. For example, the Rethinking Student Mental Wellbeing Project has delivered training and developed procedural guidelines to enable staff to support students effectively; delivered anti-stigma campaigns targeted at students; established new services where appropriate; conducted research; and produced resources for staff and students.

Subsequent academic literature on health promoting universities has largely reported on experience drawn from practice, or detailed focused research framed within the conceptual context of Healthy Universities. A number of papers have described research relating to health promotion needs assessment and implementation in German and Lithuanian universities (Meier et al., 2007; Stock et al., 2001; 2003). Lee (2002) has described the establishment of a health promoting university initiative at the Chinese University of Hong Kong, while Xiangyang et al. (2003) have reported on a study that aimed to create six health promoting universities across Beijing, concluding that the university community can benefit greatly from implementing health promotion campaigns based on the principles of the Ottawa Charter (WHO, 1986). Stock et al. (2010) have

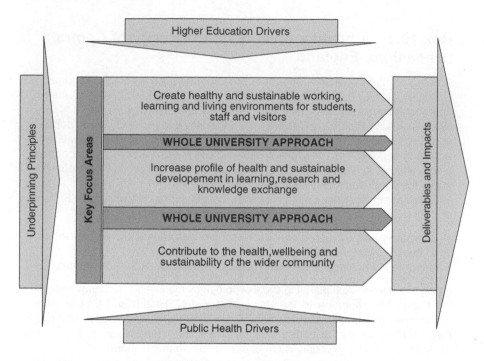

Figure 10.2 Healthy universities: a model for conceptualizing and applying the healthy settings approach to higher education (Dooris, 2010)

evaluated the German Network of Health Promoting Universities, concluding that it has worked effectively, has developed meaningful processes and structures and has formulated practical guidelines. Dooris and Doherty (2010a, 2010b) have reported on a UK national qualitative research study, investigating current Healthy University activity and exploring the potential for developing a national programme, while Orme and Dooris (2010) have explored the role of higher education as a setting for promoting health and sustainability in an integrated and coherent way, and for facilitating synergy between public health, sustainable development and climate change agendas.

The English National Network of Healthy Universities has consulted on, developed and articulated a model for applying healthy settings thinking within higher education, offering a useful means of conceptualizing the Healthy Universities approach, which is understood to aspire to create a learning environment and organizational culture that enhances the health, wellbeing and sustainability of its community and enables people to achieve their full potential (Dooris, 2010) (see Figure 10.2). The model is structured to show (Dooris, 2010):

Principles: The approach is underpinned by principles reflecting the values that characterize higher education and public health. These include equality and diversity; participation and empowerment; partnership; sustainability; holistic and whole system health; evidence informed and innovative practice; and evaluation, learning and knowledge exchange.

Drivers: Healthy Universities must take account of both higher education and public health drivers. It must therefore be guided by the distinctive culture of universities and show how it can help to deliver key institutional priorities while also anticipating, identifying and responding to key public health challenges pertinent to its population.

Whole university approach: In applying the healthy settings approach, Healthy Universities is concerned to adopt a whole system perspective (see Part II, Chapter 2 for a detailed overview of whole systems thinking). A whole university approach thus not only anticipates and responds to higher education and public health agendas, it also involves securing high level commitment and leadership, engaging a wide range of stakeholders, and combining high visibility health related projects with system level organization development and change. As illustrated in Figure 10.3, it also requires a proactive and systematic operational process that identifies entry points and catalysts; establishes appropriate governance mechanisms; designates responsibilities and accountabilities; assesses assets and needs; sets priorities; agrees, implements and monitors progress against a delivery plan; conducts wider evaluation; and celebrates achievements. This process is important in ensuring that a healthy university acts to harness and connect relevant activities and initiatives, thereby strengthening its holistic focus.

Focus areas: A whole system approach involves working within and across three key areas of activity relating to the environment of the setting, the core business of the setting, and connections to the wider community. Applying this thinking to higher education, it is evident that the Healthy Universities approach aims to:

- create healthy and sustainable learning, working and living environments (such as campus and building design; cycle planning and incentives; work–life balance policy; supportive management culture)
- integrate health and sustainable development within the mainstream activities of the university (for example, health and sustainable development as multidisciplinary cross-cutting themes in curricula, research and knowledge exchange; tools to facilitate integration within different subject areas; health as a priority in research and knowledge exchange)
- contribute to the health, wellbeing and sustainability of local, regional, national and global communities (including health and sustainability impact assessment; active role in partnerships; locally embedded research; volunteering and outreach)

Deliverables: The Healthy Universities approach has the potential to deliver tangible contributions to health, wellbeing, sustainable development and core business priorities (such as higher quality health and welfare services; healthy and sustainable food procurement processes and catering services; increased personal

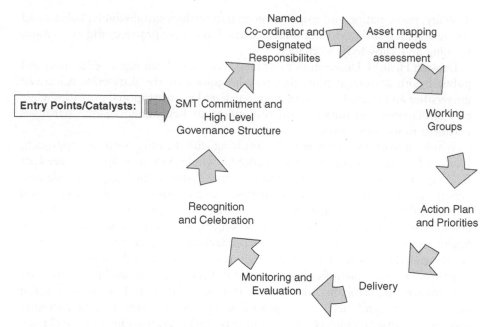

Figure 10.3   Healthy universities: an operational process (adapted from Doherty and Dooris, 2006; reproduced with permission from *Education and Health*)

responsibility for health among students and staff; strengthened institution-level commitment to practise corporate social and environmental responsibility).

   Impacts: The approach also has the potential to result in longer-term impacts within, outside and beyond the university, leading to improved business performance and productivity; strengthened capacity and capability to contribute to the pursuit of policy ambitions; and increased positive and reduced negative institutional influences on health and ecological sustainability.

Challenges and opportunities for Healthy Universities

In order to engage effectively with the Healthy Universities approach and translate it into meaningful policy and practice, it will be necessary to address a number of challenges, utilizing the three core strategies of mediation, enablement and advocacy highlighted in the Ottawa Charter (WHO, 1986).

   As with many other settings, it is demanding to introduce and integrate an understanding of and commitment to health within a sector that does not have this as a central aim and comprises free-thinking and fiercely autonomous institutions. This requires a thorough understanding of higher education, an appreciation of competing agendas and an ability to mediate for health. Such mediation must demonstrate convincingly why the university is an important setting for public health improvement by highlighting the issues of particular relevance to its community (such as alcohol and substance misuse;

mental wellbeing; obesity, food and physical activity; sexual health; climate change). It must also show how investment in student, staff and community wellbeing can impact positively on core business (including student recruitment, experience, retention and achievement; widening participation; staff recruitment, retention, performance and productivity). As highlighted by Dooris and Doherty (2009, 2010b), this challenge is particularly pertinent at a time when institutions are experiencing initiative overload and are beleaguered by continuing change and severe resource constraints. As this mediation takes effect and health begins to be embedded within policy and practice, a further challenge is to move to a position where the Healthy University initiative is seen to be mainstream rather than merely a discrete project, and understood to be a core responsibility across all schools and services.

In seeking to embed health within the core business of universities, it is essential that Healthy Universities plays an enabling role. As explored by Dooris (2001), this means:

- offering a positive and health enhancing working environment for staff, which is underpinned by empowering management styles, supportive communication systems and appropriate service provision and development opportunities
- providing secure and supportive learning and living environments for students, within which they can gain knowledge and understanding, develop skills, explore possibilities, experiment safely, make informed choices, and discover and achieve their potential
- proactively facilitating staff within and across a diversity of disciplines to raise awareness and develop professional competences, by integrating health, wellbeing and sustainable development within curricula, research and knowledge exchange
- engaging with and empowering local communities through widening access, encouraging student volunteering, participating in partnerships and demystifying research findings.

While individual universities can do much to support and improve health and wellbeing, many determinants of health are situated outside their immediate locus of control. However, recognizing the vast resource of accumulated knowledge and evidence at their disposal and the high level of respect afforded to them, this points to the importance of developing institutional and sectoral advocacy roles. By harnessing and channelling this influential voice to comment and call for action on these wider determinants, Healthy Universities can avoid parochialism and become a force for positive change, thereby helping to create conditions that support health. In so doing, it will be particularly important to connect and demonstrate synergy between key societal agendas such as community cohesion, social inclusion and sustainable development. As discussed in Part I, Chapter 2, there has been an increasing drive to develop synergy between public health and sustainable development (Griffiths and Stewart, 2008; Griffiths et al., 2009), with key public health organizations recognizing that the causes and manifestations of both ecologically unsustainable development and poor health are interrelated and frequently pose further interconnected challenges and opportunities. For example, improved land use planning can reduce carbon emissions, reduce air pollution and increase levels of physical activity. Related to this, there have been calls for the settings approach to forge closer links and become a force for a green and healthy future (Bentley 2007; Davis and Cooke, 2007; Dooris, 1999; Poland and Dooris, 2010) and Orme and Dooris (2010) have discussed this challenge in relation to higher education, suggesting that the Healthy Universities approach offers a timely mechanism for strengthening connections and realizing potential.

Within the context of these very real challenges, it is evident that there are important opportunities to harness the potential offered by the Healthy Universities approach, as highlighted in the report of national research conducted with English universities and stakeholder bodies (Dooris and Doherty, 2009). This emphasized the value of building on the experience and success of healthy schools and healthy further education by extending, tailoring and applying the settings approach to higher education, suggesting that this could help make sense of and harness the disparate health-related activities that take place in universities, thereby lending greater coherence and increasing effectiveness. There was also an appreciation that engagement with and commitment to Healthy Universities has the potential to enhance quality, reputation and distinctiveness within an increasingly competitive marketplace, and to strengthen the overall delivery of the settings approach by encouraging an integrated approach across the education sector. Building on the wealth of activity already taking place within the sector and the breadth of understandings currently located under the umbrella of Healthy Universities, the research also demonstrated a growing recognition of the value of a comprehensive whole system approach that can map and understand interactions, synergies and interrelationships within higher education settings (Dooris, 2005; Naaldenberg et al., 2009). Since this research was carried out, the Developing Leadership and Governance for Healthy Universities project funded by the Higher Education Funding Council for England (HEFCE) has nurtured the English National Network, the membership of which has rapidly expanded (www.healthyuniversities.ac.uk). At the same time, there has been increasing interest in international networking, both at European and global levels. These national and international developments demonstrate the growing interest in and engagement with the Healthy Universities agenda.

Reflecting on developments within the UK higher education sector, Steuer and Marcs (2008) have challenged what they perceive to be an overriding focus on serving the economy and fuelling individual competitiveness. They advocate a transformative approach to quality that moves beyond a narrow focus on learners as future workers, calling for a broader higher education mandate that serves the dual purpose of enhancing both personal and collective wellbeing.

Summary points

- Higher education represents a key sector in and through which to invest for public health, offering enormous potential for positive impacts on the health and wellbeing of students, staff and the wider community. Not only is it an influential setting for an increasingly diverse population of students, many undergoing a formative time of transition while at university, it also employs and contracts a large workforce, is a generator and communicator of multidisciplinary knowledge, exerts substantial corporate leverage and has a sizeable institutional footprint.

- Building on wider healthy settings theory and practice emphasizing the necessity of aligning health and core business agendas, there is a growing appreciation that investment for health within the sector can contribute to mainstream higher education priorities such as student recruitment, experience, retention and achievement; staff engagement, experience and performance; and institutional and societal productivity and sustainability. Within a context characterized by limited resources and multiple agendas, it will be important to relate Healthy Universities to ambitions set out in government policy, to evidence its contributions and benefits to higher education, and to advocate for health to form part of the offer being proposed by institutions in an increasingly competitive market place (Browne, 2010).

- Universities also shape the future through their formal and informal influences on their populations. They thus offer the possibility of building understanding of and commitment to health, sustainable development and social justice, thereby generating a throughput of engaged students and staff exerting a constructive influence as local and global citizens within families, communities, workplaces and political processes. Through these mechanisms, they can magnify their role as engines of innovation and positive social, economic and cultural change.

- A commitment to healthy universities and to harnessing the potential of the sector to contribute to public health improvement and capacity and capability building will require effective leadership and partnership development. At national and European levels, there is a clear demand for stakeholder organizations to demonstrate leadership through championing a Healthy Universities programme or framework that not only adds value within the higher education sector, but also helps to build consistency of approach across the entire spectrum of education. Significantly and optimistically, the UK Government's Strategy for Public Health in England (HM Government, 2010: 34) affirms that the Healthy Schools, Healthy Further Education and Healthy Universities programmes will continue to be developed by their respective sectors, as voluntary programmes, collaborating where appropriate and exploring partnership working with business and voluntary bodies.

Online Further Reading

Dooris, M. and Doherty, S. (2010) 'Healthy Universities: current activity and future directions – findings and reflections from a national-level qualitative research study', *Global Health Promotion*, 17(3): 6–16.

This paper provides an in-depth overview of Healthy Universities, drawing on a national research study carried out in England. The findings suggested that, while there is growing understanding of the need for a comprehensive whole system approach to improving health within higher education settings, there are a number of very real challenges, including a lack of rigorous evaluation, the difficulty of integrating health into a non-health sector and the complexity of securing sustainable cultural change.

Naaldenberg, J., Vaandrager, L., Koelen, M., Wagemakers, A., Saan, H. and de Hoog, K. (2009) 'Elaborating on systems thinking in health promotion practice', *Global Health Promotion*, 16: 39–47.

This paper explores the opportunities offered by adopting a systems perspective in health promotion, showing how such thinking can increase insight into the functioning of partnerships and facilitate processes of social learning and innovation. It concludes by suggesting that systems thinking can help to reach a more integral and sustainable approach in which the complex nature of health promotion is supported.

References

Beattie, A. (1995) 'Editorial: new agendas for student health', *Health for All 2000 News*, 31: 2–3.

Bentley, M. (2007) 'Healthy Cities, local environmental action and climate change', *Health Promotion International*, 22: 246–53.

Black, C. (2008) *Working for a Healthier Working Age Population: Dame Carol Black's Review of the Health of the Working Age Population*. Norwich: The Stationery Office.

Browne, Lord (2010) *Securing a Sustainable Future for Higher Education*. www.independent.gov.uk/browne-report (accessed 30 April 2011).

Butland, B., Jebb, S., Kopelman, P., McPherson, K., Thomas, S., Mardell, J. and Parry, J. (2007) *Tackling Obesities: Future Choices – Project Report*. London: Foresight Programme, Government Office for Science.

Crouch, R., Scarffe, P. and Davies, S. (2006) *Guidelines for Mental Health Promotion in Higher Education*. Available at: www.mhhe.heacademy.ac.uk/silo/files/uuk-student-mh-guidelines.doc (accessed 18 November 2010).

Davis, J. and Cooke, S. (2007) 'Educating for a healthy, sustainable world: an argument for integrating Health Promoting Schools and Sustainable Schools', *Health Promotion International*, 22: 346–53.

Department of Health (2004) *Choosing Health: Making Healthy Choices Easier*. London: The Stationery Office.

Department of Health (2008) *High-Quality Care for All: NHS Next Stage Review Final Report.* London: The Stationery Office.

Department of Health (2009) *NHS 2010–2015: From Good to Great: Preventative, People-Centred, Productive.* London: The Stationery Office.

Department for Work and Pensions, Department of Health and Health and Safety Executive (2005) *Health, Work and Well-Being – Caring for Our Future: A Strategy for the Health and Well-Being of Working Age People.* London: DWP/DH/HSE.

Doherty, S. and Dooris, M. (2006) 'The healthy settings approach: the growing interest within colleges and universities', *Education and Health*, 24: 42–43.

Dooris, M. (1999) 'Healthy cities and local agenda 21: The UK experience – Challenges for the new millennium', *Health Promotion International*, 14: 365–75.

Dooris, M. (1999) 'The health promoting university as a framework for promoting positive mental well-being – a discourse on theory and practice', *International Journal of Mental Health Promotion*, 1: 34–44.

Dooris, M. (2001) 'The "health promoting university": a critical exploration of theory and practice', *Health Education*, 101: 51–60.

Dooris, M. (2002) 'The Health Promoting University – opportunities, challenges and future developments', *Promotion and Education*, S1: 20–4.

Dooris, M. (2005) 'Healthy settings: challenges to generating evidence of effectiveness', *Health Promotion International*, 21: 55–65.

Dooris, M. (2010) *Healthy Universities: An Introduction.* Preston: UCLan. www.healthyuniversities.ac.uk (accessed 18 November 2010).

Dooris, M. and Doherty, S. (2009) *National Research and Development Project on Healthy Universities: Final Report.* London: Higher Education Academy Health Sciences and Practice Subject Centre.

Dooris, M. and Doherty, S. (2010a) 'Healthy Universities: time for action: a qualitative research study exploring the potential for a national programm', *Health Promotion International*, 25: 94–106.

Dooris, M. and Doherty, S. (2010b) 'Healthy Universities: current activity and future directions – findings and reflections from a national-level qualitative research study', *Global Health Promotion*, 17: 6–16.

Faculty of Public Health Medicine (1995) *Health for All 2000. News*, 31.

Grant, A. (with Kester, G., Donnelly, N. and Hale, B.) (2002) *Reducing the Risk of Student Suicide: Issues and Responses for Higher Education Institutions.* UUK Management Guidance Series. London: UUK/SCOP.

Griffiths, J. and Stewart, L. (2008) *Sustaining a Healthy Future.* London: Faculty of Public Health.

Griffiths, J., Rao, M., Adshead, F. and Thorpe, A. (eds) (2009) *The Health Practitioner's Guide to Climate Change. Diagnosis and Cure.* London: Earthscan.

Health and Safety Executive (2006) *Healthy Workplace, Healthy Workforce, Better Business Delivery: Improving Service Delivery in Universities and Colleges through Better Occupational Health.* London: HSE.

HEFCE (Higher Education Funding Council for England) (HEFCE) (2010) *Trends in Young Participation in Higher Education: Core Results for England.* Bristol: HEFCE. Available at: www.hefce.ac.uk/pubs/hefce/2010/10_03 (accessed 18 November 2010).

HESA (Higher Education Statistics Agency) (2009) *Headline Statistics.* Cheltenham: HESA. Available at: www.hesa.ac.uk/index.php/content/category/1/1/161 (accessed 18 November 2010).

HM Government (2010) *Healthy Lives, Healthy People: Our Strategy for Public Health in England.* Norwich: The Stationery Office.

Lee, S. (2002) 'Health promoting university initiative in Hong Kong', *Promotion and Education*, S1: 15.

Meier, S., Stock, C. and Krämer, A. (2007) 'The contribution of health discussion groups with students to campus health promotion', *Health Promotion International*, 22: 28–36.

Naaldenberg, J., Vaandrager, L., Koelen, M., Wagemakers, A., Saan, H. and de Hoog, K. (2009) 'Elaborating on systems thinking in health promotion practice', *Global Health Promotion*, 16: 39–47.

Orme, J. and Dooris, M. (2010) 'Integrating health and sustainability: the Higher Education Sector as a timely catalyst', *Health Education Research*, 25: 425–37.

Poland, B. and Dooris, M. (2010) 'A green and healthy future: a settings approach to building health, equity and sustainability', *Critical Public Health*, 20: 281–98.

Polymerou, A. (2007) *Alcohol and Drug Prevention in Colleges and Universities: A Review of the Literature.* London: Mentor UK.

St Leger, L., Young, I., Blanchard, C. and Perry, M. (2010) *Promoting Health in Schools: From Evidence to Action.* Paris: International Union for Health Promotion and Education. Available at: www.iuhpe.org/?page=516andlang=en (accessed 18 November 2010).

Steur, N. and Marcs, N. (2008) *University Challenge: Towards a Wellbeing Approach to Quality in Higher Education.* London: New Economics Foundation.

Stewart-Brown, S. (2006). *What Is the Evidence on School Health Promotion in Improving Health or Preventing Disease and, Specifically, What Is the Effectiveness of the Health Promoting Schools Approach?* Copenhagen: WHO Regional Office for Europe. (Health Evidence Network Report available at: www.euro.who.int/document/e88185.pdf accessed 5 March 2010.)

Stock, C., Wille, L. and Krämer, A. (2001) 'Gender-specific health behaviors of German university students predict the interest in campus health promotion', *Health Promotion International*, 16: 145–54.

Stock, C., Kücük, N., Miseviciene, I., Guillén-Grima, F., Petkeviciene, J., Aguinaga-Ontoso, I. and Krämer, A. (2003) 'Differences in health complaints among university students from three European countries', *Preventive Medicine*, 37: 535–43.

Stock, C., Milz, S. and Meier, S. (2010) 'Network evaluation: priniciples, structures and outcomes of the German working group of Health Promoting Universities', *Global Health Promotion* 17: 25–32.

Theaker, T. and Thompson, J. (eds) (1995) *The Settings-based Approach to Health Promotion: Conference Report.* Welwyn Garden City: Hertfordshire Health Promotion.

Tsouros, A., Dowding, G., Thomson, J. and Dooris, M. (eds) (1998) *Health Promoting Universities: Concept, Experience and Framework for Action.* Copenhagen: WHO Regional Office for Europe. Available at: www.euro.who.int/document/e60163.pdf (accessed 18 November 2010).

Universities UK (2000) *Guidelines on Student Mental Health Policies and Procedures for Higher Education.* London: UUK.

Universities UK (2008) *Higher Education in Facts and Figures: Summer 2008.* London: UUK.

Wanless, D. (2002) *Securing Our Future Health.* London: HM Treasury.

Wanless, D. (2004) *Securing Good Health for the Whole Population.* London: HM Treasury.

Warwick, I., Statham, J. and Aggleton, P. (2008) *Healthy and Health Promoting Colleges – Identifying an Evidence Base*. London: Thomas Coram Research Unit, University of London.

WHO (World Health Organization) (1986) *Ottawa Charter for Health Promotion*. Geneva: WHO.

World Health Organization (WHO) (1998) *Health21 – The Health for All Policy for the WHO European Region – 21 Targets for the 21st Century*. Copenhagen: WHO Regional Office for Europe.

Xiangyang, T., Lan, Z., Xueping, M., Tao, Z., Yuzhen, S. and Jagusztyn, M. (2003) 'Beijing health promoting universities: practice and evaluation', *Health Promotion International*, 18: 107–13.

11

Health Promoting Prisons: Dilemmas and Challenges

James Woodall and Jane South

Aims

- To introduce the rationale and principles underpinning the health promoting prison
- To set the health promoting prison within a political context and outline how prisons have emerged as a setting for health promotion
- To explore the conceptual and practical challenges facing the health promoting prison
- To discuss the future of the health promoting prison

Prisons have been regarded as the most problematic of the settings-based environments (Whitehead, 2006), as prisons generally work within hierarchical, disempowering and penalizing structures that are fundamentally antithetical to the core values of health promotion (Smith, 2000; Whitehead, 2006; Woodall, 2010a). While the discourse and ideology of health promotion is incongruous in a setting that curtails individual freedom and choice, there are clear opportunities for health promotion work. Prisons are, for example, an opportunity to address the health and social circumstances of prisoners and a prime setting to tackle inequalities in health (Baybutt et al., 2010). This has been reflected by strong political will, both nationally (Department of Health, 2002, 2004, 2009; HM Prison Service, 2003) and internationally (WHO, 1995, 1998, 2003a, 2007), to regard the prison as a key social setting for health promotion.

Health promoting prisons: an important public health opportunity

Currently there are a record number of people residing within prison establishments in England and Wales (Ministry of Justice, 2010) and, moreover, a body of evidence exists which shows that a high proportion of this group have complex health needs (Rutherford and Duggan, 2009). These health needs include mental health problems (Fazel and Danesh, 2002; WHO, 2008), long standing physical disorders (Plugge et al., 2006; Stewart, 2008) and drug and alcohol issues (Centre for Social Justice, 2009; Prison Reform Trust, 2009; Social Exclusion Unit, 2002). Many of those entering the criminal justice system have also been subjected to a lifetime of social exclusion, including poor educational backgrounds, low incomes, meagre employment opportunities, lack of engagement with normal societal structures, low self-esteem and impermanence both in terms of accommodation (including bouts of homelessness) and relationships with family members (Department of Health, 2009; Levy, 2005; Prison Reform Trust, 2009; Senior and Shaw, 2007). The Social Exclusion Unit (2002), in their highly cited report, claimed that prisoners were 13 times more likely to have grown up in care and more likely to have run away from home as a child. The report revealed that most prisoners had disrupted educational experiences and were less likely to have any qualifications or basic skills.

Prisons are not necessarily in the primary business of promoting health (Smith, 2000), but do provide an opportunity to access marginalized groups who would otherwise be classified as hard to reach in the wider community (Baybutt et al., 2010). For many prisoners, due to their chaotic pre-prison lives, a period of imprisonment can often be the first time they consider their health needs or contemplate accessing support and services (Woodall, 2010a). This was highlighted in the White Paper *Choosing Health* (Department of Health, 2004: 129):

> Generally speaking, people in prison have poorer health than the population at large and many of them have unhealthy lifestyles. Many will have had little or no regular contact with health services before coming into prison.

Much of the prison population can be described as transient and mobile in that they frequently shift between imprisonment and free society, serving multiple and relatively short term sentences. Health promoting prisons, therefore, have the potential to reduce health inequalities through building the physical, mental and social dimensions of prisoners' health and enabling prisoners to adopt healthy behaviours that can be taken back into the community (Department of Health, 2002; HM Prison Service, 2003). Furthermore, commentators have proposed that by improving the health of individuals confined within prison, this can positively affect the health of prisoners' immediate family and relatives (Conklin et al., 2000; Hammett et al., 2002; Sifunda et al., 2006; Whitehead, 2006). Scott et al. (2004), for example, outlined how HIV-related knowledge, acquired as part of a peer education programme in prison, was diffused to family members in the community.

Recent examples of interventions within prisons to reduce health inequalities include: Walking the Way to Prison Health, an extension of the national walking for health initiative. The rationale of the initiative is based on the premise that walking not only improves physical health, but social and mental health too. It was perhaps these latter points that aroused the particular interest of prisons

(Paterson et al., 2007). Health Trainer schemes have also been implemented that enable trained prisoners and ex-offenders to improve the health of their peers and improve their engagement with services (Sirdfield, 2006; Sirdfield et al., 2007). Innovative work has also started to address the health of older prisoners – one of the fastest growing sub-sections of the prison population (Prison Reform Trust, 2008). This has been highlighted in Box 11.1.

Box 11.1   *Music in Time* health promotion prison project

The Music in Time project was developed specifically to address a perceived gap in provision for older prisoners in the South West of England. The aim of the project was to offer older prisoners a music education programme to build confidence and self-efficacy, develop new relationships and learn new skills. An evaluation of the project suggested that an array of personal and social opportunities, including improved self confidence, self esteem, self efficacy, interpersonal and communication skills, focus and discipline, enhanced wellbeing, and improved mental health, occurred as a result of the programme (de Viggiani et al., 2010).

The prison setting is also a workplace for staff, and policies and practices should therefore ensure that staff health is promoted rather than demoted within the setting. Prison staff are vital to the running of prison establishments, yet they are often vulnerable to stress in the workplace caused by work-related pressures, including low staff to prisoner ratios (Woodall, 2010a). This has major implications, as research indicates that the stressful role of working in a prison can impact on the psychological wellbeing of the individual and can also spill into home life, potentially contaminating social and family relationships (Crawley, 2002, 2005). Moreover, it is axiomatic that in order for prisoners to be rehabilitated and released into the community as law abiding, healthy citizens, prison staff themselves need to feel valued and be able to maintain good physical, mental and psychosocial health (Bögemann, 2007).

Principles underpinning the health promoting prison

Prisoners' rights are arguably at the core of the health promoting prison. In 1966, the United Nations, in their International Covenant on Economic, Social and Cultural Rights (United Nations, 1966), stated that every citizen has the right to the highest attainable standard of physical and mental health and, in 1990, they declared that prisoners should have access to health services available in the country without discrimination based on their legal status (United Nations, 1990). More recently, it was acknowledged in England and Wales that imprisonment should not remove the rights of prisoners to receive a good level of healthcare and it should not make it more likely that they become ill or experience deterioration in their health status (HM Prison Service and NHS Executive, 1999). Linked to prisoners' rights is the principle of healthcare equivalence. The premise is that individuals detained in prison must have the benefit of care equivalent to that available to the general public (Niveau, 2007).

While the health promoting prison is a relatively new concept, a definition has been proposed that reflects the equivalence and respect agendas. It states that the health promoting prison is:

> a place of compulsory detention in which the risks to health are reduced to a minimum; where essential prison duties such as the maintenance of security are undertaken in a caring atmosphere that recognizes the inherent dignity of all prisoners and their human rights; where health services are provided to the level and in a professional manner equivalent to what is provided in the country as a whole; and where a whole-prison approach to promoting health and welfare is the norm. (Gatherer et al., 2009: 89)

The health promoting prison should include all facets of prison life, from addressing individual health need through to organizational factors and the physical environment (de Viggiani, 2009). The Ottawa Charter (WHO, 1986),

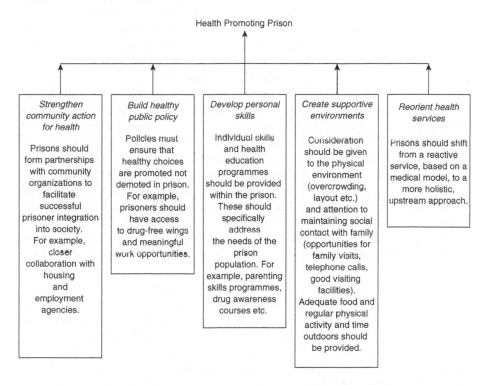

Figure 11.1   The Ottawa Charter as a framework for action within the health promoting prison

alluded to in Part I, is a useful framework to envisage these facets of prison life and has been used by others to map health promotion work in prisons (Ramaswamy and Freudenberg, 2007). Figure 11.1 attempts to demonstrate the applicability of the Ottawa Charter to the health promoting prison.

Current guidance from the WHO suggests that the health promoting prison should be underpinned by four key pillars (WHO, 2007). These pillars acknowledge that prisons should be: safe; secure; reforming and health promoting; and grounded in the concept of decency and respect for human rights. Guidance also advocates a whole prison approach to health promotion (Department of Health, 2002; WHO, 2007), which has three main components. Firstly, policies in prisons should promote rather than demote health. Secondly, the environment should actively support health. Finally, there should be a focus on prevention, health education and health promotion within the setting for both prisoners and staff. The underlying view of the health promoting prison is that health is everyone's business, it is not just for those in traditional healthcare roles.

The health promoting prison: the evolving political context

The delivery of healthcare in prison has undoubtedly had a turbulent history, particularly in England and Wales where responsibility for health has shifted in recent times from the Prison Medical Service to the NHS. Space does not permit discussion of these issues, though useful overviews can be found elsewhere (see Senior and Shaw, 2007). This section instead highlights the political backdrop concerning the emergence of the health promoting prison.

Prisons have been officially regarded as key settings for health promotion since 1995, after a meeting organized by the World Health Organization (WHO, 1995), where delegates agreed that the public health importance of prisoner health was neglected throughout Europe (Gatherer et al., 2005). Acknowledgement was given to several issues, including variations between countries in the provision of health promotion in prison and the requirement not only to address the needs of prisoners, but also prisoners' families and prison staff. The meeting endorsed prisons as settings for health promotion and concluded that health promotion in prison should include, amongst other things: the prevention of deterioration in health, enablement and empowerment, a duty of care to the whole community and be underpinned by a multidisciplinary and holistic approach.

The consensus for change generated from the meeting acted as a platform to launch the WHO's Health in Prisons Project, an initiative with a primary remit to improve all aspects of health in prison through policy change (Gatherer et al., 2005). Prior to the establishment of the Health in Prisons Project there was no formal mechanism for prisons to share good practice and prison health services were of limited interest to prison management and national health services across Europe (Gatherer and Møller, 2009; Gatherer et al., 2009).The Health in Prisons Project has a number of strategic aims but functions through creating and disseminating good practice and working towards influencing prison policy and practices in its member countries. Thirty-eight countries are now committed to the Health in Prisons Project and participating at a policy making level to reduce public health risks through improving health in prisons (Møller et al., 2009).

In 2005 Gatherer et al. appraised the substantial progress made by the Health in Prisons Project in its first decade. Notwithstanding considerable achievements, the authors suggested that formidable barriers remained. These barriers included: prison overcrowding and unhygienic facilities, rising prison populations, inherent traditions, political perspectives, the reluctance of staff to evolve their ways of working and resource restrictions. Due to these problems, experts claim that the Health in Prisons Project still has a necessary function, as major health problems continue to face those in prison (Gatherer et al., 2009). Furthermore, the Health in Prisons Project is seen as a model of practice that should expand beyond Europe into other areas of the world (Weinstein, 2010).

The health promoting prison concept has gained momentum as a conceptual framework to guide policy and practice in England and Wales (Department of Health, 2002, 2004, 2009; HM Prison Service, 2003). Indeed, some have argued that it is England and Wales that presently lead Europe in policy development and in the integration between prison and public health services (Gatherer and Fraser, 2009; Whitehead, 2006). In 2002, the strategy document *Health Promoting Prisons: A Shared Approach* (Department of Health, 2002) legitimized and championed a health promotion focus in prison healthcare, advocating the prevention of deterioration in health as well as encouraging prisoners to adopt healthy behaviours (Condon et al., 2007). It emphasized the need for a range of staff to be involved in health promotion, not just those who were seen to have a traditional healthcare role. This policy set the foundations for the introduction of a Prison Service Order (PSO 3200) on health promotion in 2003 (HM Prison Service, 2003). The PSO was a major breakthrough for health promotion within the prison setting; Baybutt et al. (2010), for example, suggest that the translation of a Department of Health strategy into an auditable prison document was a crucial step forward for health promoting prisons, providing a level of commitment to health within the offender management system. The PSO now sets out required actions for prison governors to promote health as part of a whole prison approach (Condon et al., 2008). Under the instruction of the PSO, prisons are expected to specifically address major health areas. These are: mental health promotion and well-being, smoking, healthy eating and nutrition, healthy lifestyles and drug and other substance misuse. Prison health performance indicators have also been developed which focus on the delivery of health promotion in prisons through PSO 3200 (NOMS et al., 2007). Box 11.2 summarizes the major health promotion policy developments influencing prisons in England and Wales.

Box 11.2 Health promotion policy developments influencing prisons in England and Wales

1995 A WHO meeting in London convenes to ascertain the feasibility of health promotion in prisons.

2002 *Health Promoting Prisons: A Shared Approach* is published by the Department of Health and Her Majesty's Prison Service. This legitimized and championed a health promotion focus in prison healthcare.

2003 Prison Service Order 3200 is launched outlining required actions for prison governors to promote health.

2004 *Choosing Health*, the White Paper on public health for England, makes a firm and explicit commitment to people in prison.

2009 The publication of *Improving Health, Supporting Justice* by the Department of Health moved away from a distinct focus on prison health towards a whole criminal justice perspective. The main themes of the report include: increasing the efficiency and effectiveness of systems, care pathways and continuity of care, ensuring equity of access and increasing capacity and capability.

Conceptual challenges for health promotion in prisons

Despite the promise of the health promoting prison and its potential to address health and reduce inequalities, the impact of the settings approach and the actual outcomes that health promotion policy and strategy has made to prisoners' health is unclear (Douglas et al., 2009; Woodall, 2010a). Critics of the health promoting prison have described it as a contradiction in terms (Goos, 1996; Smith, 2000), an oxymoron (McCallum, 1995; de Viggiani, 2006b), simply incompatible (Greenwood et al., 1999) and, according to de Viggiani (2006a), at best a vision and at worst, a dream. Indeed, in a study by Douglas et al. (2009), women prisoners described a prison environment that was very much at odds with the notion of the health promoting prison. As has already been stated, the environment of the prison is not always conducive to health and can sometimes conflict with the promulgation of health promotion values. As an example, prisoners are frequently deprived of outside cell contact and access to the outdoors. Prisoners are also taken away from family and friends and only permitted a limited amount of contact time with them. Research shows that this can be particularly detrimental to prisoners' mental wellbeing (Woodall, 2007; Woodall, 2010b, 2010c; Woodall et al., 2009).

In addition to the above, there are some serious conceptual challenges still facing the health promoting prison. As a starting point, the concept of health itself and how this has been historically defined and applied within the prison setting will be scrutinized.

'Prison health' is a relatively new expression. While the term has historically been aligned with a biomedical perspective, focused on the prevention of disease and illness in prison populations (Morris and Morris, 1963; Sim, 1990), defining and applying health through this biomedical lens has implications for the prison as a health promoting setting. Primarily, health is defined by its absence of disease and not the attainment of positive health and wellbeing or personal growth. Indeed, critical reviews of prison health services have described provision that is underpinned by a medical model of delivery (HMIP, 1996). The settings approach, however, as outlined in detail in Chapter 2 in Part I of this book, has clearly evolved from an ecological viewpoint which recognizes that health is determined by an interaction of environmental, organizational and personal factors within the places that people live their lives (Dooris, 2009). Yet, the application of a biomedical view within prison settings produces an emphasis on prevention that is inconsistent with the central tenets of health promotion and a settings approach. Arguably, a biomedical view has the danger of obscuring the wider political, social and environmental determinants that can impinge upon prisoners' health, such as poverty, education, employment and housing.

While not undermining the clear efforts of prisons to detach from the biomedical perspective, there are indications that a reactive, narrowly focused view of health still prevails. One concern lies in the heavy, unbalanced emphasis on disease control, eradication, screening and testing in health promotion policy and practice. Health promotion within prison has even been described as part of a clinical service (Department of Health, 2002: 2) and this has inevitably encouraged many prison governors to interpret health promotion and the health promoting prison as an exclusive issue for health professionals. Recognizing that healthcare within prisons is essential, however, it is important to position it as only one small aspect of creating health promoting prisons.

Since the introduction of PSO 3200 practical action has been taken to displace the medical model. For example, a member of the senior management team (a non-health professional) must chair health promotion committee meetings (HM Prison Service, 2003). Similarly, within health promotion performance targets, it is suggested that members of the health promotion action group are drawn from a range of prison departments, including: healthcare, catering, physical education, general education, substance misuse services, chaplaincy and mental health services (NOMS et al., 2007). Despite the fact that health promotion has been consistently couched as a whole prison matter, an evaluation of the implementation of PSO 3200 with prisons in the North West of England showed that healthcare workers still remained in control of the agenda (Baybutt, 2004).

In terms of recognizing the determinants of prisoners' health, action under the health promoting prison banner has been criticized because it remains focused on the symptoms of the problem rather than tackling the root causes of poor health (Caraher et al., 2002). Smith (2002) argues that prison-based health promotional discourse may in fact miss the point as, in reality, it is individualistic, behaviourist and victim blaming and fails to recognize that health problems experienced by prisoners are entrenched in their wider environment and their experience of inequality, poverty and disadvantage. Clearly, health promotion in prison contributes towards dealing with behaviour change, but it is only when the collective factors that produce ill-health are tackled that there will be any real health improvement (Smith, 2000). This is reiterated by Caraher et al. (2002) and Woodall (2010a), who suggest that there is a need for health promotion in prison, but also for wider social policy which addresses the broader determinants of health and illness.

Initiatives often launched under the rubric of health promotion remain reactionary and individualistic, addressing specific disease prevention targets that respond to the physical, psychological, emotional and social needs of individuals in only a partial way (de Viggiani, 2006a, 2006b). Indeed, some critics have argued that current health promotion activities within prisons signal a rather superficial commitment to the original WHO principles (de Viggiani, 2006a) (this will be discussed further in respect to empowerment). The perception that health promotion comprises one-off, short-lived events that are implemented on sporadic, ad-hoc occasions has been problematic in prison (de Viggiani, 2009), as has the notion that the health promoting prison should be solely focused on prisoners to the neglect of prison staff (Woodall, 2010a). Other settings, such as healthy schools (see Part II, Chapter 9), have acknowledged the health of teaching and other staff as an important element. Similar trends have not been as prominent in work on health in prisons, where the focus has tended to be almost exclusively on prisoners.

Practical challenges to the health promoting prison

As well as conceptual issues, there have been practical challenges that have inhibited the development of the health promoting prison. Health promotion in prisons remains under-resourced, under-funded and an activity on the periphery of the organization's priorities (Caraher et al., 2002). In addition, prison staff working closely with prisoners often view health promotion as constituting additional work, something that is perceived as being outside their professional remit or something to do when time is available from their regular daily duties (Bird et al., 1999; Caraher et al., 2002). Bird et al. (1999: 19), for example, found that mental health promotion was not seen as being a core duty of prison staff. Activities in relation to promoting mental health were seen as being nice to know rather than essential to know. Healthcare staff also perceived health promotion as a specialist activity and not part of their role.

Empowerment and the health promoting prison

Whether core values within health promotion can be applied to a prison context is highly contentious. Empowerment, for instance, has become a flagship value for health promotion and is seen as the holy grail or raison d'être of the discipline (Rissel, 1994). Prisons are undoubtedly settings of tremendous power inequalities (Bosworth and Carrabine, 2001) and, according to some (Sim, 2002), the downfall of health promotion in prison has been that it has failed to confront this power differential. As an example, policy and strategy related to the health promoting prison has rarely used the term empowerment, despite the fact that empowerment is a key principle in the formation of a healthy setting (Dooris, 2001; Denman et al., 2002; Green et al., 2000).

Originally empowerment was regarded as a key element of the health promoting prison, emphasized clearly at an international level by the WHO (WHO, 1995). In England and Wales, the policy document *Health Promoting Prisons: A Shared Approach* (Department of Health, 2002), paid no attention to empowerment despite the document endorsing the principles set out in the Ottawa Charter. Similarly, PSO 3200 (HM Prison Service, 2003) does not allude to empowerment even though its primary focus is on promoting health. While empowering prisoners has never been an accepted pursuit in prison systems, even regarded as morally questionable and politically dangerous (Aldridge Foundation and Johnson, 2008: 2), there is a growing recognition that prisons should be supportive and empowering (de Viggiani et al., 2005: 918). Though the concept of empowerment applied to the context of imprisonment is especially complex, empowerment is still a core concept for health promotion and should therefore be considered central to the development of the health promoting prison. Within the literature there are, however, two arguments on this issue.

The first position is that empowerment cannot take place within prisons as the prevailing organizational structures inhibit any expression of free will or power. Health promotion's ideology and the central values of autonomy, choice, partnership working and empowerment are deemed incongruous to prison regimes, which are disempowering, isolating and security focused (Whitehead, 2006). Indeed, Condon et al. (2008) supported the proposition that prisoners have insufficient autonomy to ensure that their health needs are met. Similarly, empowerment cannot be fostered in a setting where little choice can be sanctioned, where autonomy and personal agency are frowned upon and where prisoners are under surveillance, controlled and forced into subservience and obedience (Maeve, 1999; Smith, 2000; de Viggiani, 2006b). For this reason, health promotion values are always likely to contradict the institutional mandate to contain and punish those who are sentenced to imprisonment by the courts (Courtenay and Sabo, 2001). The second position is that there is a degree to which empowerment can be facilitated within a prison context. In a WHO publication on the essentials in prison health (Møller et al., 2007: 5) it was suggested that as much empowerment as possible be built into the prison regime. Similarly, the WHO (2003b) have also noted that opportunities should be provided in prison to strengthen feelings of personal responsibility and of empowerment within the constraints of custody.

If prisons are to embrace health promotion and support a settings approach, then empowerment is critical to attaining this. Similarly, recognizing that the majority of prisoners serve relatively short sentences, imprisonment would best serve the public by becoming a more positive, empowering experience (de Viggiani et al., 2005). Yet, power over individuals can be particularly damaging to health and contribute to a loss of control and disempowerment (Woodall, 2010b). Within the prison context, this is difficult to evade as prisons must keep the public protected. Nonetheless, this power must be proportional and kept to an absolute minimum in line with protecting the public.

Advancing the health promoting prison

The health promoting prison is, in comparison to settings such as schools, hospitals and universities, still in its infancy. Major developments have been achieved so far, mainly under the leadership of WHO Europe. If a settings approach in prison is to truly move forward, both conceptually and practically, then health promoters should seek to embed the key values of health promotion within the prison setting. Currently, health promotion in prison is still associated with acute healthcare activities, with front-line prison staff still unclear about their role within the health promoting prison. In their current guise, prisons as health promoting environments are more concerned with individually centred lifestyle interventions or disease prevention activities rather than, for example, considering wider influences like architecture, policies, structures, prisoner and staff relationships and how these impact on individuals. If a settings approach is to be fully realized in prison, then a more radical, upstream and holistic outlook is ultimately required.

Summary points

- The health promoting prison has the potential to reduce health inequalities and address the health needs of those who are often hardest to reach in the community.

- A consistent problem for the health promoting prison is that the application of health promotion values within the context of imprisonment is incongruous, as prisons work within structures that are hierarchical, disempowering and penalizing.

- Though clear ideological incompatibilities exist, there is strong political commitment, both nationally and internationally, to regard the prison as a key social setting for health promotion.

- In comparison to other settings, such as schools, it is clear that more needs to be done to reconfigure prisons towards the health promoting settings movement.

Online Further Reading

Condon, L., Hek, G. and Harris, F. (2008) 'Choosing health in prison: prisoners' views on making healthy choices in English prisons', *Health Education Journal*, 67: 155–66.

Drawing on empirical findings from a number of prisons in England, this paper argues that political developments within the health promoting prisons movement have not resulted in prisoners being able to make consistently healthy choices. The paper highlights a range of barriers that exist in the setting which limit prisoners' abilities to maintain and improve their health.

Woodall, J. (2007) 'Barriers to positive mental health in a Young Offenders Institution: a qualitative study', *Health Education Journal*, 66, 132–40.

This paper shows how the prison regime acts as a barrier to promoting positive mental health with young offenders. It shows how isolation from family and friends can be detrimental to health, but also how prisoner–staff relations can positively and negatively impact on mental wellbeing. The paper argues that promoting health and dealing with the needs of offenders in prison is a complex task.

References

Aldridge Foundation and Johnson, M. (2008) *The User Voice of the Criminal Justice System*. London: The Aldridge Foundation.

Baybutt, M. (2004) *PSO 3200 Health Promotion Baseline Audit. Report of Findings*. Preston: University of Central Lancashire.

Baybutt, M., Hayton, P. and Dooris, M. (2010) 'Prisons in England and Wales: an important public health opportunity?', in J. Douglas, S. Earle, S. Handsley, L. Jones, C. Lloyd and S. Spurr (eds), *A Reader in Promoting Public Health: Challenge and Controversy*, 2nd edn. Milton Keynes: Open University Press.

Bird, L., Hayton, P., Caraher, M., McGough, H. and Tobutt, C. (1999) 'Mental health promotion and prison health care staff in Young Offender Institutions in England', *International Journal of Mental Health Promotion*, 1: 16–24.

Bögemann, H. (2007) 'Promoting health and managing stress among prison employees', in L. Møller, H. Stöver, R. Jürgens, A. Gatherer and H. Nikogosian (eds), *Health in Prisons*. Copenhagen: WHO Regional Office for Europe.

Bosworth, M. and Carrabine, E. (2001) 'Reassessing resistance. Race, gender and sexuality in prison', *Punishment & Society*, 3: 501–15.

Caraher, M., Dixon, P., Hayton, P., Carr-Hill, R., McGough, H. and Bird, L. (2002) 'Are health-promoting prisons an impossibility? Lessons from England and Wales', *Health Education*, 102: 219–29.

Centre for Social Justice (2009) *Breakthrough Britain: Locked Up Potential*. London: The Centre for Social Justice.

Condon, L., Hek, G. and Harris, F. (2007) 'A review of prison health and its implications for primary care nursing in England and Wales: the research evidence', *Journal of Clinical Nursing*, 16: 1201–9.

Condon, L., Hek, G. and Harris, F. (2008) 'Choosing health in prison: prisoners' views on making healthy choices in English prisons', *Health Education Journal*, 67: 155–66.

Conklin, T.J., Lincoln, T. and Tuthill, R.W. (2000) 'Self-reported health and prior health behaviors of newly admitted correctional inmates', *American Journal of Public Health*, 90: 1939–41.

Courtenay, W.H. and Sabo, D. (2001) 'Preventive health strategies for men in prison', in D. Sabo, T.A. Kupers and W. London (eds), *Prison Masculinities*. Philadelphia: Temple University Press.

Crawley, E. (2002) 'Bringing it all back home? The impact of prison officers' work on their families', *Probation Journal*, 49: 277–86.

Crawley, E. (2005) 'Surviving the prison experience? Imprisonment and elderly men', *Prison Service Journal*, 160: 3–8.

de Viggiani, N. (2006a) 'A new approach to prison public health? Challenging and advancing the agenda for prison health', *Critical Public Health*, 16: 307–16.

de Viggiani, N. (2006b) 'Surviving prison: exploring prison social life as a determinant of health', *International Journal of Prisoner Health*, 2: 71–89.

de Viggiani, N. (2009) *A Healthy Prison Strategy for HMP Bristol. Project Report.* Bristol: University of the West of England.

de Viggiani, N., Mackintosh, S. and Lang, P. (2010) *Music in Time: An Evaluation of a Participatory Creative Music Programme for Older Prisoners.* Bristol: University of the West of England.

de Viggiani, N., Orme, J., Powell, J. and Salmon, D. (2005) 'New arrangements for prison health care provide an opportunity and a challenge for primary care trusts', *British Medical Journal*, 330: 918.

Denman, S., Moon, A., Parsons, C. and Stears, D. (2002) *The Health Promoting School: Policy, Research and Practice.* London: Routledge.

Department of Health (2002) *Health Promoting Prisons: A Shared Approach.* London: Crown.

Department of Health (2004) *Choosing Health: Making Healthier Choices Easier.* London: The Stationery Office.

Department of Health (2009) *Improving Health, Supporting Justice: The National Delivery Plan of the Health and Criminal Justice Programme Board.* London: Department of Health.

Dooris, M. (2001) 'The "Health Promoting University": a critical exploration of theory and practice,' *Health Education*, 101: 51–60.

Dooris, M. (2009) 'Holistic and sustainable health improvement: the contribution of the settings-based approach to health promotion', *Perspectives in Public Health*, 129: 29–36.

Douglas, N., Plugge, E. and Fitzpatrick, R. (2009) 'The impact of imprisonment on health. What do women prisoners say?', *Journal of Epidemiology and Community Health*, 63: 749–54.

Fazel, S. and Danesh, J. (2002) 'Serious mental disorder in 23,000 prisoners: a systematic review of 62 surveys', *The Lancet*, 359: 545–50.

Gatherer, A. and Fraser, A. (2009) 'Health care for detainees', *The Lancet*, 373: 1337–8.

Gatherer, A. and Møller, L. (2009) 'Social justice, public health and the vulnerable: health in prisons raises key public health issues', *Public Health*, 123: 407–9.

Gatherer, A., Møller, L. and Hayton, P. (2005) 'The World Health Organization European health in prisons project after 10 years: persistent barriers and achievements', *American Journal of Public Health*, 95: 1696–700.

Gatherer, A., Møller, L. and Hayton, P. (2009) 'Achieving sustainable improvement in the health of women in prisons: the approach of the WHO Health in Prisons Project', in D.C. Hatton and A. Fisher (eds), *Women Prisoners and Health Justice*. Oxford: Radcliffe.

Goos, C. (1996) 'Perspectives on healthy prisons', in N. Squires and J. Strobl (eds), *Healthy Prisons: A Vision for the Future*. Liverpool: The University of Liverpool, Department of Public Health.

Green, L.W., Poland, B.D. and Rootman, I. (2000) 'The settings approach to health promotion', in B.D. Poland, L.W. Green and I. Rootman (eds), *Settings for Health Promotion: Linking Theory and Practice*. Thousand Oaks, CA: Sage.

Greenwood, N., Amor, S., Boswell, J., Joliffe, D. and Middleton, B. (1999) *Scottish Needs Assessment Programme. Health Promotion in Prisons*. Glasgow: Office for Public Health in Scotland.

Hammett, T.M., Harmon, M.P. and Rhodes, W. (2002) 'The burden of infectious disease among inmates of and releasees from US correctional facilities, 1997', *American Journal of Public Health*, 92: 1789–94.

HM Prison Service (2003) *Prison Service Order (PSO) 3200 on Health Promotion*. London: HM Prison Service.

HM Prison Service and NHS Executive (1999) *The Future Organization of Prison Health Care*. London: Department of Health.

HMIP (1996) *Patient or Prisoner? A New Strategy for Health Care in Prisons*. London: Home Office.

Levy, M. (2005) 'Prisoner health care provision: reflections from Australia', *International Journal of Prisoner Health*, 1: 65–73.

Maeve, M.K. (1999) 'Adjudicated health: incarcerated women and the social construction of health', *Crime, Law and Social Change*, 31: 49–71.

McCallum, A. (1995) 'Healthy prisons: oxymoron or opportunity?', *Critical Public Health*, 6: 4–15.

Ministry of Justice (2010) *Prison Population and Accommodation Briefing for 23rd July, 2010*. London: Ministry of Justice.

Møller, L., Gatherer, A. and Dara, M. (2009) 'Barriers to implementation of effective tuberculosis control in prisons', *Public Health*, 123: 419–21.

Møller, L., Stöver, H., Jürgens, R., Gatherer, A. and Nikogosian, H. (2007) *Health in Prisons*. Copenhagen: WHO Regional Office for Europe.

Morris, T. and Morris, P. (1963) *Pentonville: A Sociological Study of an English Prison*. London: Routledge.

Niveau, G. (2007) 'Relevance and limits of the principle of "equivalence of care" in prison medicine', *Journal of Medical Ethics*, 33: 610–13.

NOMS, HM Prison Service & Department of Health (2007) *Prison Health Performance Indicators*. Guidance Booklet. London: Offender Health.

Paterson, S., Moore, S. and Woodall, J. (2007) 'Exercise referral and offender management in relation to mental health: an example from HMP Everthorpe', *Journal of Mental Health Training, Education and Practice*, 2: 23–4.

Plugge, E., Douglas, N. and Fitzpatrick, R. (2006) *The Health of Women in Prison*. Oxford: Department of Public Health, University of Oxford.

Prison Reform Trust (2008) *Doing Time: The Experiences and Needs of Older People in Prison*. London: Prison Reform Trust.

Prison Reform Trust (2009) *Bromley Briefings. Prison Factfile*. London: Prison Reform Trust.

Ramaswamy, M. and Freudenberg, N. (2007) 'Health promotion in jails and prisons: an alternative paradigm for correctional health services', in R.B. Greifinger, J. Bick and J. Goldenson (eds), *Public Health Behind Bars: From Prisons to Communities*. New York: Springer.

Rissel, C. (1994) 'Empowerment: the holy grail of health promotion?', *Health Promotion International*, 9: 39–47.

Rutherford, M. and Duggan, S. (2009) 'Meeting complex health needs in prison', *Public Health*, 123: 415–18.

Scott, D.P., Harzke, A.J., Mizwa, M.B, Pugh, M. and Ross, M.W. (2004) 'Evaluation of an HIV peer education program in Texas prisons', *Journal of Correctional Health Care*, 10: 151–73.

Senior, J. and Shaw, J. (2007) 'Prison healthcare', in Y. Jewkes (ed.), *Handbook on Prisons*. Cullompton: Willan Publishing.

Sifunda, S., Reddy, P.S., Braithwaite, R., Stephens, T., Ruiter, R.A.C. and van den Borne, B. (2006) 'Access point analysis on the state of health care services in South African prisons: a qualitative exploration of correctional health care workers' and inmates' perspectives in Kwazulu-Natal and Mpumalanga', *Social Science and Medicine*, 63: 2301–9.

Sim, J. (1990) *Medical Power in Prisons*. Milton Keynes: Open University Press.

Sim, J. (2002) 'The future of prison health care: a critical analysis', *Critical Social Policy*, 22: 300–23.

Sirdfield, C. (2006) 'Piloting a new role in mental health – prison based health trainers', *Journal of Mental Health Workforce Development*, 1: 15–22.

Sirdfield, C., Bevan, L., Calverley, M., Mitchell, L., Craven, J. and Brooker, C. (2007) *A Guide to Implementing the New Futures Health Trainer Role Across the Criminal Justice System*. Lincoln: University of Lincoln.

Smith, C. (2000) '"Healthy prisons": a contradiction in terms?', *Howard Journal of Criminal Justice*, 39: 339–53.

Smith, C. (2002) 'Punishment and pleasure: women, food and the imprisoned body', *Sociological Review*, 50: 197–211.

Social Exclusion Unit (2002) *Reducing Re-offending by Ex-prisoners*. London: Crown.

Stewart, D. (2008) *The Problems and Needs of Newly Sentenced Prisoners: Results from a National Survey*. London: Ministry of Justice.

United Nations (1966) *International Covenant on Economic, Social and Cultural Rights*. Geneva: Office of the United Nations High Commissioner for Human Rights.

United Nations (1990) Basic Principles for the Treatment of Prisoners. Adopted and Proclaimed by General Assembly Resolution 45/111 of 14 December 1990. New York: United Nations.

Weinstein, C. (2010) 'The United States needs a WHO health in prisons project', *Public Health*, 124: 626–8.

Whitehead, D. (2006) 'The health promoting prison (HPP) and its imperative for nursing', *International Journal of Nursing Studies*, 43: 123–31.

WHO (World Health Organization) (1986) *Ottawa Charter for Health Promotion*. Geneva: WHO.

WHO (World Health Organization) (1995) *Health in Prisons. Health Promotion in the Prison Setting.* Summary report on a WHO meeting, London 15–17 October 1995. Copenhagen: WHO Regional Office for Europe.

WHO (World Health Organization) (1998) *Mental Health Promotion in Prisons.* Report on a WHO meeting. Copenhagen: WHO Regional Office for Europe.

WHO (World Health Organization) (2003a) *Moscow Declaration: Prison Health as Part of Public Health.* Copenhagen: WHO Regional Office for Europe.

WHO (World Health Organization) (2003b) *Promoting the Health of Young People in Custody.* Copenhagen: WHO Regional Office for Europe.

WHO (World Health Organization) (2007) *Health in Prisons. A WHO Guide to the Essentials in Prison Health.* Copenhagen: WHO Regional Office for Europe.

WHO (World Health Organization) (2008) Background Paper for Trenčín Statement on Prisons and Mental Health. Copenhagen: WHO Regional Office for Europe.

Woodall, J. (2007) 'Barriers to positive mental health in a Young Offenders Institution: a qualitative study', *Health Education Journal*, 66, 132–40.

Woodall, J. (2010a) 'Control and choice in three category-C English prisons: implications for the concept and practice of the health promoting prison'. Unpublished PhD thesis, Faculty of Health. Leeds: Leeds Metropolitan University.

Woodall, J. (2010b) 'Exploring concepts of health with male prisoners in three category-C English prisons', *International Journal of Health Promotion and Education*, 48: 115–22.

Woodall, J. (2010c) 'Working with prisoners and young offenders', in D. Conrad and A.K. White (eds), *Promoting Men's Mental Health*. Oxford: Radcliffe.

Woodall, J., Dixey, R., Green, J. and Newell, C. (2009) 'Healthier prisons: the role of a prison visitors' centre', *International Journal of Health Promotion and Education*, 47: 12–18.

Part 3

The Workplace Setting

Introduction to Part III

Workplaces as a Setting for Health Promotion

Margaret Hodgins

There are principally two reasons why the workplace has been identified as a priority setting for health promotion. Firstly, it offers an opportunity to support the promotion of health in a large audience and secondly, being employed and having good working conditions are now recognized as significant determinants of health at both individual and population levels.

At the level of the population, a healthy workforce contributes to the maximization of the production of goods and services and reduces the costs of work-related morbidity and mortality. At an individual level, work has the potential to promote health and wellbeing. Primarily, it provides income that enables people to purchase goods and services but work also allows people to develop and use skills, offers opportunities for a sense of personal control and achievement, social contact and interpersonal relationships. Conversely, adverse working conditions can lead to both physical and psychosocial health hazards. While fatalities (estimated at 2 million per year) have decreased in recent years, work-related illnesses have increased. Illnesses associated with working conditions may be linked to the more subtle aspects of working conditions such as long hours culture, incivility in relationships or organizational injustice. For example, the risk of coronary heart disease is increased by 50% by work-related stress, and this is consistently associated with high demand and low decision latitude in the workplace. This argues strongly for taking a settings approach to workplace health, which is explored in depth in Chapter 12.

Treating the workplace as a setting conceals the fact that workplaces are very diverse. Variation in size is the most obvious dimension, but workplaces also vary greatly according to their purpose, structure and culture. It is interesting to see here that three very different workplaces – a multinational manufacturing enterprise, a multisite public service organization and a medium-sized medical supplies firm – all describe successful settings-based approaches to health management. There are a number of similarities across all three case studies.

Firstly, all employed an approach that integrated three core elements of good workplace health promotion practice, often described in comprehensive models of workplace health promotion. Occupational health and safety, which is primarily concerned with health protection through the reduction of the physical and chemical hazards of the work environment, is a statutory requirement. Many organizations fail to take their health activities beyond this point. Specific behaviour change programmes that encourage individual workers to give up high-risk behaviours and engage in healthier behaviours in order to avoid specific diseases are common enough, especially where organizations pay health insurance premiums for employees. However, the significant addition to these two sets of activities, that distinguishes the setting approach, is the investment in interventions that address organizational sources of worker ill health. The preparedness of a workplace to address its own work practices, management structures, or the explicit and implicit expectations of workers is evidence that a whole system approach is being taken. The case studies in this section illustrate a mindset that sees health as something the organization or the company should be nurturing, rather than just something individual employees should adopt. This is exemplified in Royal Mail's Dignity and Respect At Work programme which addresses organizational practices that lead to employees being exposed to bullying and harassment, and in Williams Medical Supplies (WMS) the implementation of the Management Standards Approach to stress, which addresses organizational level determinants of stress. In all cases, health was understood to embrace physical, mental and social aspects.

Participation and employee involvement is described in all three cases, whether it is through formal surveys, health circles, or less formal listening times, and 'departmental huddles'. Organizations displayed an openness to employee ideas about health and wellbeing and suggestions for projects and programmes. Small and medium-sized enterprises, often described as having multiple barriers to adopting health promotion, are as well placed as large organizations in respect of participation.

Monitoring of health programmes through the measuring of outcomes and process, and feeding evaluative material back into planning structures is also evident in the three case studies. However, the difficulty in identifying how positive organizational outcomes are tracked specifically to health promotion programmes is acknowledged at Volkswagen, and highlights the complexity of evaluating settings work, discussed in earlier sections of the book.

Stakeholder conflict, the perceived clash between the business goals of production and profit, and the costs, both cash and opportunity, of activities to protect and promote health, is often seen as a difficulty for the workplace setting. The alternative view, however, is that protecting and promoting the health of workers makes good business sense, and the three organizations that describe their programmes in this part of the book, clearly subscribe to the latter view. Each refers to their conviction that protecting and promoting the health of employees is a sound corporate strategy. Maintaining the health of employees is an investment in the future.

It is interesting to note that in Chapters 14 and 15 external initiatives, designed to facilitate and encourage health promotion in workplaces, were engaged with to good effect. In the case of Royal Mail the company faced a crisis of survival, with loss of monopoly in a competitive marketplace and as a result new leadership championed a recovery plan. This led the company to link in with the 'great place to work' initiative which gave them impetus to consider health more widely in terms of both the health of the organization and its business methodologies, as well as at the level of individual employee health improvements. In Williams Medical Supplies, the Welsh Assembly Government-funded workplace health promotion accreditation programme Health at Work: the Corporate Standard, was discovered, which afforded the opportunity to develop a coherent, corporate health programme, with external consultation, feedback and support. Both external programmes have an award-based approach, a factor that perhaps could be exploited more in workplace settings work.

Analysis of the settings approach elsewhere in this book, (see, for example, Chapter 2, Chapter 3) refers to the interconnectedness of settings. Workplace settings are part of the community setting in which they reside, to whom they provide goods, services and employment. Corporate social responsibility (CSR) refers to an organization's willingness to embrace responsibility for their actions, to encourage community growth and development, and to voluntarily eliminate practices that may cause harm in the wider community. Volkswagen AG outlines positive practice in this regard, with support for global HIV/AIDS projects, sharing of occupational health and safety training resources with suppliers and involving dealerships in health protection and health promotion activities. Royal Mail is also very active in supporting charity and volunteering initiatives, encouraging employees to identify and develop a relationship with a nationwide major supported charity initiative. As well as generating fund-raising for the partner charity, employees are enabled to engage in volunteering opportunities and development projects.

Conclusions

Despite the primacy of the workplace setting, it has been observed that many workplaces either do not adopt health promotion programmes, or confine activities to one or two initiatives that focus on a health behaviour (for example, campus walking routes, healthy options on the canteen menu), rather than taking a whole system, settings approach. However, the case studies in this section, although very different from one another, have demonstrated that if the organization takes the view that protecting and promoting the health of employees is a sound corporate strategy, and applies a comprehensive model that integrates occupational health and safety, voluntary health behaviour changes and organizational level initiatives, positive health management can be developed and maintained.

Participation with employees and an openness to monitoring and evaluating all elements of a health management programme emerge as critical success factors. External support structures, such as those found in award-based initiatives, seem also to contribute to engaging workplaces with health protection and promotion.

Perhaps what is most noteworthy about the cases outlined in this section is that health promotion or health management has become an integral part of the organization, in such a way that it recedes, and as a discrete entity becomes more remote. As such, the organization is a healthy organization and the setting truly has become one where that health is created and lived by people.

12

Healthy Workplaces: Balancing Employee Health and Economic Expediency

Paul Fleming

Aims

- To explore the context within which healthy workplaces contribute to improving the health of populations from national to local level
- To explore the role of the Healthy Workplace concept in promoting employee health and strengthening economic potential of enterprises and national economies
- To examine the World Health Organization perspective on the concept of the Healthy Workplace
- To discuss the role of partnership approaches in developing Healthy Workplace initiatives

The context for healthy workplaces

In describing the context for healthy workplaces it is important that we first acknowledge that the health and wellbeing of the global community is inextricably linked with the health of the global workforce which, according to the International Labour Organization (ILO), represents some 60% of the world's population (ILO, 2010). In 2008, the 18th World Congress on Safety and Health at Work, which generated the Seoul Declaration on Safety and Health at Work, indicated that, globally, workplaces suffered some 2.3 million work-related fatalities annually (both accidents and disease) with 337 million reports of accidents requiring more than four days' absence from work (Al-Tuwaijri et al., 2008). Hämäläinen et al. (2009) have noted that while the total number of accidents in the workplace and work-related disease fatalities has increased, fatality rates per 100,000 workers have decreased. They further observe that the daily reality of such statistics is that more than 5,000 people die each day because of work-related diseases and over 960,000 workers are injured in work-related accidents. These statistics represent a loss of some 4% of global Gross Domestic Product (GDP) (Al-Tuwaijri et al., 2008), which is approximately the same scale as the predicted increase in global GDP for 2011 (IMF, 2010; World Bank, 2010).

In the United Kingdom (UK) 30 million working days are lost annually to occupational illnesses and injuries at a cost to the economy of £30 billion, which is approximately 3% of the GDP (Institute of Directors, 2006). In 2006, the Confederation of British Industry (CBI) estimated that 175 million days of sickness absence were being recorded each year, this representing seven days per employee. Several other measures of the same issue in 2006 came to somewhat different conclusions: the Chartered Institute of Personnel and Development (CIPD) showed 8.4 days of sickness absence and the Office for National Statistics' Labour Force Survey (LFS) estimated six days per worker per year, representing a total of approximately 150 million working days lost annually (Office for National Statistics, 2006). Whichever figure is used, the burden of illness and injury associated with work activity is such that the losses at a national level are considerable. A statistical picture of the state of health in the UK workplace is outlined in Box 12.1.

Box 12.1   The state of health in UK workplaces

In 2009–10 (the most recent figures available), the Health and Safety Executive's statistics for the UK (excluding Northern Ireland) showed that:

- 1.3 million people who had worked in the previous year were suffering from an illness, whether new or of long standing, which they believed had its origins or had been exacerbated by their current or past work.
- 555,000 were new cases; 152 workplace fatalities were recorded (0.5 per 100,000 workers).
- 121,430 (473 per 100,000) other injuries to employees were reported under RIDDOR (Reporting of Injuries, Diseases and Dangerous Occurrences Regulations 1995), the system which required formal reporting of defined workplace illnesses and injuries (Health and Safety Executive, 2010).
- 28.5 million working days were lost overall (1.2 days per worker); of these, 23.4 million days were due to work-related ill health and 5.1 million due to workplace injury (Health and Safety Executive, 2010).

These figures represent challenges for government and for employers from the most modest SME to the largest corporate or public sector employer. It is clear from the statistics that the maintenance of a healthy workforce makes sound economic sense and that the role of a healthy workplace is important in this process. Indeed, a healthy workforce has been deemed by the World Health Organization (WHO) to be:

> of paramount importance to the productivity, competitiveness and sustainability of enterprises, communities, and to national and regional economies. (WHO, 2010a: 1)

This is reflected in the ILO recognition of the global magnitude of occupational injuries, diseases and deaths, and the need for further action to reduce them. It also acknowledges that occupational injuries, diseases and deaths have a negative effect on productivity and on economic and social development (ILO, 2006).The question must be asked, however, is economic expediency the only driver for seeking to maintain a healthy workforce? It is the purpose of this chapter to show that a healthy workforce, working in a healthy workplace, has benefits to employers, employees and their families, communities and national populations which go beyond pure economic expediency into issues of the quality of life of individuals and communities.

In the United Kingdom context, where the costs associated with absence from work through illness or injury is of the order of £100 billion per year, the importance of good employee health has been recognized at national level by the Department of Health for England. It has viewed being in employment as a key contributor to good health status in both the physical and mental health domains (Department of Health, 2008). Recent government thinking has indicated that:

> Enabling more people to work, safeguarding and improving their health at work, and supporting disabled people or people who have health conditions to enter, stay in or return to work are critical components of our public health challenge. (Department of Health, 2010: 44).

This perspective is drawn from Dame Carol Black's seminal report on the health of working age people in England, *Working for a Healthier Tomorrow* (Black, 2008). Here, she indicated that while economic costs of ill health in the workplace can be calculated, the human costs which go far beyond the individual worker are significant and much less easy to quantify (Department for Work and Pensions, 2008). This has implications for any government that seeks to improve the health of its population through working towards appropriate public health targets.

Having established the link between the health of workers and the overall health status of the global and national populations, it is also necessary to have a clear understanding of the concept of health that underpins the concept of the Healthy Workplace. The WHO founding definition of health as being a state of complete physical, mental and social health and not merely the absence of disease or infirmity (WHO, 1948) has been somewhat superseded in recent years. Key documents such as the Alma Ata Declaration (WHO, 1978) and the Ottawa Charter for Health Promotion (WHO, 1986) built a foundation for a much stronger emphasis on the social determinants of health (WHO, 2008). The WHO Commission on the Social Determinants of Health (WHO, 2008: 1) described the social determinants of health as:

> ... the conditions in which people are born, grow, live, work and age, including the health system. These circumstances are shaped by the distribution of money, power and resources at global, national and local levels, which are themselves influenced by policy choices. The social determinants of health are mostly responsible for health inequities – the unfair and avoidable differences in health status seen within and between countries.

In order to address these inequities, the Commission made three recommendations. The first two recommendations required action through, firstly, improving daily living conditions and secondly, through tackling the inequitable distribution of money, power and resources. Underpinning these recommendations was a third that focused on measuring and understanding the problem of health inequity and assessing the impact of the action (WHO, 2008). Within its recommendations, the Commission was clear that a major factor in reducing inequities in health was the provision of fair employment and decent work. Fair employment was seen, from a public health perspective, to be a multifactorial concept that contributed to an employer–employee relationship which was infused with the ethical principle of justice (Beauchamp and Childress, 2008). Decent work was cast as employment where opportunities were afforded for:

> work [that] is productive and delivers a fair income, security in the workplace, and social protection for families; better prospects for personal development and social integration; freedom for people to express their concerns, organize, and participate in the decisions that affect their lives; and equality of opportunity and treatment for all women and men. (WHO, 2008: 76)

When the Commission on the Social Determinants came to a detailed examination of the issue of work related to health, three recommendations were made in relation to reducing inequities in health. These were:

- Make full and fair employment and decent work a central goal of national and international social and economic policy making.
- Achieve health equity by ensuring safe, secure, and fairly paid work, year-round work opportunities, and healthy work–life balance for all.
- Improve the working conditions for all workers to reduce their exposure to material hazards, work-related stress, and health-damaging behaviours.

Such recommendations were seen as taking in a raft of considerations, including the needs of vulnerable populations (notably women and children), the quality of working conditions, the rights and representation of workers, adequate income, training and health and safety in the workplace. It is interesting to note that the Commission's overall approach to the social determinants of health was again adopted by its Chair, Sir Michael Marmot, in his Strategic Review of

Health Inequalities in England post-2010, *Fair Society, Healthy Lives* (Marmot et al., 2010). Among the policy objectives indicated in this review was the creation of fair employment in good jobs. The review recognized that unemployment in all social classes was linked with higher mortality than the employed population. It also recognized that the lower the status of a worker, the less control they had over their working environment and that this in turn increased the risk of lower health status. It is in this context that we now consider the development, over time, of the Healthy Workplace Initiative.

Healthy workplaces: a developing concept

Given that the case for workplace health promotion in the global economy is strong, it is no surprise that the WHO has been at the forefront of international development of the Healthy Workplace. New impetus was introduced in the final years of the twentieth century. At the 1996 World Health Assembly's *Global Strategy for Occupational Health for All*, the WHO sought to set the agenda for health at work through:

> The promotion of a healthy work environment, healthy work practices, and health at work; the strengthening of occupational health services; the establishment of appropriate support services for occupational health; the development of occupational health standards based on scientific risk assessment; the development of human resources; the establishment of registration and data systems and information support; and strengthening of research. (WHO, 1996: 1)

While the effect of achieving greater productivity and thus economic benefit underpinned this agenda, it is clear that the health and wellbeing of employees was central to the strategy.

Ten years on, the *Stresa Declaration on Worker's Health* (WHO, 2006) developed the Global Strategy in the context of globalization and the development of national initiatives in workplace legislation and the continuing growth of economic and social inequalities between the richest and poorest in societies across the globe. This reflected the previous year's *Bangkok Charter for Health Promotion* (WHO, 2005) where it was acknowledged that other factors that influence health include rapid and often adverse social, economic and demographic changes that affect working conditions. In the decade between the Global Plan and the Stresa Declaration (1996–2006) much work was undertaken to develop workplace health promotion at international and national level. At the international level, the European Network of Health Promoting Workplaces (ENHPW) generated both the *Luxembourg Declaration on Workplace Health Promotion in the European Union* (ENHPW, 1997) and the *Barcelona Declaration on Developing Good Workplace Health Practice in Europe* (ENHPW, 2002). In the UK, examples of similar settings-based initiatives included England's *Health, Work and Wellbeing – Caring for Our Future* (Department for Work and Pensions, 2005) and Northern Ireland's *Working for Health* (HSENI, 2003).

At the Sixtieth World Health Assembly, WHO created a Global Plan of Action on Workers' Health 2008–2017. The plan had five key objectives, specifically:

- To devise and implement policy instruments on workers' health
- To protect and promote health in the workplace
- To improve the performance of, and access to, occupational health services
- To provide and communicate evidence for action and practice
- To incorporate workers' health into other policies

(WHO, 2007: 4).

In themselves, these objectives were neither innovative nor novel. It is interesting, however, to note a subtle shift from the Global Plan of Action of ten years before (WHO, 1996). The terms 'policy', 'improve performance' and 'access' denoted a strengthening of an evidence-based approach. Further, the intention of integrating workers' health into policy beyond health and employment policy indicated a move towards a joined-up government approach.

Defining and modelling the Healthy Workplace

It was in 2010 that the WHO produced its *Healthy Workplaces: A Model for Action – For Employers, Workers, Policy Makers and Practitioners* (WHO, 2010a). This model encapsulated much of the thinking captured in previous workplace health models. A Healthy Workplace is defined as:

> one in which workers and managers collaborate to use a continual improvement process to protect and promote the health, safety and wellbeing of all workers and the sustainability of the workplace by considering the following, based on identified needs:
>
> - health and safety concerns in the physical work environment;
> - health, safety and wellbeing concerns in the psychosocial work environment, including organization of work and workplace culture;
> - personal health resources in the workplace; and
> - ways of participating in the community to improve the health of workers, their families and other members of the community. (WHO, 2010a: 6)

The development of this definition includes several markers as to the requirements for relationships within the workplace environment. In the first instance, the need for partnership between management and workforce is stressed, reflecting the need to optimize employee commitment which is critical to optimal performance in the workplace (Boxall and Purcell, 2003; Seymour and Dupré, 2008). Towards the end of the twentieth century, however, the nature of the employer/employee relationship in many countries travelled an interesting and at times troubled and fragmented path. This was particularly so in the UK where, by 1998, the previously strong position of unions in collective bargaining had diminished to a point where the emphasis of their activity had shifted dramatically towards representation of workers in grievance procedures (Cully et al., 1999). In the UK, while employers have reported more positively on employee relations than have employees, formal joint consultative committees in the workplace had declined in advance of the Information and Consultation of Employees Regulations, 2005 (Kersley et al., 2006) and employees have reacted negatively to management control strategies (Danford et al., 2005). The overall effect, which has been observed over a much longer period, is to provide a weakened base for positive partnerships between employers and employees (Karnes, 2008). This effect has been reinforced in the international arena in recent years through the failure of a number of large multinational corporations. The weaknesses exposed in the banking and financial services sector in the global financial crisis of 2008 have raised many questions for employees in these sectors (Alexis and Pressman, 2010). Such a loss of confidence highlights the need for a renewed emphasis on corporate social responsibility (Lowe, 2004).

A second consideration in the defining of the Healthy Workplace is the acknowledgement that continual improvement is basic to strategic development in a more coherent planning environment. All of the countries in the OECD and increasing numbers in the developing world have developed occupational health or workplace health strategies that encourage continual improvement measures. Early work on continual quality improvement in health promotion (Kahan and Goodstadt, 1999; Tindill and Stewart, 1993) is reflected in a recent definition of continual improvement in public health which has been has been identified as:

> having the ability to improve public health practice through the use of a deliberate and defined improvement process such as Plan-Do-Check-Act, which is focused on activities that are responsive to community needs and improving population health. It refers to a continuous and ongoing effort to achieve measurable improvements in the efficiency, effectiveness, performance, accountability, outcomes, and other indicators of quality in services or processes which achieve equity and improve the health of the community. (Riley, 2010: 6)

This approach can be adopted at a range of levels, but is more often effective at the point where planning and delivery of programmes and initiatives occurs. The WHO has itself developed a framework for continual improvement in large and small enterprises (WHO, 2010b).

A third component of the definition is the need to link sustainability to the promotion of health in the workplace. Sustainability was seen by the World Summit on Sustainable Development in South Africa as encompassing:

> the interdependent and mutually reinforcing pillars of sustainable development – economic development, social development and environmental protection, at the local, national, regional and global levels. (United Nations, 2002: 1)

In terms of the Healthy Workplace, partnership in decision making for sustainability is integral to the development of the health promoting setting (Ennals,

2002). At local level, therefore, the implications are that sustainability involves the generation of a sound economic base which is inextricably linked with the development of the people in the workplace and the provision of an environmentally sensitive working environment. This again reinforces the synergies between employee health and wellbeing and the generation of appropriate wealth for enterprises and economies. Issues such as energy use and conservation, recycling policy, use of sustainable materials in administrative and production processes and protection of the environment in which the workplace is situated are all part of the sustainability agenda. Workers may become more ready partners with their employers in the endeavour to optimize sustainability.

The Healthy Workplace is also based on identified needs. Needs assessment takes account of the perspectives of both the employee and employer. The size of the workplace can pose a range of challenges in health needs assessment with SMEs and large employers posing different challenges, whether located in the private or public sectors. Thus SMEs may require a more naturalistic approach involving observation of individual workers' behaviours and qualitative enquiry

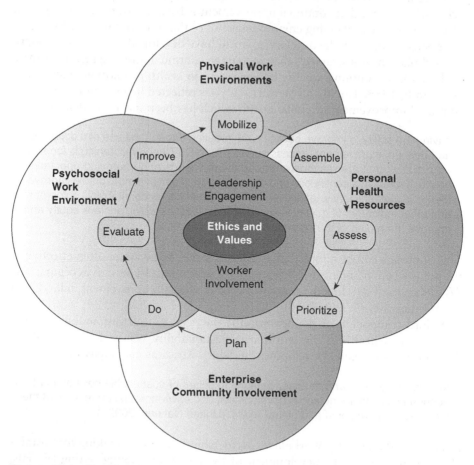

Figure 12.1 Healthy Workplace Model

relating to perceived health needs of employee and employer in the workplace (Moore et al., 2011). Corporate employers, on the other hand, need an equally sensitive evidence base but this may involve a more eclectic mix of quantitative and qualitative data. This may include the assessment of trends in, for example, sickness absence data, health and safety incidents and near misses and compensation claims mixed with focus group findings on worker perspectives on workplace health issues (Harvey and Fleming, 2004).

When considering the Healthy Workplace Model (see Figure 12.1) it is interesting to note that four avenues of influence are identified, namely: the physical work environment, the psychosocial environment, personal health resources and enterprise community involvement. Each of these avenues is defined in Box 12.2. In terms of the physical work environment in most contemporary Healthy Workplace initiatives in the developed world, the facilitation of a safe and healthy environment where physical hazards are reduced, or where possible eliminated, is a strong foundation of the setting, based on legislative imperatives (Harvey and Fleming, 2004). However, as recognized in the preamble to the *Luxembourg Declaration on Workplace Health Promotion*, occupational health and safety by itself cannot address the full range of health issues encountered in the workplace (ENHPW, 1997).

Box 12.2   Avenues of influence in the Healthy Workplace

The Physical Work Environment is … the part of the workplace facility that can be detected by human or electronic senses, including the structure, air, machines, furniture, products, chemicals, materials and processes that are present or that occur in the workplace, and which can affect the physical or mental safety, health and wellbeing of workers. If the worker performs his or her tasks outdoors or in a vehicle, then that location is the physical work environment. (WHO 2010b: 91)

The Psychosocial Work Environment is … the organization of work and the organizational culture; attitudes, values, beliefs and practices that are demonstrated on a daily basis in the enterprise/organization, and which affect the mental and physical wellbeing of employees. These are sometimes generally referred to as workplace stressors, which may cause emotional or mental stress to workers. (WHO, 2010b: 92)

Personal Health Resources are … the supportive environment, health services, information, resources, opportunities and flexibility an enterprise provides to workers to support or motivate their efforts to improve or maintain healthy personal lifestyle practices, as well as to monitor and support their ongoing physical and mental health (WHO 2010b: 93).

Enterprise Community Involvement … comprises the activities, expertise, and other resources an enterprise engages in or provides to the social and physical community or communities in which it operates; and which affect the physical and mental health, safety and wellbeing of workers and their families. It includes activities, expertise and resources provided to the immediate local environment, but also the broader global environment. (WHO, 2010b: 94)

A point worthy of note is that in a number of jurisdictions, not least the UK, health and safety in the workplace has been brought into disrepute in recent years (IOSH, 2009) due to a number of well publicized cases where health and safety measures have been at best over-zealous and at worst ridiculous. This led to an early act of the UK Coalition Government, elected in 2010, in commissioning Lord Young to report on how health and safety could regain lost credibility and regain its accessible and defensible status. Young's aim in reappraising health and safety in the workplace was:

> to free businesses from unnecessary bureaucratic burdens and the fear of having to pay out unjustified damages claims and legal fees. Above all it means applying common sense not just to compensation but to everyday decisions once again. (Young, 2010: 9)

Of equal importance to the physical environment is the pervasiveness of the psychosocial work environment (Kelloway et al., 2008). This element of the workplace environment will undoubtedly affect the attitudes of workers to their work outcomes, those with whom they interact in the workplace and also their perceptions of the place in society that they achieve through their work. Issues of poor leadership can have an effect on the health of workers (Kivimaki, 2005; Shain and Kramer, 2004). Key problems in managing the psychosocial environment include a poor organizational culture which may lack structure and purpose and fail to accord all workers their basic rights. Poor organization of actual work tasks and practices may also bring stress and uncertainty, as can a top-down style of management which reduces workers' control through disempowering management styles (WHO, 2010b).

The third avenue of influence is that of personal health resources (see Box 12.2 for a definition). Such issues include low levels of physical inactivity; dietary issues that result in either obesity or specific deficiencies; substance use, including alcohol and tobacco; sleep issues; undiagnosed/untreated illness; lack of knowledge/resources to prevent key conditions such as STIs including HIV. These issues, while important, can often be selectively targeted by employers and health professionals as the focus of what they call health promotion (Moore et al., 2011). An information-giving strategic approach is developed which can have victim-blaming aspects (Tones and Tilford, 2001), placing responsibility on the individual without providing the contextual support. In order to address these issues in a holistic manner, health education needs to be accompanied by structural supports such as access to fitness facilities and appropriate transport; provision of healthy food choices (subsidized where necessary), substance use policies (including smoke free environments) and flexible working (WHO, 2010b).

The final avenue of interest is enterprise community development. The definition in Box 12.2 clearly highlights the fact that workplaces are a part of wider communities and environments. They can be affected by poor indicators in the physical environment that differ across countries, with the UK and Ireland having issues, for example, including air quality, and congested roads (Mitchell, 2005). The more lacking a community is in infrastructure, the more likely it is to have health and safety deficits, poorer literacy rates and less capacity to fund its own non-profit enterprises. In addressing the ways in which workplaces can be involved in the community, it is clear that an eclectic range of voluntary, regulatory, legislative, fiscal and other financial measures needs to be adopted to enable enterprises from SME to large employers to promote the health of their workers through community engagement.

The process: initiating and sustaining a programme

The Healthy Workplace Model has as a central tenet: the concept of a sound ethical and values base (Kriger and Hanson, 1999). The need for the dynamic development of ethical principles for health promotion has been identified as an ongoing concern in the international debate relating to the Bangkok Charter for Health Promotion (WHO, 2005). The Bangkok Charter saw a shift in emphasis from the socio-ecological, communitarian approach of the Ottawa Charter (WHO, 1986) to an investment-led, macro-factor global approach to health promotion policy and planning (Mittelmark, 2007). Given that the principle of health equity has been central to health promotion since the Ottawa Charter (WHO, 1986), it is no surprise that the WHO Model recognizes the need for equal contributions of key players in the Healthy Workplace through the engagement of employers and involvement of workers. The tension for employers in ensuring a healthy working environment for their employees, while at the same time ensuring optimization of the profitability of their business, is very real. Employers need to balance a range of considerations, including the need to contain operating costs through optimizing staffing efficiencies. At the same time, however, they need to recognize that the costs associated with providing an optimally healthy workplace can be recouped through increased productivity, decreased staff turnover and reduced sickness absence rates. Evidence shows that there is a sound business case for the development of the Healthy Workplace (WHO, 2010b).

Advocacy with employers can be strengthened to encourage them to move from a do no harm approach of fulfilling only their basic health and safety requirements, on the grounds that workers' health is their personal concern, to a more fulsome development of a healthy workplace (Bevan, 2010). It is also useful for employers to be aware that their reputation for taking account of workers' welfare can be a deciding factor in good employees deciding to work for a specific employer (Highhouse and Hoffman, 2001). Workers also need to be fully involved in the development of the Healthy Workplace and employers therefore need to be committed to the empowerment of workers (WHO, 1986). This involves equal status being accorded to management and workforce (Grawitch et al., 2009).

Agreeing a partnership approach between management and workers and the values base underpinning that partnership fulfils the 'Mobilize' phase, which is the first element of the process cycle (see Figure 12.1). (Partnership in settings is discussed in more detail in Chapter 4.) The cycle actually describes the steps necessary for using the Healthy Workplace Model in creating a Healthy Workplace

Programme. Mobilization entails obtaining commitment from employers, employees, unions and other interested parties through the development of agreed policies for the development of a healthy workplace. 'Assemble' involves bringing to reality the investment of resource (human, financial and physical) needed in the development of a healthy workplace (Downie and Sharpe, 2007). This also sets in place committee structures which will recognize both statutory and non-statutory responsibilities in developing a healthy workplace while at the same time ensuring that all relevant groups are represented, for example, women and disabled workers (Hart, 2008). This goes beyond mere agreement to participate, involving agreement to fund, discuss, innovate and be open to change.

'Assess' involves employing an effective needs assessment strategy (Fleming, 1999), which draws together the knowledge base necessary to both describe the current situation in the workplace and also the desired situation towards which the Healthy Workplace initiative is travelling. This will involve a range of enquiry designs, both qualitative and quantitative, which are contextually appropriate. Having obtained the necessary knowledge, the next phase of the cycle, 'Prioritize', entails setting the criteria with which the order of addressing those issues identified in the assessment phase can be undertaken. These criteria need to be agreed by both workers and management and also be ranked in order of importance according to a framework such as Maslow's Hierarchy of Need (Maslow, 1970) or Bradshaw's dimensions of need (Bradshaw, 1972). The seriousness of the issue in terms of both severity and likelihood of risk, the ability to provide a remedy and the cost effectiveness of specific interventions should be taken into account here. Gaining agreement at this point may be challenging in that employers and employees may bring very different perspectives to the prioritization process.

'Plan' seeks to develop a strategic Healthy Workplace plan that would have a timeline of some 3–5 years. The plethora of health promotion planning models would provide the necessary tools to bring a coherent approach to this phase (see, for example, Ewles and Simnett, 2003). This would then spawn annual operational plans which would themselves generate specific topic plans, for example a healthy eating plan or a risk management plan derived from risk audit. The penultimate stage is self-explanatory. 'Do' means just that: implement the strategic plan through the ongoing actions of its operational and topic plans. This could nonetheless provide a range of logistical challenges and need careful planning. The final stage, 'Evaluate', needs to be operationalized from the outset of the 'Do' phase and is seen as vital to the credibility and integrity of the health promoting settings approach (Dooris, 2006). As with the planning phase, a range of evaluation strategies is available (Dugdill and Springett, 2001) although it must be recognized that evaluating complex settings such as workplaces can, like the 'Do' phase, present a range of challenges.

So what are the implications of implementing the Healthy Workplace Model for employers, employees, governments and communities? As will become clear in Chapters 13–15, the Healthy Workplace concept offers interesting and unique possibilities to organizations as diverse as a large multinational vehicle manufacturing company, a large public sector organization in the UK in the form of Royal

Mail and, on a much smaller and focused scale, SMEs. It is clear that a business case can be made for the viability of the Healthy Workplace and that a growing number of such settings would be to the benefit of local and national economies. It must be asked, however, if the economic imperative should be the principal driver for developing healthy workplaces. It would seem that a much more pressing motivator is the improvement in the working lives of millions of those employed in the global workforce. The great benefit of the Healthy Workplace Model is that it can be adapted to create a 'best fit' to any workplace situation and is a dynamic process that can respond to changing conditions within an organization or SME. Further, returning to where this chapter started, the ability for a growing cadre of healthy workplaces to address the numbers of days lost through work-related illness, injury or death could have a significant positive effect on national and global economies. With the potential for gains to be made by both workers and their employers it can be argued that healthy workplaces can have the potential, and the responsibility, to balance employee health with economic expediency.

Summary points

- The burden of work-related disease, injury and fatalities at the national and global levels is such that strategies such as the Healthy Workplace are necessary to improve the health of workers.

- Governments consistently include being in work as a key element of improving both personal and public health thus contributing to national economic growth.

- The WHO Healthy Workplace Model provides a useful framework within which large employers and SMEs can promote the health of workers and enhance the economic prospects of employers and communities.

- Healthy workplaces need to be developed through a genuine partnership between employers and employees, with organizational support being balanced with workers' taking personal responsibility for their own health in a favourable workplace environment.

Online Further Reading

Moore, A.B., Parahoo, K. and Fleming, P. (2011) 'Managers' understanding of workplace health promotion within small and medium-sized enterprises: A phenomenological study', *Health Education* Journal, 70: 92-101.

Moore et al.'s article explores SME managers' perspectives on the interconnectedness of workplace health promotion and business development. The role that managers perceive themselves to play in creating healthy workplaces is key to the development of Healthy Workplace strategies.

References

Al-Tuwaijri, S., Feitshans, I., Fedotov, I., Gifford, M., Gold, D., Machida, S., Nahmias, M., Niu, S. and Sandi, G. (2008) XVIII World Congress on Safety and Health at Work Introductory Report. *Beyond Death and Injuries: The ILO's Role in Promoting Safe and Healthy Jobs*. Geneva: International Labour Organization.

Alexis, G.Y. and Pressman, S. (2010) 'After shame; before corporate moral obligation (CMO): ethical lag and the credit crisis', *International Journal of Management Concepts and Philosophy*, 4 (3/4): 244–66.

Beauchamp, T.L. and Childress, J.F. (2008) *Principles of Biomedical Ethics*. Oxford: Oxford University Press.

Bevan, S. (2010) *The Business Case for Employee Health and Wellbeing*. London: The Work Foundation.

Black, C. (2008) *Working for a Healthier Tomorrow – Review of the Health of Britain's Working Age Population*. London: The Stationery Office.

Boxall, P. and Purcell, J. (2003) *Strategy and Human Resource Management*. Basingstoke: Palgrave.

Bradshaw, J.(1972) 'A taxonomy of social need', *New Society* (March), 640–3.

Cully, M., Woodland, S. and O'Reilly, A. (1999) *Britain at Work: As Depicted by the 1998 Workplace Employee Relations Survey*. London: Routledge.

Danford, A., Richardson, M., Stewart, P. and Tailby, S. (2005) 'Voice in the UK: comparative studies of union strategy and worker experience', *Economic and Industrial Democracy*, 26: 593–620.

Department of Health for England (2008) *Health Inequalities: Progress and Next Steps*. London: Department of Health.

Department of Health for England (2010) *Healthy Lives, Healthy People*. London: Department of Health.

Department for Work and Pensions (2005) *Health, Work and Wellbeing – Caring for Our Future*. London: Department for Work and Pensions. www.dwp.gov.uk/docs/health-and-wellbeing.pdf (accessed 26 November 2010).

Department for Work and Pensions (2008) *Working for a Healthier Tomorrow*. London: Department for Work and Pensions. Available at: www.dwp.gov.uk/docs/hwwb-working-for-a-healthier-tomorrow.pdf (accessed 26 November 2010).

Dooris, M. (2006) Healthy Settings: Challenges to generating evidence of effectiveness. *Health Promotion International*, 21 (1): 55–65.

Downie, A.M. and Sharpe, D.J. (2007) 'Why do managers allocate resources to workplace health promotion programmes in countries with national health coverage?', *Health Promotion International*, 22: 102–111.

Dugdill, L. and Springett, J. (2001) 'Evaluating health promotion programmes in the workplace', in I. Rootman, M. Goodstadt, B. Hyndman, D. McQueen, L. Potvin, J. Springett and E. Ziglio, E. (eds), *Evaluation in Health Promotion: Principles and Perspectives*. Copenhagen: WHO Regional Office for Europe.

Ennals, R. (2002) *Partnerships for Sustainable Healthy Workplaces*. Derby: British Occupational Hygiene Society. Available at: www.worldstp.com/WSP/RichardEnnals.pdf (accessed on 3 December 2010).

ENHPW (European Network of Health Promoting Workplaces) (1997) *Luxembourg Declaration on Workplace Health Promotion in the European Union (updated 2007)*. Luxembourg: ENHPW.

ENHPW (European Network of Health Promoting Workplaces) (2002) *Barcelona Declaration on Developing Good Workplace Health Practice in Europe*. Barcelona: ENHPW.

Ewles, L. and Simnett, I. (2003) *Promoting Health A Practical Guide*, 5th edn. London: Bailliere Tindall.

Fleming, P. (1999) 'Health promotion for individuals, families and communities', in Long, A. (ed.) (1999) *Interactions for Practice in Community Nursing*. Basingstoke: Macmillan. pp 228–59.

Grawitch, M.J., Ledford, G.E., Ballard, D.W. and Barber, L.K. (2009) 'Leading the healthy workforce: the integral role of employee involvement', *Consulting Psychology Journal: Practice and Research*, 61: 122–35.

Hämäläinen, P., Saarela, K.L. and Takala, J. (2009) 'Global trend according to estimated number of occupational accidents and fatal work-related diseases at region and country level', *Journal of Safety Research*, 40: 125–39.

Hart, S. (2008) *A Critique of the Business Case for Corporate Social Responsibility: Equality and Workplace Health and Safety*. Halifax, Nova Scotia: Memorial University.

Harvey, H.D. and Fleming, P. (2004) *Impacting Health at Work*. London: Chadwick House Publishing.

HSENI (Health and Safety Executive for Northern Ireland) (2003) *Working for Health*. Belfast: Health and Safety Executive for Northern Ireland.

Health and Safety Executive (2010) *Health and Safety Executive Statistics 2009/10*. London: HSE.

Highhouse, S. and Hoffman, J.R. (2001) 'Organizational attraction and job choice', in C. Cooper and I.T. Robertson (eds), *International Review of Industrial and Organizational Psychology*. Chichester: John Wiley and Sons.

ILO (International Labour Organization) (2006) *ILO Convention 187: Promotional Framework for Occupational Safety and Health Convention*. Geneva: ILO.

ILO (International Labour Organization) (2008) *Global Employment Trends*. Geneva: ILO.

ILO (International Labour Organization) (2010) *Global Employment Trends*. Geneva: ILO.

Institute of Directors and the Health and Safety Commission (2006) *Leading Health and Safety at Work*. Available at: www.corporateaccountability.org (accessed 24 November 2010).

IMF (International Monetary Fund) (2010) *World Economic Outlook, October 2010: Recovery, Risk and Rebalancing*. Washington, DC: IMF.

IOSH (Institute of Occupational Safety and Health) (2009) *The Value of Health and Safety: 2009*. Leicester: IOSH.

Kahan, B. and Goodstadt, M. (1999) 'Continuous quality improvement: can CQI lead to better outcomes?', *Health Promotion International*, 14: 83–91.

Karnes, R.E. (2008) 'A change in business ethics: the impact on employer–employee relations', *Journal of Business Ethics*, 87: 189–97.

Kelloway, K.E., Teed, M. and Kelley, E. (2008) 'The psychosocial environment: towards an agenda for research', *International Journal of Workplace Health Management*, 1: 50–64.

Kersley, B., Alpin, C. and Forth, J. (2006) *Inside the Workplace: Findings from the 2004 Employment Relations Survey*. Abingdon: Routledge.

Kivimaki, M., Ferrie, J.E., Brunner, E., Head, J., Shipley, M.J., Vahtera, K. and Marmot, M. (2005) Justice at work and reduced risk of coronary heart disease among employees: the Whitehall II study. *Archives of Internal Medicine*, 165: 2245–51.

Kriger, M.P. and Hanson B.J. (1999) 'A value-based paradigm for creating truly healthy organizations', *Journal of Organizational Change Management*, 12: 302.

Lowe, G. (2004) *Healthy Workplace Strategies: Creating Change and Achieving Results*. Ottawa: Health Canada.

Marmot, M., Allen, J., Goldblatt, P., Boyce, T., McNeish, D., Grady, M. and Geddes, I. (2010) *Fair Society, Healthy Lives: A Strategic Review of Health Inequalities* in England post-2010 (The Marmot Review). London: The Marmot Review.

Maslow, A.H. (1970) *Motivation and Personality*, 2nd edn. New York: Harper and Row.

Mitchell, G. (2005) 'Forecasting environmental equity: air quality responses to road user charging in Leeds, UK', *Journal of Environmental Management*, 77: 212–26.

Mittelmark, M.B. (2007) 'Setting an ethical agenda for health promotion', *Health Promotion International*, 23: 78–85.

Moore, A.B., Parahoo, K. and Fleming, P. (2011) 'Managers' understanding of workplace health promotion within small and medium-sized enterprises: a phenomenological study', *Health Education Journal*, 70: 92–101.

Office for National Statistics (2006) *Labour Force Survey*. London: Office for National Statistics.

Riley, W. (2010) 'Defining quality improvement in public health', *Journal of Public Health Management Practice*, 16: 5–7.

Seymour, A. and Dupré, K. (2008) 'Advancing employee engagement through an employee workplace strategy', *Journal of Health Services Research and Policy*, 13 (suppl 1): 35–40.

Shain, M. and Kramer, D.M. (2004) 'Health promotion in the workplace: Framing the concept, reviewing the evidence', *Occupational and Environmental Medicine*, 61: 643–8.

Tindill, B.S. and Stewart, D.W. (1993) 'Integration of total quality and quality assurance', in A.F. Al-Assaf and J.A. Schmele (eds), *The Textbook of Total Quality in Healthcare*. Delray Beach, FL: St Lucie Press.

Tones, K. and Tilford, S. (2001) *Health Promotion: Effectiveness, Efficiency and Equity*. Cheltenham: Nelson Thornes.

United Nations (2002) *Report of the World Summit on Sustainable Development*. New York: United Nations.

WHO (World Health Organization) (1948) Preamble to the Constitution of the World Health Organization as adopted by the International Health Conference, New York, 19–22 June, 1946; signed on 22 July 1946 by the representatives of 61 States (Official Records of the World Health Organization, no. 2, p. 100) and entered into force on 7 April 1948. Geneva: WHO.

WHO (World Health Organization) (1978) *Declaration of Alma Ata on Primary Health Care*. Geneva: WHO.

WHO (World Health Organization) (1986) *Ottawa Charter for Health Promotion*. Geneva: WHO.

WHO (World Health Organization) (1996) *Global Strategy for Occupational Health for All*. Geneva: WHO.

WHO (World Health Organization) (2005) *Bangkok Charter for Health Promotion in a Globalised World*. Geneva: WHO.

WHO (World Health Organization) (2006) *Stresa Declaration on Workers' Health*. Geneva: WHO.

WHO (World Health Organization) (2007) *Global Plan of Action on Workers' Health 2008–2017*. Geneva: WHO.

WHO (World Health Organization) (2008) *Closing the Gap in a Generation: Health Action on the Social Determinants of Health*. Geneva: WHO.

WHO (World Health Organization) (2010a) *Healthy Workplaces: A Model for Action*. Geneva: WHO.

WHO (World Health Organization) (2010b) *WHO Healthy Workplace Framework and Model: Background and Supporting Literature and Practices*. Geneva: WHO.

World Bank (2010) *Global Recovery Faces Fiscal Headwinds*. Washington, DC: World Bank.

Young, D. (2010) *Common Sense, Common Safety*. London: Cabinet Office.

13

Volkswagen: A Comprehensive Approach to Health Promotion in the Workplace

Uwe Brandenburg

Aims

- To demonstrate how a comprehensive workplace health promotion approach is realized in a large multinational company
- To describe the health management system at Volkswagen
- To provide examples of health promotion and rehabilitation programmes and corporate social responsibility
- To explore the costs and benefits of the health management system

---

The Volkswagen Group operates 60 production plants in 15 European countries and a further six countries in the Americas, Asia and Africa. Around the world, more than 370,000 employees produce almost 26,000 vehicles or are involved in vehicle-related services each working day. The challenges for corporate workplace health promotion are significant, and have been addressed in the development of a health management system, outlined and discussed below.

The basic value position of an organization is a key to understanding the culture and the organization's commitment or otherwise to health promotion. The people, the workers and their families are valued highly at Volkswagen, not just as a means of production but as an investment for the future. The health, fitness, competence and motivation of a company's workers determine its competitiveness and whether or not it succeeds:

> A company's value lies not in its buildings or machines, nor in its bank accounts. [...] The true value of a company lies entirely in the people who work for it, and in their spirit of cooperation.

These words were spoken over forty years ago by the then General Director of Volkswagen, Heinrich Nordhoff (1966: xx). Drucker (2009) highlights that a business enterprise has only one true resource: people. Especially in a knowledge economy, human resources, rather than financial and physical capital, are an organization's competitive edge (Crawford, 1991). Companies who want to be competitive and successful in the global market need able-bodied, highly motivated workers. The economic success of a company, particularly a global player, depends to a large extent on the optimal use and sustained nurturing of its human capital.

Workers are the most important source of creativity. It follows therefore that investing in workers' health is investing in potential (Ulich and Wülser, 2004), although the gains in terms of economic success may only be seen in the mid to long term. However, the protection and promotion of health are not rooted merely in the economic imperative. They are also a social obligation and an expression of corporate culture.

A variety of internal and external conditions significantly influence how a company supports the health of its employees. External factors include globalization, economic trends, and statutory requirements, and internal factors include ideas about the nature of work and workers, approach to or philosophy of management, concepts of health, expertise in occupational health and in health promotion, as well as the specific illnesses and risk factors that are associated with the core occupations of the company (Brandenburg et al., 1990, 1996, 2000; European Agency for Safety and Health at Work, 2007, 2010; European Foundation for the Improvement of Living and Working Conditions, 2007; Murray and Lopez, 1997; Scheuch, 1997; Statistisches Bundesamt, 2010; WHO, 2005; World Economic Forum, 2007, 2008).

Consideration of these conditions creates special challenges for a company that manufactures products at 60 locations worldwide. The countries where Volkswagen Group products are manufactured (for example Spain, Poland, Portugal, Brazil, Mexico, South Africa, India, Russia) present at times radically different conditions, for example; living conditions, cultural values, types of diseases, economic situation, and statutory requirements (European Foundation for the Improvement of Living and Working Conditions, 2007; Lopez et al., 2006; Mathers and Loncar, 2005; WHO, 2005; WHO Europe, 2009), which require specific approaches to health protection and promotion. The motto 'think global, act local' is the key to handling such differences. Local and regional particularities of the production sites are taken into account when considering group-wide standards and operating procedures.

The approach taken to workplace health at Volkswagen

At Volkswagen health protection and health promotion are future-orientated concepts which support and nurture employees in a sustainable way and contribute to human resource and organizational development. They are integral components of HR policy and are part of general company policy. They find expression in the *Values and Guidelines of the Volkswagen Group* (Volkswagen AG, 2006b), in the *Declaration on Social Rights and Industrial Relationships at Volkswagen* (Volkswagen AG, 2002a), the Volkswagen Group requirements for sustainable development with regard to the relationships and business partners (2009a), as well as in the *Volkswagen Group Code of Conduct* (2010a). The Group is committed to guaranteeing healthy working conditions at all sites. The corporate philosophy in Volkswagen can be found in *The Guidelines on Health Protection and Health Promotion* (Volkswagen AG, 2010a, 2010b) within the Volkswagen Group. These guidelines, which in 2010 were revised and adapted to reflect changed circumstances, apply to all Volkswagen sites and brands. Mandatory standards, operating procedures and general recommendations ensure appropriate healthcare for all employees in the Volkswagen Group. A group-wide health audit also serves to verify whether the guidelines are being followed. Counselling and support services are offered in conjunction with this. In order to provide these services in an optimal manner, a pool of experts has been recruited from throughout the group and their specialized knowledge and skills have been systematically recorded and made available to everyone in Group Occupational Health Services.

At Volkswagen, the health management system adheres closely to the six quality criteria for the planning and implementation of successful high quality health measures in the workplace, devised by the partners within the European Network for Workplace Health Promotion (ENWHP, 1999). The criteria are outlined in Box 13.1.

Traditional occupational health and safety services, while essential, cannot alone address the wide range of issues that affect employee health and wellbeing (ENWHP, 2007). To promote health in a large multinational group requires not only a comprehensive approach, characterized by addressing prevention of occupational illness and the support and promotion of optimal physical and mental health, but that the approach be coherent at a corporate level while also locally flexible.

Box 13.1   Quality Criteria for Workplace Health Promotion

⇒ The organization has a written corporate philosophy on workplace health promotion. The executive team is fully behind this philosophy and actively contributes towards implementing it.

⇒ The health promotion measures are properly integrated into the existing structures and processes of the organization.

⇒ The organization provides enough resources (budget, staff, rooms, further training etc.) for workplace health promotion.

⇒ The executive team/company management regularly monitors the progress of health promotion measures.

⇒ Workplace health issues are an integral part of training and retaining, especially regarding the executive team.

⇒ All staff have access to important health-related facilities, for example break, and rest rooms, canteen and sports amenities.

(ENWHP, 1999)

This is achieved at Volkswagen in the context of an integrated health management system, as outlined in Figure 13.1. The health management system is a corporate strategy, which aims at both preventing ill health at work and enhancing health promoting potential and wellbeing in the workforce.

The physical and mental health of workers, as well as their motivation, must be maintained and fostered in the long term. Health management entails the reduction of health risks as well as the creation and reinforcement of health promoting resources.

In pursuing health management goals, the organization adheres to the principles of personal responsibility and solidarity. The individual worker is expected to share responsibility for their health with the company. The company helps and supports workers when an individual has reached the limit of what she or he can reasonably do on their own. The principles reflect an image of a worker who is willing to take independent action and who wants to contribute, have a say in decisions and take joint responsibility. Such a worker wishes neither to be spoon-fed nor to be deprived of his or her free will.

Health Management at Volkswagen

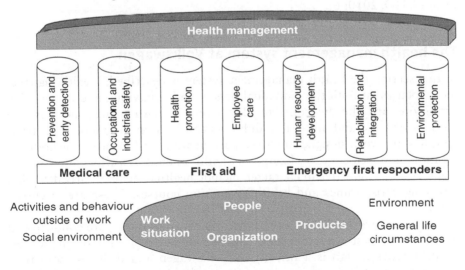

Figure 13.1   The integrated health management system at Volkswagen

In designing programmes for health management, key questions are posed, to ascertain the appropriateness of the programme in terms of legality, ethics, effectiveness, and feasibility:

- Is the activity or programme legally permissible? Does it invade privacy? How can data protection requirements be fulfilled?
- Is the activity or programme ethical? Will all participants be treated respectfully?
- Is the programme effective? What evidence is available regarding impact and outcome?
- Is the activity or programme economically feasible? What are the costs and benefits?
- Is the company responsible for the programme?

Health management is an ongoing process that includes workers and their work situations, the company as a whole, the company's products, as well as the social environment and ecological aspects. The conceptual structure and practical tools of health management are constantly being reviewed.

In keeping with the principle of health promotion, to involve populations as a whole in the context of their everyday life, rather than just at-risk groups (WHO, 1984), the target group for health management includes all workers; healthy workers with healthy lifestyles, workers with illnesses and healthy or unhealthy lifestyles, as well as workers who are healthy (or feel healthy) but have unhealthy habits. Healthcare programmes can also be opened up to workers' family members, as far as possible and allowed by statutory provisions, and to workers at the dealerships/workshops of the group brands and suppliers, a feature of workplace health promotion termed enterprise community involvement (WHO, 2010: 6).

The health management system at Volkswagen

In this section the health management system is described. Health management focuses on both the individual person and behaviour, and on working conditions and the environment. The overall health management system consists of basic and add-on modules, as can be seen in Figure 13.2. Basic modules are work design, employee participation and information/communication, and medical care. Examples of add-on modules, which are complementary and supportive in character, include health coaching, early detection screening programmes and health promotion courses. These are discussed below.

Structuring work and the work environment so that they are conducive to health is the best way to protect and promote the health of employees. Healthy work design is a priority at Volkswagen and includes more than ergonomic workplace design, inspection and risk assessment. Work design embraces innovative work models, new forms of work organization and

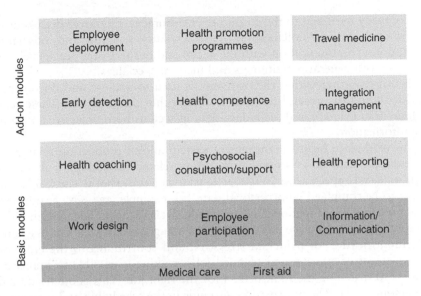

Figure 13.2 Modules in the health management system

design of working time, involvement in procurement decisions, compatibility of family and work/work–life-balance, and protection from bullying, discrimination and sexual harassment.

Ergonomic workplace design that integrates ergonomic principles throughout the entire product creation process guarantees that the health aspects of the workplace receive consideration throughout, starting with the design and planning phase. This includes application of ergonomic structural principles, advice on occupational medicine, and final ergonomic approval for new machines, facilities and equipment (Jacob et al., 2010; Loth et al., 2010; Marschall et al., 1998; Toledo-Munoz and Lins, 2010). Examples of ergonomic workplace design are swinging/swivelling component positioners, mobile assembly line conveyor work seats, automated component handling tools, height-adjustable skids, manipulators, mobile conveyor belts and swinging/swivelling work seats.

At Volkswagen, employees are involved as much as possible in matters that directly or indirectly affect their health. At the root of this lies the conviction that employees are capable of participating in deciding such matters, that they wish to participate, and that they must be given the opportunity to do so (for more about participation as a principle of health promotion, see Chapter 4). Participation encourages commitment, mobilizes knowledge and skills, builds competence and helps to improve structures and processes. Opportunities for participation include extended workplace inspections, special workshops, health circles, employee surveys, employee suggestions system, quality circles, continuous improvement process and group work.

Communication and information are integral parts of the health management system and occur in various forms and at different levels. This applies to both the company itself and to the corporate environment. Employee discussions are a part of this, as are collaboration with scholarly, scientific and international institutions, communication with the social and health insurance agencies, and dialogue with general practitioners and medical specialists.

Health reporting within the company is used to analyse and document the workload and the general health situation within the company. These reports include both primary and secondary data as well as both objective and subjective information.

The workplace health management system allows production related data, for example data on ergonomic and safety related technology, pollution and environmental impact, as well as data related to preventive health check-up requirements to be combined with personal data (for example, age, sex, health restrictions, results of occupational health medical check-ups). The system delivers comprehensive workplace information, including standardized risk assessments and identification of principal stressors, and contributes to the ergonomic improvement of existing and planned jobs, making it possible to improve the process of matching the right person for the right job. This is often referred to as person–job-fit. The information also aids in the scheduling and management of occupational health check-ups. Moreover, the system generates a database that can then be used to analyse the connections between workload and diseases (Nöring et al., 2010).

The Health Coaching allows specific groups of employees to benefit from an integrated approach to healthcare. The programme has several stages. It includes a health check-up as well as several training offers and individual coaching sessions (Brandenburg and Marschall, 2000).

Health promotion programmes form another add-on module. These are aimed at specific health problems and target groups, and aim to facilitate behaviour change, foster health awareness, reduce health risk factors, and increase general fitness. In each plant in Germany there is a Fitness-Centre/Health-Park used for fitness and rehabilitation. Examples of such health promoting courses and seminars are:

- Back training
- Sitting, lifting and carrying training
- Relaxation techniques
- Gymnastics
- Fitness training
- Muscle structure training
- Smoking cessation programmes
- Early detection programmes
- Diet counselling
- Addiction prevention
- Stress management seminars

Various opportunities for information and counselling are made available to employees. These include heart attack risk assessment, substance abuse counselling, psychological counselling, travel medicine, and nutritional counselling. These options are communicated to employees in various ways: special consultation hours, special campaigns, exhibitions, lectures, intranet pages, brochures and articles in the factory newspaper.

Early identification of counselling for employees with health risk factors and health disturbances can take place both during occupational medical check-ups and through special screening programmes in which employees may participate on a voluntary basis.

In 2009, it was decided to introduce a general health check-up facility with the aim of maintaining and promoting employee health and fitness, which included assessment of current individual health and fitness and early identification of risk factors for chronic diseases. This can be seen in Figure 13.3. This high quality medical examination allows for the detection of important health risk factors and health disturbances (for example, physical inactivity, smoking, hypertension, alcohol consumption, cholesterol, overweight and malnutrition) (BKK Bundesverband, 2007; Mathers and Loncar, 2005; Robert Koch-Institut, 2007; Schauder et al., 2006; WHO and World Economic Forum, 2008; World Economic Forum, 2007, 2010; Yusuf et al., 2004). The check-up also assists in the task of managing demographic change that is taking place (Brandenburg and Domschke, 2007; Stork and Mann, 2010). The check-up facility is intended for all employees. It has been introduced in the plants in Germany and will gradually be introduced in the plants abroad.

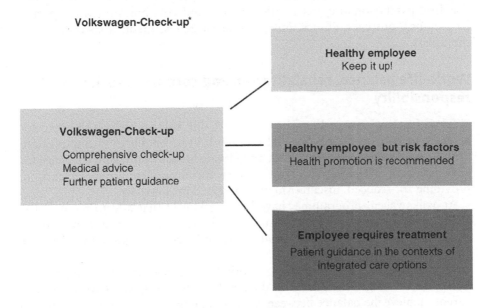

*<45 years old every five years; 45 years and older every three years

Figure 13.3 Volkswagen check-up facility

The check-up consists of a basic module as well as supplementary and add-on modules. A fitness test can also be added as an option. The check-up generates an individual health profile. This health profile then serves as the basis for suggesting health-related follow-up measures as the next step. These follow-up offers, which are discussed during the medical consultation, include such options as:

- Health promotion programmes (courses, workshops)
- Health coaching
- Cardio-training, gymnastics
- Special week with fitness and health activities
- Information meetings (health competence)
- Follow-up medical measures
- Ongoing patient care

Given the growing significance of psychological and psychosomatic disturbances and diseases (Berufsverband Deutscher Psychologinnen und Psychologen, 2008; BKK Bundesverband, 2008; Murray and Lopez, 1997; Robert Koch-Institut, 2007, 2010), the psychological health and care of employees with psychological or psychosomatic illnesses is becoming increasingly important. This entails disease prevention and promotion of psychological health, early detection and de-escalation of psychological disorders, diagnosis and intervention, and reintegration of people with mental illnesses into the working life. The healthcare options available include medical consultation, psychological services, social coaches, psychosomatic consultation hours, and collaboration with specialized clinics, outreach clinics, independent surgeries, medical specialists and therapists.

Work–life balance, rehabilitation and corporate social responsibility

Work is just one part of life. The term work–life balance reflects the need for workers to balance their work and non-work lives. Enabling its employees to find the right balance between work and private life is a permanent challenge for any successful company. The right balance encourages employee satisfaction, providing for reduced absenteeism and increased productivity.

At Volkswagen, programmes have been developed that add to the modular health management system to ensure that health protection and promotion endeavours go beyond the factory gates, and embrace families and the enterprise community.

The company offers a number of work–life balance projects to support its staff in reconciling time spent with the family with time spent at work. To help parents achieve the balance between work and family, some factories are able to offer special childcare facilities, Employees who do not have family responsibilities also have their own individual ideas about harmony between work and private life, and want their employer to take their interests into account. Creative employment solutions with flexible, individual working time models have been available for all members of staff for many years.

Reintegration programmes are an important element of a comprehensive approach to workplace health promotion, although few examples exist compared to more traditional lifestyle-orientated programmes. In cooperation with external partners, the Volkswagen plant in Wolfsburg has developed an intervention and reintegration programme that permits quick, optimal and individualized reintegration of workers with psychological and psychosocial impairments. Job rehabilitation at Volkswagen involves the combined efforts of both the employer and employee to return to work. Based on a systematically applied algorithm, each individual is offered a healthcare module tailored to his or her personal situation. In the course of implementation, it is possible to adapt the module dynamically so that it better fits with the individual employee's particular life and working conditions (Lamberg et al., 2010).

For employees who return to work after a long illness or accident, all responsible parties both within and outside the company develop an individual rehabilitation plan jointly. The goal of this is for the employee to re-enter the work process in a systematic way and as early as possible. The package of measures available to aid in this process includes assignment of the worker to his or her former job, the reconfiguration of the workplace for disabled accessibility, work trial runs for a few hours at a time, changes in work organization, targeted adaptations, retraining and various other forms of rehabilitation. These could include outpatient rehabilitation, inpatient rehabilitation at a clinic on a contractual basis, job-related training, or visits to the Volkswagen plant's own internal rehabilitation centre on site in Wolfsburg.

A workplace-orientated approach has been specially developed for employees with musculoskeletal disorders, called the JobReha programme. The JobReha programme is characterized by the interweaving in a practical way of both internal company and external health measures, the coordination of the specific needs of the employee with workplace-related musculoskeletal complaints, continuous adjustment of therapy and rehabilitation goals to reflect the employee's individual needs, and workplace-specific prevention. A recent evaluation of the programme has documented its success (Teumer et al., 2010).

In cooperation with health insurance and other partners, a prevention and health promotion programme has been developed, called RehaFit. It includes a number of health measures that can be used by employees. The aim is to avoid health disturbances and to promote health and wellbeing. The special feature of RehaFit is that the waiting times for employees who want to take part in programmes are very short. For example, in the rehabilitation centre one can arrange a time within three days.

The Work2Work programme is an innovative HR concept made available to employees who, because of serious health impairments, have been medically certified as having altered work capabilities. They are offered meaningful work in a way commensurate with their abilities and are thus prepared for reintegration into the primary internal labour market within Volkswagen. This is done by special workplace design and structuring of work processes, as well as through supplementary care. Employees must also actively participate in improving their own health.

Corporate social responsibility features in Volkswagen's corporate health management strategy (Volkswagen AG, 2006b, 2009b). Health is considered a responsibility that goes beyond the factory gate. Volkswagen AG is a member of the Global Business Coalition on HIV/AIDS. For many years, Volkswagen has been strongly committed to the battle against HIV/AIDS in South Africa and Brazil. The company has already been recognized numerous times for its HIV/AIDS jobs programme, which ranges from educational and counselling services to medical care and medication. When implementing such programmes, Volkswagen also supports its suppliers.

During a multi-year programme conducted in cooperation with, *inter alia*, the International Labour Organization (ILO), suppliers in Brazil, Mexico and South Africa were given in-depth training in occupational health and safety. The occupational health and safety service was improved through this cooperative effort. The experiences have been incorporated into a supplier management system. It is used as a reference resource for achieving minimum global standards in the production processes and labour relations of Volkswagen suppliers. The standards that Volkswagen practises at its own plants are the yardstick by which these global standards are measured, and this includes specific occupational health and safety standards. At the present time the Volkswagen Health Service is involved in a pilot scheme that integrates dealerships in health promotion activities. The idea is health within the entire chain: supplier, producer and dealership.

The costs and benefits of health management

Evaluation plays an increasingly important role in contemporary health promotion. Interventions and programmes need to evaluated, with a view to short, medium and long term indicators. (Evaluation principles are discussed in more detail in Chapter 5.)

> Company health promotion measures are implemented under the condition that they not only improve employee health, but also have a positive influence on direct, illness-related costs, as well as on absenteeism and productivity. (Kramer and Bödeker, 2008: 5)

Statements pertaining to the costs and benefits of health management are, however, especially problematic given the numerous challenges associated with operationalization and measurement of inputs and outcomes. While the direct costs can to some degree be reliably calculated, determining the indirect costs is fraught with difficulty. It is also much more difficult to measure and assess the benefits (Badura et al., 2009; Brandenburg et al., 1996; Chenoweth, 2002; Fritz, 2006; Günther and Albers, 2009; Lowe, 2003). The benefits derived from health promoting activities and programmes often cannot be defined in terms of a direct causal relationship, quantified exactly or assigned a monetary value. Here, only the plausibility argument remains; logic and experience argue in favour of the benefits.

Numerous studies, especially those conducted in the Anglo-American sphere (see, for example, Aldana, 2001; Chapman, 2003; Fulmer et al., 2003; Kreis and Bödeker, 2003; Lowe, 2003; Pelletier, 2001; Sockoll et al., 2008), have some general applicability and substantiate the economic benefits of disease prevention and health promotion. Volkswagen's experience has demonstrated that a comprehensive health management system produces positive outcomes, also in economic terms (Brandenburg, 1998; Brandenburg and Marschall, 1997). This can be seen in the form of:

- Improvement of the status of employees' health
- Reduced onset of occupational diseases
- Increase in health consciousness
- Changes of health behaviour
- Improvement in wellbeing
- Better working atmosphere
- Better communication and cooperation among employees
- Reduction of risk factors that affect health

Critical success factors

Ensuring that health management is embedded within the everyday practice of a company, a key feature of a settings approach, presents a challenge to workplaces. At Volkswagen success is attributed to a number of interrelated factors.

Firstly, a holistic view of health underpins heath protection and promotion activities. Health is understood to encompass wellbeing as well as illness prevention. Psychological and social aspects of health are taken into account as much as occupational and influences and potential risks to health.

Secondly, health protection and health promotion are carried out with a view to the future; they are an integral part of goal setting, planning and decision making processes. This can be best described as a pro-active, foresighted approach, and it takes precedence over retro-active correction. This is in keeping with health promotion principles, as is the commitment to monitoring and evaluation. The systems that maintain health are seen as continuous processes that must be constantly improved and innovatively developed.

Finally, health protection and health promotion are achieved by creating a work environment that is conducive to health. Creating a healthy workplace always has priority over measures that focus only on the individual. For this a multidisciplinary approach is essential and accordingly Volkswagen requires that those working in health management possess competences in some areas of medicine, ergonomics, psychology, physiology, and economic and social science. There is a commitment to further health-related training and education for staff.

Summary points

- An integrated health management system can contribute significantly toward the maintenance and promotion of employee health and fitness.
- Workplace health promotion should not be limited to person/behaviour-orientated measures. It must also include work design, the working conditions and must pay attention to the interdependency between an individual's behaviour and his or her working circumstances.
- A balance must be struck between the company's responsibility to prevent work-related health risks and to promote worker health and fitness through adequate working and performance conditions, and the worker's individual responsibility and willingness to maintain and improve his or her own health.
- A company is only ever as healthy and productive as its workforce. For this reason, Volkswagen follows this maxim: if you want performance from your workers, you must protect and promote their health as well. Health, fitness and competence are preconditions for top performance.

Online Further Reading

Hunt, M.K., Lederman, R., Stoddard, A.M., LaMontagne, A.D., McLellan, D., Combe, C., Barbeau, E. and Sorensen, G. (2005) 'Process evaluation of an integrated health promotion/occupational health model in WellWorks-2', *Health Education and Behaviour*, 32: 10–26.

The approach to health management outlined in this chapter could be described as an integrated approach. The results of a process evaluation of a randomized, controlled study comparing the effectiveness of an integrated health promotion/occupational health programme (HP/OHS) with a standard intervention (HP) are reported in this paper. While a similar number of activities were offered in both conditions, in the HP/OHS condition there were higher levels of worker participation using three measures, thus indicating the value of employing an integrated approach.

References

Aldana, S. (2001) 'Financial impact of health promotion programs: a comprehensive review of the literature', *American Journal of Health Promotion*, 15: 296–320.

Badura, B., Schröder, H. and Vetter, C. (eds) (2009) *Fehlzeiten-Report 2008. Betriebliches Gesundheitsmanagement: Kosten und Nutzen.* Heidelberg: Springer.

Berufsverband Deutscher Psychologinnen and Psychologen (eds) (2008) *Psychische Gesundheit am Arbeitsplatz in Deutschland.* Berlin: BDP.

BKK Bundesverband (ed.) (2007) *Hearts and Minds at Work in Europe.* Essen: BKK BV.

BKK Bundesverband (ed.) (2008) *Seelische Krankheiten prägen das Krankheitsgeschehen.* BKK Gesundheitsreport 2008. Essen: BKK BV.

Brandenburg, U. (1998) 'Rechnen sich Gesundheitsschutz und Gesundheitsförderung für das Unternehmen?', in A. Schröer (ed.), *Blickpunkt Krankenstand – Wettbewerbsvorteil Gesundheitsförderung.* Bremerhaven: Wirtschaftsverlag NW.

Brandenburg, U. and Domschke, J.-P. (2007) *Die Zukunft sieht alt aus.* Wiesbaden: Gabler.

Brandenburg, U. and Marschall, B. (1997) 'Using health protection and health promotion to increase economic efficiency', in J. Mossink and F. Licher (eds), *Costs and Benefits of Occupational Safety and Health.* Amsterdam: NIA TNO B.V.

Brandenburg, U. and Marschall, B. (2000) '"Gesundheitscoaching" für Führungskräfte', in B. Badura, M. Litsch and C. Vetter (eds), *Fehlzeiten-Report 1999. Psychische Belastung am Arbeitsplatz.* Berlin: Springer.

Brandenburg, U., Kollmeier, H., Kuhn, K., Marschall, B. and Oehlke, P. (eds) (1990) *Prävention and Gesundheitsförderung im Betrieb.* BAU Tb 51. Bremerhaven: Wirtschaftsverlag NW.

Brandenburg, U., Kuhn, K., Marschall, B. and Verkoyen, C. (eds) (1996) *Gesundheitsförderung im Betrieb.* BAU Tb 74. Bremerhaven: Wirtschaftsverlag NW.

Brandenburg, U., Nieder, P. and Susen, B. (eds) (2000) *Gesundheitsmanagement im Unternehmen.* Weinheim: Juventa.

Chapman, L.S. (2003) 'Meta-evaluation of worksite health promotion economic return studies', *American Journal of Health Promotion*, 6: 1–10.

Chenoweth, D.H. (2002) *Evaluating Worksite Health Promotion.* Champaign, IL: Human Kinetics.

Crawford, R. (1991) *In the Era of Human Capital: The Emergence of Talent, Intelligence and Knowledge as the Economic Force and What It Means.* New York: Harper Business.

Drucker, P.F. (2009) *Management*, Vol. 1. Frankfurt/Main: Campus.

European Agency for Safety and Health at Work (2007) *Expert Forecast on Emerging Psychosocial Risks Related to Occupational Safety and Health.* Luxembourg: European Union.

European Agency for Safety and Health at Work (2010) *European Survey of Enterprises on New and Emerging Risks.* Luxembourg: European Union.

European Foundation for the Improvement of Living and Working Conditions (2007) *Fourth European Working Conditions Survey.* Dublin: European Foundation for the Improvement of Living and Working Conditions.

ENWHP (European Network for Workplace Health Promotion) (1999) *Healthy Employees in Health Organizations. Good Practice in Workplace Health Promotion (WHP) in Europe – Quality Criteria of Workplace Health Promotion.* Essen: European Network for Workplace Health Promotion.

ENWHP (European Network for Workplace Health Promotion (2007) *Luxembourg Declaration on Workplace Health Promotion in the European Union.* Essen: European Network for Workplace Health Promotion.

Fritz, S. (2006) *Ökonomischer Nutzen 'weicher' Kennzahlen*, 2nd edn. Zürich: vdf Hochschulverlag.

Fulmer, I.S., Gerhart, B. and Scott, K.S. (2003) 'Are the 100 best better? An empirical investigation of the relationship between being a "great place to work" and firm performance', *Personnel Psychology*, 56: 965–93.

Günther, T. and Albers, C. (2009) 'Kosten und Nutzen des betrieblichen Arbeits- und Gesundheitsschutzes', *Controlling*, 21: 388–95.

Jacob, H., Toledo Munoz, B., Busche, C. and Jendrusch, R. (2010) 'Durchgängige Ergonomieabsicherung im Produktentstehungsprozess bei Volkswagen', in GfA (eds), *Mensch- and prozessorientierte Arbeitsgestaltung im Fahrzeugbau*. Dortmund: GfA Press.

Kramer, I. and Bödeker, W. (2008) *Return on Investment im Kontext der betrieblichen Gesundheitsförderung und Prävention*. IGA-Report 16. Essen/Dresden/Siegburg: BKK BV/DGUV/ AOK-BV/AEV.

Kreis, J. and Bödeker, W. (2003) *Gesundheitlicher and ökonomischer Nutzen betrieblicher Gesundheitsförderung und Prävention*. IGA-Report 3. Essen/Dresden: BKK BV/HVBG.

Lamberg, J., Göldner, R., Strunk, S., Kuhr, A., Schmid-Ott, G. and Simon, A. (2010) *Neue Strategien zur Versorgung psychosozial beeinträchtigter Mitarbeiterinnen und Mitarbeiter am Beispiel des Interventions- and Reintegrationskonzeptes des Gesundheitswesens der Volkswagen AG am Standort Wolfsburg*. Manuskript. Wolfsburg: Volkswagen Gesundheitswesen.

Lopez, A.D., Mathers, C.D., Ezzati, M., Jamison, D.T. and Murray, C.J. (2006) 'Global and regional burden of disease and risk factors, 2001: systematic analysis of population health data', *The Lancet*, 367: 1747–57.

Loth, S., Schatt, N., Pietsch, R. and Linsenmayer, J. (2010) 'Ergonomie in der Fertigung', in GfA (eds), *Mensch- and prozessorientierte Arbeitsgestaltung im Fahrzeugbau*. Dortmund: GfA Press.

Lowe, G.S. (2003) *Healthy Workplaces and Productivity: A Discussion Paper*. Quebec: Minister of Public Works and Government Services Canada.

Marschall, B., Brandenburg, U. and Lippmann, K. (1998) 'Projective ergonomische Arbeitsplatzgestaltung bei Volkswagen', in K. Landau (eds), *Mensch-Maschine-Schnittstellen*. Stuttgart: IfAO.

Mathers, C.D. and Loncar, D. (2005) *Updated Projections of Global Mortality and Burden of Disease, 2002–2030: Data Sources, Methods and Results*. Geneva: WHO.

Murray, C.J. and Lopez, A.D. (1997) 'Alternative projections of mortality and disability by cause 1990–2020: global burden of disease study', *The Lancet*, 349: 1498–504.

Nordhoff, H. (1966) 'Festvortrag', *Verhandlungen der Deutschen Gesellschaft für Arbeitsschutz*, vol. 9. Kongress für Arbeitsschutz und Arbeitsmedizin 1965. Darmstadt: Steinkopff.

Nöring, R., Dubian, C., Göldner, R., Klobes, F., Stumpf, J. and Thiemich, J. (2010) 'Arbeitsplatzmanagementsystem–Ein Beitrag zur Steigerung der Wettbewerbsfähigkeit', in GfA (eds), *Mensch- and prozessorientierte Arbeitsgestaltung im Fahrzeugbau*. Dortmund: GfA Press.

Pelletier, K.R. (2001) 'A review and analysis of the clinical- and costeffectiveness studies of comprehensive health promotion and disease management programs at the worksite: 1998–2000', *American Journal of Health Promotion*, 16: 107–16.

Robert Koch-Institut (ed.) (2007) *Gesundheit in Deutschland*, 2nd edn. Berlin: RKI.

Robert Koch-Institut (ed.) (2010) *Depressive Erkrankungen*. Gesundheitsberichterstattung des Bundes. Berlin: RKI.

Schauder, P., Berthold, H., Eckel, H. and Ollenschläger, G. (eds) (2006) *Zukunft sichern: Senkung der Zahl chronisch Kranker*. Köln: Deutscher Ärzte-Verlag.

Scheuch, K. (1997) 'Psychomentale Belastung und Beanspruchung im Wandel von Arbeitswelt und Umwelt', *Arbeitsmed. Sozialmed. Umweltmed.*, 32: 289–96.

Sockoll, I., Kramer, I. and Bödeker, W. (2008) *Wirksamkeit und Nutzen betrieblicher Gesundheitsförderung und Prävention.* IGA-Report 13. Essen/Dresden/Bonn/Siegburg: BKK BV/DGUV/AOK-BV/AEV.

Statistisches Bundesamt (2010) *Qualität der Arbeit.* Wiesbaden: Statistisches Bundesamt.

Stork, J. and Mann, H. (2010) 'Neue Aspekte betrieblicher Gesundheitsvorsorge und Gesundheitsberichterstattung als Beitrag zur Bewältigung des Demografischen Wandels', in GfA (eds), *Mensch- und prozessorientierte Arbeitsgestaltung im Fahrzeugbau.* Dortmund: GfA Press.

Teumer, F., Wassmus, A.-K., Cyganski, L., Teichler, N., Gutenbrunner, C. and Schwarze, M. (2010) 'Gesundheitsökonomische Evaluation der JobReha bei Volkswagen Nutzfahrzeuge Hannover', *Arbeitsmed. Sozialmed. Umweltmed.* 45: 102–4.

Toledo Munoz, B. and Lins, F. (2010) 'Ergonomie im Volkswagen Konzern: Gewappnet für die Zukunft', in GfA (eds), *Mensch- und prozessorientierte Arbeitsgestaltung im Fahrzeugbau.* Dortmund: GfA Press.

Ulich, E. and Wülser, M. (2004) *Gesundheitsmanagement in Unternehmen.* Wiesbaden: Gabler.

Volkswagen AG (2002a) Declaration on Social Rights and Industrial Relationships at Volkswagen. Available at: http://www.volkswagenag.com/vwag/vwcorp/info_center/en/publications/2010/01/social_charter.-bin.acq/qual-BinaryStorageItem.Single.File/Download_4_Social_Charta_.pdf (accessed 23 May 2011).

Volkswagen AG (2002b) *Global Compact. Aufbruch. Zukunft. Verantwortung.* Wolfsburg: Volkswagen AG Regierungsbeziehungen.

Volkswagen AG (2006a) *Eins und eins gleich drei. Corporate Social Responsibility bei Volkswagen.* Wolfsburg: Volkswagen AG.

Volkswagen AG (2006b) Values and Guidelines of the Volkswagen Group. Available at: www.volkswagenag.com/vwag/vwcorp/info_center/en/publications/2006/12/Values_and_Guidelines_of_the_Volkswagen_Group.-bin.acq/qual-BinaryStorageItem.Single.File/werte_und_leitlinien-english.jpg (accessed 23 May 2011).

Volkswagen AG (2009a) Volkswagen Group requirements for sustainable development with regard to the relationships with business partners. Available at: www.volkswagenag.com/vwag/vwcorp/info_center/en/publications/2011/04/volkswagen_group_requirements.-bin.acq/qual-BinaryStorageItem.Single.File/sustainability_requirements.file.pdf (accessed 23 May 2011).

Volkswagen AG (2009b) *1:0 für Volkswagen. Corporate Social Responsibility in Südafrika.* Wolfsburg: Volkswagen AG.

Volkswagen Group Code of Conduct (2010a) www.volkswagenag.com/vwag/vwcorp/info_center/en/publications/2010/07/Verhaltensgrundsaetze_des_Volkswagen_Konzerns.-bin.acq/qual-BinaryStorageItem.Single.File/The%20 Volkswagen%20Group%20Code%20of%20Conduct.pdf (accessed 23 May 2011)

Volkswagen AG (2010a) *Leitlinien zum Gesundheitsschutz und zur Gesundheitsförderung im Volkswagen Konzern.* Wolfsburg: Volkswagen AG.

Volkswagen AG (2010b) *Verhaltensgrundsätze des Volkswagen Konzerns.* Wolfsburg: Volkswagen AG.

World Economic Forum (2007) *Working Towards Wellness.* Geneva: World Economic Forum.

World Economic Forum (2008) *Working Towards Wellness: The Business Rationale.* Cologne/Geneva: World Economic Forum.

World Economic Forum (2010) *Global Risks 2010. A World Economic Forum Report.* Cologne/Geneva: World Economic Forum.

WHO (1984) *Health Promotion: A Discussion Document on Concepts and Principles.* Geneva: WHO.

WHO (2005) *Preventing Chronic Diseases: A Vital Investment.* Geneva: WHO.

WHO Europe (2009) *The European Health Report 2009.* Copenhagen: WHO Regional Office for Europe.

WHO (2010) *Healthy Workplaces: A Model for Action.* Geneva: WHO

WHO and World Economic Forum (2008) *Preventing Non-communicable Diseases in the Workplace through Diet and Physical Activity.* Geneva: WHO.

Yusuf, S., Hawken, S., Ounpuu, S., Dans, T., Avezum, A., Lanas, F., McQueen, M., Buday, A., Pais, P., Varigos, J. and Lisheng, L. (2004) 'Auswirkung der potentiell beeinflussbaren Risikofaktoren des Myokardinfarkts in 52 Ländern (die INTERHEART-Studie): eine Fall-Kontroll-Studie', *The Lancet*, 364: 937–53.

14

Promoting Health and Wellbeing at the Royal Mail Group, UK

Steven Boorman

Aims

- To provide an example in practice of a comprehensive approach to workplace health promotion in a large, multisite organization
- To illustrate how contextual factors can act as a trigger for a cultural change that embraces health and wellbeing
- To demonstrate how workplace health can be part of a corporate strategy
- To provide examples of innovative approaches to workplace health promotion

Royal Mail is one of the largest UK businesses, and the largest UK employer of men. Although its workforce has downsized considerably from nearly 250,000 at the turn of the century, it remains a large multisite organization with approximately 173,000 employees. The profile of the workforce makes traditional health promotion a challenge; it is 80% male, predominantly manual blue collar, ethnically diverse and strongly unionized. The scale of the organization also presents particular operational challenges in respect of reaching and communicating with all employees about health matters. There are many thousands of offices and Internet access is not universal. The Royal Mail has risen to these challenges and has devised an extensive, comprehensive, integrated health improvement programme, which is well received by employees and demonstrates positive health outcomes. The organization takes a serious and strategic approach to improving the health of the workforce, moving in recent years to a broad-based health improvement programme that is both comprehensive and innovative. It is based on a win–win situation; both employees and employers win by creating the conditions for good health and wellbeing in the workplace.

Contextual factors influencing the approach taken to improving health and wellbeing at Royal Mail

The approach taken to health and wellbeing at Royal Mail is consistent with generic health promotion principles, as articulated by the World Health Organization (WHO, 1984); it addresses the entire workforce, not just employees at specific risk, it addresses determinants of health in the workplace which are beyond the control of individuals, it combines diverse methods and approaches and it is participatory, including employees in intervention design. Improving health in the workplace has traditionally involved addressing hazards through risk assessment and preventive programmes. Recent years have seen a movement toward greater consideration of psychosocial health matters and an acknowledgement of the need to develop comprehensive models of workplace health promotion. Comprehensive models include giving attention to safety and physical working conditions, facilitating voluntary health behaviours, provision of health screening services and addressing broader psychosocial health matters through interventions that alter organizational processes or procedures.

Organizations that embrace this comprehensive approach go beyond the statutory imperative (Harvey and Fleming, 2004) and aim to improve health by addressing the factors that determine health in the workplace in addition to prevention of accidents and promotion of healthy lifestyles (discussed in more detail in Chapter 12). The development of workplace health promotion at Royal Mail reflects these broad trends, in addition to responding to factors particular to the sector and within the organization itself.

As an organization Royal Mail has long recognized the value of investing in the health of its staff, employing its first workplace doctor over 150 years ago and having developed a comprehensive staff welfare service in the middle of the twentieth century. Although health promotion activities had been common in the 1980s and 1990s, it was clear that financial pressures in the business had resulted in occupational health approaches becoming more reactive and centred on sickness management. An approach to workplace health promotion using a mixture of traditional and less conventional approaches evolved strongly in the organization in the latter part of the twentieth century. However, a much more strongly integrated and strategic approach to health and wellbeing has evolved within the past ten years, seeing the development of health promotion and occupational health services as part of, and indeed embedded within, a major strategic transformation plan.

The approach was born during a period of significant business commercial challenge, when the organization faced loss of a monopoly in a highly competitive marketplace and during a period when employee morale had fallen sharply. Across a broad range of human resources (HR) measures – staff satisfaction, attendance, grievances, industrial action, accidents and so on – it was evident that employee engagement was poor and impacted significantly on quality of service, which in turn resulted in significant loss making. The organization, despite a history of 350 years, faced a crisis of survival and it was clear that significant change was needed to build business success. A new leadership team developed a very simple recovery plan for the organization, highlighting the need to return to profit, linking financial success to the need to improve the quality of service to customers and recognizing that these two simple aims could be underpinned or enabled by making the organization a better place to work in. This approach is consistent with the idea that improving health and wellbeing is a corporate strategy (ENWHP, 2005), and with Lowe's observation that employee wellbeing is an organization performance issue and not just a matter of personal health (Lowe, 2010).

Becoming a 'Great Place to Work' took equal importance to the goals of quality and financial improvement and allowed Royal Mail to consider health more widely in terms of both the health of the organization and its business methodologies, as well as at the level of individual employee health improvements. Creating a healthy workforce was therefore understood as a broad and far-ranging concept rather than within the confines of a medically dominated occupational health programme.

Specific business challenges at the time (including, for example, changes in competition and technology, changes in working methods and practices, rising expectations of customers) led to downsizing. At times like this it can be easy for companies to focus on supporting those leaving an organization. However, a feature of the approach at the Royal Mail was, while ensuring good support for leavers, also to target specifically improvement for those on whom the company's future success would rely.

Alongside developing and improving its health programmes, detailed below, the organization began by addressing courageously issues of poor leadership, management practice and working conditions through developing a series of cultural change programmes within the Great Place to Work approach. Cultural change is a key feature of whole system change within workplaces. Culture is usually understood as the shared meanings members of an organization have about the organization, what is valued and what matters. A positive culture, that engages workers and supports changes that create a benign working environment, is one of the building blocks of a healthy organization. The approach taken overall is consistent with the definition of a healthy workplace offered by the World Health Organization, quoted in Box 14.1 (this concept is discussed in more detail in Chapter 12). It is comprehensive, integrating a range of elements, and is in keeping with the main theme of this book – the settings approach, looking to the whole system to improve health (a systems approach to health promotion is discussed in more detail in Chapter 3).

Box 14.1   The Healthy Workplace as defined by the World Health Organization

A Healthy Workplace is one in which workers and managers collaborate to use a continual improvement process to protect and promote the health, safety and wellbeing of all workers and the sustainability of the workplace by considering the following, based on identified needs:

- health and safety concerns in the physical work environment
- health, safety and wellbeing concerns in the psychosocial work environment, including the organization of work and workplace culture
- personal health resources in the workplace; and
- ways of participating in the community to improve the health of workers, their families and other members of the community. (WHO, 2010: 6)

Some programmes can be described as multicomponent, addressing simultaneously a number of health issues and employing several methodologies, while others are more focused, for example health screening. Some initiatives are similar to those found in other organizations, while others are innovative, demonstrating the need to adapt ideas to the particular circumstances of a workforce or occupational group. These programmes and initiatives are outlined below.

Fostering engagement through health promotion: the Feeling First Class programme

A good example of change in the approach taken at Royal Mail can be found in the Feeling First Class programme. The Feeling First Class programme was among a series of linked programmes supporting the wider Great Place to Work cultural change initiative. It addressed employee wellbeing. The title is intended to link health to the business of successful postal operations. Employee engagement is one of the building blocks for a healthy organization (Lowe, 2010), and a key aim of this programme was to foster employee engagement using positive health promotion as a tool. In a more traditional approach, health promotion initiatives may be offered to employees in the hope of engaging them in health matters. Royal Mail took a more innovative pathway. In order to facilitate employee engagement more generally, health promotion activities were devised in a participative way with employees.

Developing the Feeling First Class programme started with the aim of rebalancing reactive initiatives with a focus on broader health promotion and wellbeing activities. A health board, consisting of senior managers, specialists, local managers, unions and shop floor employees, was created and, based on widespread consultation and involvement, a comprehensive workplace wellbeing programme was developed.

While the programme deliberately included traditional elements associated with health promotion such as nutrition, exercise, smoking and other lifestyle factors, the programme was broadened to encompass elements such as involvement in job design, review of priorities around psychological and physical health support, and social needs. Also included within the programme design were elements of communications, evaluation (and use of data to inform changing priorities) and a strand that included seeking partnerships with health promoting partners, for example, third sector organizations with interest in health or resources available via public health or primary care initiatives. This latter approach was successful in accessing specialist information and health promotional materials, for example working with the Roy Castle Foundation on lung cancer awareness, or the Men's Health Forum on tackling the issue of providing health promotion materials to a predominantly male workforce. This strand did require considerable investment of time in administration as often resources were available on a local basis, requiring multiple contacts to develop regional or national services. It also required some lateral thinking or flexibility in terms of what may constitute suitable inclusion. A wide contact network enabled, for example, Lottery-funded sports initiatives to be promoted to Royal Mail employees within the overarching framework of the programme. Subsequent evaluation included individual health and organizational outcomes. In terms of health, smoking cessation rates, lifestyle age scores and intention to change scores displayed improvement. At the organizational level, significant improvements in quality of service to customers, commercial sales and return to business profitability were evident.

Addressing the psychosocial work environment: the Dignity and Respect at Work programme

The psychosocial environment includes organizational culture, often expressed in the daily practices that affect the mental and physical wellbeing of employees. Determinants of psychosocial health include work organization, command and control issues, work–life balance and policy and practice in respect of bullying, discrimination and harassment (WHO, 2010).

In attempts to identify priorities for health improvement with employees, feedback placed dignity and respect at work as a key issue, including the need to tackle complaints of bullying and harassment. Many and various programmes supporting improvements to dignity and respect were started, including company-wide diversity and inclusion training to all staff at all levels. The organization pulled this together under the banner of the Dignity and Respect at Work programme (DRAW). Groups were initiated at local and national level to act as stakeholder coordinating groups, with the aim of surfacing issues and ideas for resolving them.

A zero tolerance approach to bullying and harassment was adopted, with resources being allocated to ensure prompt and well-managed investigation of allegations or complaints. Further, an external independent 24/7 helpline specifically dedicated to supporting those needing advice and support in relation to such incidents was made available to employees. The approach, however, went beyond tertiary level intervention, that is, addressing problems caused by bullying for individual targets. The programme also aimed to identify and address organizational practices that led to employees being exposed to bullying and harassment. The external helpline was very carefully structured to ensure complete confidentiality, but also allowed where necessary use of anonymized data (and only in such circumstances that such data would protect the confidentiality of users) to identify areas of organizational practice that needed change. A senior leader (the chairman of Royal Mail) personally championed this issue and monitored at a board level the effectiveness of complaint handling and resolution. Where allegations were substantiated a strong line was taken, leading in some cases to dismissal of the perpetrator. Dismissal of a perpetrator can only underscore the commitment of the organization to protecting employees from bullying and aggressive behaviour and to promoting their health, given that the literature on workplace bullying indicates that targets of bullying often perceive that nothing is done following allegations and investigation of incidents of bullying.

Changing work practices: the Work Time Learning and Listening programme

Simply having a forum to raise and discuss issues with a practical focus on addressing problems can contribute greatly to creating a positive corporate culture. Postal operations require complex working arrangements, sometimes changing shift patterns, and with many workers constantly out delivering or collecting mail, the simple issue of inconsistent contact with managers was identified as a concern through in-house research. For some workers the only time they saw or spoke to their managers was when they became sick or had a grievance or conduct issue. Key to a supportive and changed working environment was an improved and supportive, trusting relationship between workers and management. Lowe (2010) places considerable emphasis on trust in his model of healthy organizations, describing it as driven by management credibility, respect and fairness. Simple approaches again were adopted to enable this, beginning with a mandated short team meeting once a week. The style and approach to this meeting was also considered carefully. Instead of it simply being used for a management led briefing it is styled to be a Work Time Learning and Listening (WTLL) session. The sessions are structured to allow two-way dialogue and provide opportunity for employees to raise and discuss solutions for workplace issues as well as allowing managers to improve information flows, avoiding the need to rely on notice boards and notes. For major business issues, significant changes, issues of competition, health promotion and a range of other topics specific briefing packs, called *Talkabout*, were developed. Thus the WTLL sessions facilitated discussion and debate on key topics. These changes to working practices helped to address some of the psychological stressors impacting on individuals and contributed an improved organizational morale.

Improving physical working conditions: the First Line Fix programme

Physical working conditions remain a significant determinant of health and wellbeing in the workplace. The physical working environment refers to the structure, air, machinery, furniture, products, chemicals, materials and production processes in the workplace (WHO, 2010). Listening to employees revealed that the quality of local workplaces was a significant influence on morale. Employee feedback particularly indicated frustration with many simple issues in local working environments, a matter seen to be due to restricted money for investment and often complicated commissioning arrangements. This was tackled with a programme called First Line Fix. This programme gave managers a small budget that was available to local employee control for prioritizing issues they wanted improved. Issues could vary from providing TV facilities in a rest room through to repainting a toilet, but significantly, local employees made the decision about how they wanted the money spent. Initial concerns about health and safety or procurement issues fortunately proved groundless and the scheme proved successful and popular. It gives employees more autonomy or control in determining their local environment. In this, the Royal Mail demonstrates adherence to the key principles of health promotion. Participation, involvement and responsibility of the people in the workplace is critical for the achievement of the goal of healthy people in healthy organizations, as articulated by the European Network of Workplace Health Promotion (Hanson, 2007).

Safety issues were prioritized also by employees at Royal Mail. This secured management attention and action and resulted in steady reduction in accidents from the beginning of the programme, reversing a rising trend. Accident and incident data were used to highlight areas for improvement and major changes to handling mail (to reduce manual handling of loads), dealing with dog attacks and addressing issues of safety in vehicle yards showed benefit in reducing reported accidents.

Personal health resources in the workplace

Acknowledging that the provision of health information has limits as a health promotion strategy, it is important also to acknowledge that, if organized and presented in a manner that engages and empowers workers, information can contribute to health gain. Personal health resources include services and information that allow workers to support their efforts to improve or maintain healthy personal lifestyles and to monitor their physical and mental health (WHO, 2010).

The issue of dealing with the particular demographic profile of the Royal Mail workforce was briefly highlighted in the early part of this chapter. Men use primary care facilities less than women (Men's Health Forum, 2009) and men are often forgotten in health promotion messages (Kickbusch et al., 2005). Early in the approach taken at Royal Mail it was established that distributing traditional health education literature was not always effective. It was perceived that men were likely to discard it or to fail to read its contents. A number of different approaches were considered to help improve retention of health information and to improve awareness of health matters.

Firstly, approaches that enabled health education information to be sent to employees' homes were piloted, where often other family members would not only benefit from informing themselves, but would also act as the conduit to raise health awareness in their partners or fathers. As there were some concerns about whether the approach would be felt inappropriate (for example for highly personal issues such as testicular cancer), a pilot was undertaken to explore the use of health education materials informing partners and encouraging them to perform checks with their men. Surprisingly, feedback on this campaign was universally positive, although curiously when a cervical screening programme had been promoted to women previous to this initiative it received a number of less positive comments! It may be that the approach via a partner allows a distance from the workplace, necessary for this sensitive issue.

Secondly, redesigning health education materials was undertaken and found to be of significant benefit. While there is always a risk in using humour, cartoons or flippant slogans, it transpired that the target audience within the workforce was more receptive and more likely to retain information in such formats. Working with a third sector organization, the Men's Health Forum, delivering personal health messages to men on the walls and mirrors of washrooms and toilets was trialled. One manager remarked on the surprising lack of graffiti on posters targeted in this way. Formal evaluation confirmed awareness after such a campaign was significantly higher than using simple health education leaflets.

The charity the organization worked with used this experience to pilot other innovative ways of delivering health messages to men. For example, converting health messages into a workshop manual format was one such successful approach. Men used to seeing this format of material being associated with car repairs, found similar style books and short manuals, which included cartoons, diagrams and humorous analogies, a readable and useful form of communication. Evaluation suggested higher rates of retention and the approach has been continued over many years with manuals targeting health issues for families as well as men, and for cancer, obesity and many other topics. This has prompted the development of a range of mini-manuals on specific issues such as hypertension, stress, back pain or lifestyle issues such as smoking. The approach displays elements of best practice in respect of engaging men in health promotion, for example: using opportunistic and innovative methods, finding a hook that will appeal to men, maintaining a positive and non-threatening focus (Department of Health and Children (Ireland), 2008).

Across an organization on the scale of Royal Mail, with many thousands of offices, the challenge of distributing such materials is not insubstantial. While simply posting is one obvious option (!), this is not without cost and in the early days of developing approaches the access across the workforce to electronic communication materials was comparatively poor. This was initially tackled with mobile vehicles, health buses of a variety of sizes and shapes that could visit workplaces. These vehicles were highly visible, with colours and branding designed to contrast and stand out alongside the regular red operational vehicles. The Royal Mail was fortunate to obtain funding for development of some bespoke trailers and vehicles, enabling the provision of on-site health screening facilities. A national touring programme was developed using either occupational health staff or health promotion trained staff. The touring programme reached a remarkable proportion of employees and proved very popular. At one site attendance records confirmed uptake of 110%, suggesting that some staff attended more than once in a day! Alongside providing simple screening for risk factors such as weight, blood pressure, cholesterol or diabetes it was also feasible to target issues relevant to personal and organizational safety such as eyesight testing (for drivers particularly). This allowed the Royal Mail to collate anonymized statistical data to understand the comparative health and lifestyle risk factors that existed in the workforce, which in turn enabled further planned programmes to be targeted to needs.

Physical activity and other health-related issues are also actively promoted through Royal Mail's employee benefits programme. As a large public service Royal Mail staff may access discounts with some providers for a range of benefits, including access to gym membership, tax effective means of cycle purchase, health insurance and cash plan schemes amongst many others.

Screening for health: the QHealth and Health Check-in programmes

The health buses described above were also deployed to play a role in health screening. As well as carrying specialist staff and health education literature, space was used to provide access to computer and other media (for example, video cassette or DVD-based materials). Given a prevalence of 6.5% for coronary heart disease in England (British Heart Foundation, 2010), it is an obvious target for an intervention. An early coronary risk assessment programme, called Heartshape, using lifestyle risk factors to calculate potential coronary risk and provide individualized health advice on the basis of inputted responses, proved popular with the workforce. This early precursor was later followed by more widely available commercial programmes and several different lifestyle health promotional approaches were offered. One called QHealth uses a postal questionnaire to provide a personal health risk appraisal and advice, and then feeds into an Internet-based tool to enable personal health checks. QHealth is described in Box 14.2.

As information technology use and access has improved over time, online versions of this approach have been utilized. In 2008 Royal Mail launched its online Health Check-in. This health risk appraisal tool may be accessed from the employee's home using a password login and allows users to track progress once an initial health risk appraisal has been completed. The programme provides for email updates and coaching reminders, encouraging staff to maintain positive change. It also provides advice on nutrition including sample menus for healthier meals, tailored exercise programmes, and other health risk areas. These are accessible to other family members to enable positive reinforcement of health promoting behaviours.

It is commonly recommended that evaluation of health promotion interventions includes impact, process and outcome measures. Evaluation of these programmes has deliberately collated information across a number of metrics: uptake, employee satisfaction, impact on engagement scores and also more targeted research such as follow-up on levels of health awareness, retention of health messages and intention to change health behaviours.

Box 14.2   The QHealth health screening programme

Royal Mail developed a personal Health Risk Appraisal, QHealth, in partnership with BUPA, who provided the administration and analysis as an independent provider. A postal health and lifestyle questionnaire was sent to those requesting it, and responses generated a personal health assessment with personalized advice and high quality health promotion materials. Nearly 60,000 staff responded, demonstrating the appeal of this approach. QHealth provides individuals with relevant personal health data and the organization with a valuable source of anonymized health intelligence data for planning and prioritizing future health initiatives.

The Royal Mail employee assistance programme

Many organizations provide their workers with access to assistance and support for personal issues. Royal Mail had offered its employees access to a telephone-based helpline called Connect since the mid-90s. It was used to access sources of advice for personal issues, such as financial debt or relationship issues. During the design of the Feeling First Class programme this service was reviewed and careful consideration was given to the psychosocial needs of employees during a period of high workplace change.

It was recognized that unmet psychological or social needs outside the workplace impact on employee performance both as risk factors for sickness absence, but also as stressors resulting in sick presence. Attending work when distracted by health symptoms may result in mistakes and an increased risk of accident, or generate interpersonal behavioural issues. A decision was made to review the range of issues involved and to extend significantly the support that the helpline approach could provide. The old helpline was re-branded, maintaining an independent and confidential support that could be accessed direct by an employee without management involvement.

In developing the new approach employees were involved in the design and this led to the identification of the need to ensure a comprehensive support resource covering the spectrum of physical, mental and social advice needs. The new programme was called HELP (health, employment, legal and practical). Based on employee needs assessment it seeks to be a one-stop shop providing employees with advice across the topics contained within its acronym. It is described in Box 14.3.

To ensure truly integrated support this employee support facility has a comprehensive database of Royal Mail employment practices and procedures and also linkage to sources of charitable funding for those in financial distress (for example, the Benevolent Fund). Practitioners providing the support helpline can help employees through the application or administrative processes involved, which at time of distress can be a significant support. Ensuring that advice is accurate, up to date and in line with Royal Mail practices and policies requires regular updating, training and ensuring seamless access to business sources of information, such as human resource data.

Box 14.3   The HELP employee assistance programme

In 2002 Royal Mail extended its employee assistance support to develop a service called HELP (health, employment, legal and practical). Care was taken to develop a brand and identity for this service reinforcing its independence and confidentiality. HELP provides a very broad-based employee assistance approach on a confidential basis available every hour of every day. Where necessary employees can be directed to the occupational health practitioner support or can receive face-to-face support or counselling. A Web portal supports the HELP service, and there are podcast and downloadable materials to support employees. Tracking the anonymized usage of this service enables warning of emerging issues which can enable Royal Mail to provide additional support service when needed, for example after natural disasters such as flooding.

Corporate social responsibility at Royal Mail

The activities that an organization might engage in, or the expertise and resources it can provide to support the social and physical wellbeing of the broader community in which it operates is an important element of contemporary workplace health promotion. Alongside the changes in approach for physical working conditions, psychosocial and personal health matters, a comprehensive Corporate Social Responsibility (CSR) approach was created, building in many instances from existing programmes but seeking to improve areas of health, safety, sustainability and social action. CSR is best described as the integration of social and environmental concerns in business operations and in interactions with their stakeholders on a voluntary basis. CSR is gaining currency within workplace health promotion. It is recommended that it goes beyond a public relations exercise, including a programme of actions that instils pride and fosters team spirit among employees (Lowe, 2010).

Royal Mail's staff have unique contact with the communities they work within and the organization was already very active in supporting charity and volunteering initiatives. While continuing to support these activities, the business sought to encourage employees to identify and develop a relationship with a nationwide major supported charity initiative. The charity was chosen by employee vote. As well as generating significant fund raising for the partner charity, this approach enabled volunteering opportunities, development projects and opportunities for employees to raise their own and the business' profile in the community. Other social action projects included publicizing the benefits of payroll giving to charity (with remarkable uptake) and a broad-ranging programme working with schools.

Dealing with challenges

Few businesses can afford to invest in health promotion programmes without question. The programmes described in this chapter were developed in Royal Mail during a period of major business change, financial uncertainty and major commercial pressure. There are a number of critical success factors that are seen to be key to the success of the health promotion programme at Royal Mail. Senior leadership commitment and support was deemed essential. This was secured by developing a clear business case, including key metrics such as attendance levels, employee engagement and satisfaction with the initiative. It was important to ensure that health promoting initiatives were incorporated within the new ways of working adopted within the business and that they did not appear as a separate, additional requirement, and it is in this that the settings approach within health promotion is most evident. Managers and employees were involved in developing initiatives in order to avoid a top-down approach and operational staff identified priority needs. This not only fostered participation, it allowed early successes to be identified. Union or employee cynicism was addressed by involvement in design, and open, frank discussions on issues during planning stages. Innovative approaches were adopted, recognizing that traditional health promotion methods need adaption to the demographic profile and geographic needs of a diverse and widespread workforce. Partnership working, another important success factor, was expressed in the recognition of opportunities for partnership with third sector and publicly available resources. This enabled programmes to be delivered without huge investment or logistic challenges. Success was celebrated, ensuring internal communications regularly featured news of successful initiatives, with personalized stories featuring individuals. Finally, in measuring benefit and the incorporation of health data into regular management reports, the commercial value of a healthy workforce was promoted, allowing management to appreciate the value of investing in employee health and wellbeing.

Summary points

- The approaches described constitute a comprehensive, broad approach to workplace health promotion and support.
- Royal Mail employees benefit from well-planned and coordinated initiatives, designed to be accessible and easily available.
- The services are cost effective and provide a return on the investment by helping to ensure a healthy workforce that maximizes quality and productivity and supports the high standards of customer service the organization aspires to maintain.
- The approach has been effective in improving employer brand and customer confidence has been gained as a result.

Further Online Reading

Lomas, L. and McLuskey, J. (2005) 'Pumping up the pressure: a qualitative evaluation of a workplace health promotion initiative for male employees', *Health Education Journal* 64: 88–95.

An initiative to encourage male employees to participate in blood pressure screening is evaluated in this paper. The initiative took place in NHS Trust workplaces, and the evaluation was qualitative, involving interview with 14 male participants. The men liked the convenience of the workplace location as it provided a forum for discussion of other health issues with a health professional.

References

British Heart Foundation (2010) www.heartstats.org/datapage.asp?id=1584 (accessed 1 December 2010).

Department of Health and Children (Ireland) (2008) *National Men's Health Policy 2008–2013*. Dublin: Stationery Office.

ENWHP (European Network for Workplace Health Promotion) (2005) *The Luxembourg Declaration on Workplace Health Promotion in the European Union*. Essen: ENWHP.

Hanson, A. (2007) *Workplace Health Promotion: A Salutogenic Approach*. Milton Keynes: Author-House.

Harvey, H. and Fleming, P. (2004) *Impacting Health at Work*. London: Chadwick House Publishing.

Kickbusch, I., Wait, S. and Maag, D. (2005) *Navigating Health: The Role of Health Literacy*. London: Alliance for Health and the Future.

Lowe, G. (2010) *Creating Healthy Organizations*. Toronto: University of Toronto Press.

Men's Health Forum (2009) www.menshealthforum.org.uk/mhw-2009/19524-national-mens-health-week-2009-statistics (accessed 9 February 2011).

WHO (World Health Organization) (1984) Health Promotion: Concepts and Principles. Report of a Working Group. Available at: http://whqlibdoc.who.int/euro/-1993/ICP_HSR_602__m01.pdf (accessed 7 February 2011).

WHO (World Health Organization) (2010) *Healthy Workplaces: A Model for Action*. Geneva: WHO.

15

Workplace Health Promotion in SMEs: An Example of Good Practice

Margaret Hodgins, John Griffiths and Rob Whiting

Aims

- To outline why small and medium-sized enterprises (SMEs) are a priority for workplace health promotion
- To explore the particular context of SMEs as settings for workplace health promotion
- To showcase an example of good practice in an SME, Williams Medical Supplies
- To outline challenges for workplace health promotion in SMEs

---

Small and medium-sized enterprises (SMEs)

SMEs make up a very significant proportion of the global economy and are identified as a priority area for action by the European Network of Workplace Health Promotion (ENWHP, 2007). However, their situation with respect to health and safety is less favourable than that of larger enterprises (EASHW, 2003) due at least in part to the fact that SMEs are underserved in terms of workplace health promotion and/or occupational health services (ENWHP, 2001a). SMEs differ in many respects from larger enterprises and therefore require different considerations in the protection and promotion of health, an idea consistent with the principles of a settings approach, in particular the importance of context.

SMEs: a priority for workplace health promotion

The need to consider the special case of the health of workers in SMEs has been identified on a number of occasions, both internationally and in specific jurisdictions (see, for example, Black, 2008; ENWHP, 1998, 2002, 2005; Health and Safety Authority, 2008). Within the EU, enterprises are classified as micro if they have fewer than 10 employees, small if they have between 10 and 50 employees and medium if they have between 50 and 250 employees (European Commission, 2003), although this categorization is not uniformly applied in the research literature. SMEs make up a very significant proportion of the global economy. Together, micro, small and medium-sized enterprises represent 99% of all enterprises in the EU, although there is considerable variation across states (ENWHP, 2001a). Only 15% of workers work in companies with over 250 employees (EFIWLC, 2007). In general, SMEs provide around 90 million jobs and therefore are both socially and economically important (European Commission, 2003).

The health of workers in SMEs has been signalled as a matter of concern. Eakin et al. (2001) report that many studies find higher levels of risk factors, hazardous conditions and work-related injury in SMEs. Within EU states, occupational accident risk is much higher for small and medium-sized enterprises. Fatal accidents are twice as likely in companies with fewer than 50 employees compared to those with more than 250 (ENWHP, 2001a) and more accidents generally occur in small workplaces than large (MacEachen et al., 2010). There is also the possibility that small companies are more likely to fail to report accidents or injuries (Champoux and Brun, 2002). Conversely, sickness absence is lower in SMEs than larger organizations (EFIWLC, 2007).

Comprehensive models of workplace health promotion not only acknowledge the role of prevention of injury and illness but the potential of work and the workplace to enhance mental health and to contribute to feelings of wellbeing, inclusion and participation. Interestingly, there is virtually no information on positive health in small enterprises.

Occupational health services and workplace health promotion in SMEs: the importance of context

SMEs are generally agreed to be underserved in terms of workplace health promotion and/or occupational health services. The smaller the enterprise, the less likely it is that occupational health services will be available. For example, safety risk assessments were conducted in only 30–50% of small enterprises compared to 90% in larger companies (ENWHP, 2001a). There is also a significant correlation between company size and perceptions of being informed about workplace health risk; employees in larger companies report higher levels of information (EFIWLC, 2007). One UK survey found that only 18% of companies with fewer than 25 employees had two or more health-related initiatives, compared to 74% of companies with more than 500 employees (Gee et al., 1997).

The particular features of SMEs, for example, the dominance of the owner/manager, the need for flexibility around tasks or roles, employment relations and their potential economic instability, form the context for their health management. Appreciation of context is critical to taking a systems approach, which in turn underpins the settings approach (see Chapter 3 for a lengthier discussion on systems and settings). Promoting health in this setting requires an understanding of how the system operates and connects with the wider environment.

Lack of safety or workplace health services and programmes can be understood somewhat in terms of financial resources. Small and even medium-sized enterprises may work from a narrow profit margin, prohibiting investment in dedicated personnel to develop health promotion programmes. Lack of technical knowledge on the part of owner–managers, and not being connected well with trade unions or trade associations have also been suggested as reasons for low levels of health management in SMEs (Eakin and Weir, 1995; MacEachen et al., 2010).

A number of studies suggest, however, that finance and expertise only partially explain the absence of health initiatives and services. Champoux and Brun (2002), interviewing 223 small-sized enterprises in Quebec, found that economic obstacles were less important than expected in implementing OHS (Occupational Health and Safety); only one-third of respondents felt that costs of prevention were an obstacle and only 10% that prevention was not profitable. An obvious response to the difficulty of affording dedicated internal resources for health promotion is for third parties, for example statutory agencies, to provide occupational and workplace health supports and services to SMEs. Available evidence indicates that take-up is very poor, even when such supports and expertise are offered at no charge to companies. In an initiative providing a free health and safety starter pack and a free OHS inspection to 600 SMEs in Liverpool, only 123 actually took the pack, and less than half availed themselves of an inspection (EASHW, 2002). A similar project, Workplace Health Connect, which aimed to provide practical advice on workplace health, safety and return to work issues to SMEs, fared equally poorly in terms of uptake. A more comprehensive, needs-based approach, Fair Chance to Work, which included visits, the devising of a seminar programme based on identified needs within organizations along with consultancy and small grants, failed to attract more than a handful of SMEs (Griffin et al., 2005) (see Boxes 15.1 and 15.2. for more detail on these projects).

Box 15.1   The Workplace Heath Connect initiative for SMEs

Workplace Health Connect (WHC) is a confidential service designed to give free, practical advice on workplace health, safety and return to work issues, to

(Continued)

(Continued)

smaller businesses (with 5–250 workers) in England and Wales. The WHC scheme exists at three levels:

- Level 1: a free, national **advice line** taking calls from both employers and employees, offering detailed and tailored practical advice. This is supported by a dedicated website. The Level 1 service also acts as a referral point for Level 2.
- Level 2: free problem solving **visits** from qualified advisers for employers calling via Level 1. Pathfinders (contractors that are often based on regional partnerships) deliver this service, with a telephone follow-up three months later.
- Level 3: **signposting** to approved local specialists, by the advice line and pathfinders, for employers requiring further support (Institute of Employment Studies, 2007)

The Health and Safety Executive (HSE) commissioned an independent evaluation of the Workplace Health Connect (WHC) pilot in terms of customer-related outcomes. Findings indicated that while WHC met its targets for the visit service, the advice line received fewer calls than anticipated. Users preferred to take up the offer of face-to-face support. Overall, demand for support with health issues was low. SMEs using the service were primarily interested in meeting legal requirements. Using the service did not impact on sickness absence but did lead to improvements in a range of health and safety practices. These in turn were linked to a reduction in accident rates. Users, although receiving the service well, considered costs to outweigh benefits (Health and Safety Executive, 2010).

Box 15.2   The Fair Chance to Work project

This health promotion initiative, Fair Chance to Work, was targeted at SMEs in the North East of England. Letters endorsed by organizations seen as credible to SMEs and flyers about the initiative were sent to 480 organizations. Following further targeted recruitment activities, 17 organizations responded and 15 agreed to participate, representing a response rate of 2.7%. All 15 organizations were visited and a seminar programme was put together based on identified needs within organizations. Additionally, consultancy and small grants were made available to assist organizations with their chosen activities. On-going support and contact was maintained. Six of the organizations attended none of the seminars, nor took up the offer of consultancy or grants, reducing the response rate to 1.6%. Griffin et al. (2005) concluded that the initiative failed to attract more than a handful of SMEs, despite considerable support (for example, the offer of free, multidisciplinary services, support tailored to individual needs etc.). Those that did participate reported high levels of satisfaction with an increased awareness of health at work issues. An initial audit provided to the health promotion personnel in the area, a survey and the seminars were well received, providing access to information and to networks (Griffin et al., 2005).

From this it appears that the direct costs of workplace health activities are only partially prohibitive to health and safety practice. A much more nuanced perspective, in keeping with notions of context, is in order. For example, few studies have explored the role of opportunity costs in the context of developing health protection and promotion programmes. Even if cash costs are low or negligible, opportunity costs of employees and managers being involved in activities may appear prohibitive. Perhaps, as Griffin et al. (2005) suggest, participation in any initiative that involves a longer term vision may be problematic for SMEs. Although a coherent business case may be accepted for workplace health promotion, investment in a programme may tie up financial resources that are needed in the immediate term for service or production. There may be concerns about the continued cost, even if services are provided free in the context of a special project or programme.

Champoux and Brun (2002), in their study of small-sized enterprises in Quebec, concluded that owner–managers denied, neglected or did not recognize occupational health problems in their companies. This may be an overly negative and castigatory position. There is evidence that both employers and employees in SMEs engage in trade-offs, which may make sense in the context of their day-to-day work, but ultimately leave them, as a population, exposed to risk. MacEachen et al. (2010), in the context of health and safety practice, report examples of trade-offs where the use of protective equipment slows down production or reduces service quality, and where the general or on-going investment in protection against hazards are set against the costs of an illness or injury to one person, or where proxy behaviours (for example washing hands rather than wearing gloves) are adopted as a compromise in the context of physical or economic constraints. They find that employers are often not ignorant of regulations, but rationalize safety breaches to augment economic survival.

Another contextual factor is the increased likelihood of SMEs being family or community enterprises (ENWHP, 2001a). This creates a set of social relationships that can be close, and either mutually supportive or destructive. Either situation may compromise health and safety practice, as MacEachen found. Where social relations are poor, workers may distrust any health and safety recommendations made by their employer, or conversely, when social relationships were positive, supportive and empathic, workers tended to under-recognize workplace health hazards and downplay risks, focusing on economic survival for all (MacEachen et al., 2010). Strong commitment, both to the company and to survival, in turn, may lead to resistance to external people or services. Commitment and loyalty may lead to enhanced mental health and wellbeing, a topic considerably under-researched in relation to SMEs. Mutual support between employers and workers may explain why sickness absence is lower in SMEs.

The relational context of SMEs may also underpin the tendency in SMEs to attribute responsibility for health and safety of the employee. This has been observed on the part of employers (Champoux and Brun, 2002; Fine et al., 2004), although employees, too, can share this perception, expecting that they should be the ones to navigate risks and to become more educated about risk

(MacEachen et al., 2010). The employer in a small company is personally known to employees, perhaps a friend or family member, not a remote, faceless managerial committee or HR department. Employees may feel a need to protect their employer from official or legal investigation, either through a sense of personal loyalty or simply to protect their own job.

Much of the research literature on health in SMEs is focused on what doesn't happen and why. Also, much focuses on occupational health and safety practice, which having an ethos of being perceived as prohibitive, coercive and negative (Harvey and Fleming, 2004), may explain the disapproving emphasis in the literature. As noted above, few studies explore positive health, wellbeing and aspects of health promotion practice such as participation and empowerment, which could be more easily facilitated in small organizations. Surprisingly few studies explore good practice in order to understand how to emulate it. Despite the difficulties noted, SMEs can engage well with the concept of health improvement and display good practice. The ENWHP, in an initiative launched in 1999, focused on occupational health and safety and workplace health promotion in small and medium-sized enterprises. Forty-eight examples of good workplace health promotion practice in SMEs were identified within this initiative (ENWHP, 2001b). The following section presents a more detailed case study of workplace health promotion in a company in Wales – Williams Medical Supplies.

Williams Medical Supplies: an example of good practice

Williams Medical Supplies (WMS) was established in 1986 by Robin Williams to supply general medical practitioners nationally with a wide range of medical products, including vaccines and injectables. Originally based in Northfleet, Kent, the company transferred its main administrative, purchasing and central warehouse functions to Rhymney in 1992.

During 1998 WMS invested in further development of its office and warehouse facilities with the purchase of new premises in Rhymney, a move that proved to be highly beneficial. Six years later the company's growth meant that new, larger premises were needed again. In January 2004, the company fully utilized warehousing space on an industrial estate in Rhymney. Following a major refurbishment, the new 76,000 sq ft warehouse opened in 2005. The following year saw the opening of the new headquarters on the site.

The company currently employs 160 people and is the largest supplier to general practice in the United Kingdom, with a wide range of products, including surgical instruments and medicines. The Medical Services division tests and calibrates medical equipment, and undertakes health and safety audits and electrical PAT testing.

In 2005 Williams Medical Supplies was voted one of the Sunday Times Best 100 Small Companies to Work For and has been recognized as an Investors in People (IiP) Company since 2000.

In 2009, the company was ranked 69 in the Sunday Times Deloitte Buyout Track 100, a ranking that recognizes Britain's top private equity-backed companies with the fastest-growing profits over the previous two-year period.

Rhymney is a small town at the head of one of the South Wales valleys. In the early twentieth century almost all employment in the town and the surrounding area was devoted to the mining of coal. However, as the century wore on coal production fell and by the 1980s all except one of the deep mines in Wales had ceased production. Those areas of Wales in which heavy industry and mining had been predominant, such as the Rhymney Valley, were faced with different challenges, with unemployment being a significant one of these. It was into this environment in 1992 that Williams Medical Supplies relocated when Robin Williams decided to locate his business closer to his family roots.

The company began to develop its wellbeing programme for staff in 2003/4, and this emerged as a result of the desire of the then owners to increase the level of engagement between the company and the local community. Given that the majority of employees lived within the local community, promoting their health and wellbeing was seen as a natural extension of the company's desire to invest in the community.

Investors in People recognition had already been achieved and in wanting the best for its people the company was exploring initiatives and activities that it felt would contribute to this goal. An invitation to a breakfast seminar at a local golf club afforded the opportunity to learn about a Welsh Assembly Government-funded workplace health promotion accreditation programme entitled Health at Work, The Corporate Standard. Developed in the mid-1990s (and revised several times since then) the Corporate Standard is a national mark of quality for health promotion in the workplace and offers recognition for an organization's commitment to a healthy workforce (WAG 2011). The process is seen as contributing to organizational development and so consultation and feedback is available to all applicants on any or all aspects of their application and validation visit.

Two members of staff were nominated by WMS to take the process forward: one was the communications coordinator and the other the health and safety manager. Contact was made with the Corporate Standard team and an initial visit was quickly followed by a scoping exercise/situation analysis to determine what was already in place for the promotion of employee wellbeing. This initial audit showed that many aspects of a wellbeing programme were already in place and that all that was needed was some fine tuning of the then current activity and the filling of several gaps in the approach. The fine tuning and filling of the gaps took a year to complete.

The company's approach to workplace health promotion (and the achievement of the accreditation) was based from the outset on a whole company approach. At the centre of this is the high value that the company places on its staff, recognizing that their wellbeing is central to the company's performance.

The promotion of employee health and wellbeing could be traced through many of the general management processes of the company, with these complimented by specific initiatives on health topics identified as needing to be addressed. Following the Corporate Standard process provided the company with a framework for the development of the health and wellbeing programme. Key steps included:

Organizational support: Although delegating the development of the wellbeing programme to others, the management team remained engaged in the process; maintaining awareness of the programme, being prepared to be seen to be actively supporting initiatives and activities and being involved in reviewing progress. The allocation of financial resources to the programme was key in enabling rapid progress to be made from the outset.

Communication: Communication within the company was seen as a major corporate priority and an intranet site was established, with great benefit to the wellbeing programme as it was included in the intranet pages. At this time the company employed around a hundred people so an intranet site was somewhat unusual in a company of this size. Of note is that PCs were placed in rest rooms for staff who would not normally have access to a PC as part of their role. Tremendous effort was made to communicate with staff in other innovative ways: departmental 'huddles', monthly updates, the establishment of an employee forum and a colleague communication board.

The involvement of employees: One of the critical factors underpinning the success of a workplace health promotion scheme is the way in which employees respond to it in terms of their active participation in the initiative and their ownership of it. The company recognized this from the outset, and placed a high priority on involving staff in the life of the company, therefore extending this approach to the wellbeing programme was relatively straightforward.

The Employee Forum provided an opportunity for members of staff to put forward ideas and contribute to the planning of wellbeing activities. Sports and physical activity programmes were run and promoted, with staff taking on the responsibility for these.

Monitoring, assessment and review: Health promotion activities were carefully monitored. Activities ranged from simple measurements such as the evaluation of training events and levels of participation to more complex measurements using survey tools to identify levels of morale and staff perception of their work experience. Sickness absence data were routinely collected and used to provide additional feedback to managers; for example, following the introduction of the new sickness absence policy and return to work interviews absence fell from 3.25 days to 2.14 days. On its own this might indicate the introduction of these new tools had an immediate and positive effect, but without any additional data it could be argued that the new approach made employees concerned about absence and so some were in work when in fact they should not have been. However, the surveys on staff morale and staff perception remained positive, indicating that this was not the case.

Policy development and implementation: A corporate policy sets out an organization's position on a particular topic and legitimizes action taken to achieve the goals of the policy. Having a comprehensive range of policies in place is therefore a key step in the development of a workplace wellbeing programme. In 2004 WMS had developed and implemented a wide range of corporate policies, accessing ACAS (Advisory, Conciliation and Arbitration Service) advice during their development. The range of policies included a number that impacted on the health and wellbeing of staff, including harassment and bullying, equal opportunities, HIV/Aids, alcohol and substance misuse and others. The family-friendly policy in particular addressed the needs of the staff, with shift patterns being introduced to best meet employees' requirements.

The company was also addressing a number of specific health topics at this time. Pressure management and stress had been recognized as an area of importance and information was made available to staff through the intranet site and library. Support for staff through counselling was available. At the time of the initial **Corporate Standard Assessment** (a Silver Award in June 2004), a number of recommendations were made to the company on how the company's approach to pressure and stress could be developed further.

By the time of the next assessment (June 2006, Gold Award) stress risk assessments were being undertaken and access to counselling services had been enhanced. In addition, the company was clearly taking note of the HSE Management Standards Approach (MSA), with one of the assessors noting that the HSE's Management Standards on Stress at Work were being adhered to. Risk assessments on stress were being undertaken for staff returning to work following absence, and by 2006 questions relating to stress and pressure were being included in the staff survey (see also Chapter 3 for more detail on the MSA).

In terms of lifestyle-related issues, the company actively promoted smoking cessation. In addition, and several years prior to the smoke-free legislation, the company put in place a very comprehensive smoking policy which was underpinned by a robust development process supported by extensive consultation and support for smokers wanting to stop smoking. The end result was the move to a completely smoke-free site that extended to company vehicles.

The company developed a clear nutrition statement that underpinned all catering activities. Free fresh fruit was available to staff on a daily basis and vending machines offered healthy choices.

On alcohol, the company moved to a position where the consumption of alcohol was prohibited during the working day, and for corporate functions only soft drinks were served. Support was made available to any member of staff who felt they needed help with an alcohol or drug issue.

Participation in physical activity, such as walking, cycling and five-a-side football was strongly promoted. The company negotiated the purchase and opening of a footpath at the rear of the new site to enable staff to walk/cycle safely to work. Cycle racks were put in place and showers were available for staff to use. Car sharing arrangements were in place and an environmentally friendly pool car had been purchased.

A wellbeing clinic for staff was held every six months, rehabilitation and return to work procedures were in place and links had been made with a local primary care trust, who provided an occupational health service to the company. Such an approach was unusual for a company of this size, in both its scope and depth.

The management of health and safety was identified as a key corporate activity at a very early stage and by 2002 the company had employed a dedicated, full-time health and safety officer. His participation in the health and wellbeing working group ensured full health and safety input to the team. The weekly audits of each work area ensured that risks were reviewed by the employees working in those areas, created a real sense of ownership of the management of those risks and ensured that controls introduced would be more likely to be accepted. A monthly health and safety team meeting involved employees/representatives of teams in all aspects of risk assessment and accident investigation, and minutes were communicated to the whole staff via the intranet, briefings and hard copy.

In the years after 2006, the company faced several challenges, notably a management buyout in 2007 and, in common with many other businesses, the downturn in the global economy from 2008/9. The company was restructured, losing 19 members of staff in the process. The new Chief Executive Officer and Executive team have shown a high commitment to health and safety, the environment and community engagement, and as part of this the wellbeing programme has been maintained, but with a lower emphasis. One of the major emphases today is on building morale within the company, and the wellbeing programme is an integral element of this.

Now that the major changes within the company are completed a more proactive approach to health and wellbeing is emerging. The company intends to seek accreditation for its wellbeing programme within 2011, a member of staff has been identified to lead this process and activities are under way to identify the strengths and areas of development in the current programme. The company has declared itself to be committed to achieving a Gold level of award.

Williams attributes the success of its approach to the following :

1. Although actively promoting the health and wellbeing of its staff, the company benefited from an external accreditation programme which provided the company with a clear template for action. The accreditation process caused things to happen and enabled them to continue (assessments in 2004, 2006, and again in 2011).
2. The support of the senior management team has been critical in maintaining the approach, especially so in times of financial constraint, with managers' awareness of the benefits of the process being a key factor.
3. The promotion of wellbeing is seen within the company as an essential component of good corporate practice.

Engagement: the key challenge for workplace health promotion in SMEs

Small and medium-sized enterprises, employing approximately two-thirds of the workforce, constitute an enduring challenge for health promotion and prevention systems (MacEachen et al., 2010). The levels of injury and accident in SMEs and the lack of health promotion programmes point to substantial challenges for the protection and promotion of health in this setting. However, the identification of examples of practice on the part of the ENWHP and the detailed case study described here imply that it is possible to meet these challenges.

A key challenge is clearly engagement with the concept of workplace health promotion. If there is engagement, then there are measurable benefits. In the Workplace Health Connect initiative (Box 15.1), although demand was low, involvement did lead to improvements in a range of health and safety practices, which in turn were linked to a reduction in accident rates (Health and Safety Executive, 2010). Similarly, with the Fair Chance to Work (see Box 15.2), those who participated reported high levels of satisfaction with the project and an increased awareness with health at work issues (Griffin et al., 2005). Griffin et al. conjecture that those who engaged with the project saw the benefits at an early stage, and shared the same values as the health promotion staff with regard to health at work. In other words, they were already converted. In this vein, Lansdown et al. (2007), employed Prochaska and DiClimente's stage of change model in their survey of health and safety activity in SMEs in the UK. They report:

> The model has been useful in discriminating SME readiness to engage in health and safety activity. In both [surveys], with respect to health and safety activity, two distinct groups were identified. (i) Those businesses clearly not engaged and (ii) those demonstrating good engagement. Survey data indicates significantly more time allocated to health and safety by organizations in the more advanced stages of change. The distinction implies interventions may be meaningfully targeted to organizations according to their Stage of Change. (Lansdown et al., 2007: 59)

Assessing the stage of readiness and allowing for investment of time in presenting a convincing business case for SMEs, taking their contextual situation into account (for example, possibility of managers engaging in trade-offs) may be the first step to engagement.

In the case study, it is interesting to note that the initial stimulus for WMS was a desire to invest in the community. The possibility of approaching the workplace from this perspective and focusing both support and resources at the level of the community could be explored as a way to foster engagement.

WMS found that the external accreditation programmed offered by the Welsh Assembly, an external third party, encouraged the development of activities, giving them a template to work from and a process of assessment and review. Award-based programmes differ in a number of ways from initiatives discussed earlier in the chapter. While expecting that workplaces develop policies, practices and programmes for health, they also offer an immediate incentive beyond the long term benefits of employee health protection and promotion. An evaluation of a settings-based health promotion intervention in youth organizations (the Health Quality Mark, found it to be very well received by participating organizations, leading to a raised awareness of health matters, engendering a sense of pride in the organization, and raising the profile of the organization in the local community (Hodgins and Swinburne, 2008). These latter gains are likely to be consistent with business objectives, representing added-value for engagement with health promotion.

Summary points

- Protecting and promoting health in SMEs is a priority given the fact that SMEs represent a high proportion of workplaces, yet have poorer engagement with health and safety and workplace health promotion than larger organizations.

- The settings approach in health promotion advocates taking context into account for the promotion of health. Contextual factors in SMEs include the limited availability of financial resources for dedicated health promotion work and the need for third party support at a regional or community level. Economic survival, while a priority for all businesses, is more precarious in SMEs, and therefore long term health benefits may be traded off against short term production or service costs. The community or family-based nature of SMEs may contribute to low engagement with health and safety matters, including resistance to external agents, but potentially could be a positive force in SMEs in terms of mental health.

- Once engaged, there is evidence that SMEs benefit from health promotion initiatives, demonstrating that engagement in the first instance is crucial.

- Presenting the business case bearing in mind the trade-off SMEs managers may engage in, and exploring the potential of award-based initiatives are two suggested ways forward for successful engagement with health promotion.

Online Further Reading

Hodgins, M., Battel-Kirk., B. and. Asgeirsdottir, A. (2010) 'Building capacity in workplace health promotion: the case of the Healthy Together e-learning project', *Global Health Promotion*, 17(1): 60–8.

This paper reports on the evaluation of an easily transferable e-learning course for health practitioners, occupational health and safety specialists and relevant others, to promote workplace health in small and medium-sized enterprises in rural communities. The e-learning method of education and training delivery was selected to suit the context of small workplaces since it required minimal travel cost and time to and from a course venue, and a flexible scheduling of course work around personal and professional work demands.

References

Black, C. (2008) *Working for a Healthier Tomorrow – Review of the Health of Britain's Working Age Population*. London: The Stationery Office.

Champoux, D. and Brun, J-P. (2002) 'Occupational health and safety management in small size enterprises: an overview of the situation and avenues for intervention and research', *Safety Science*, 41: 301–18.

Eakin, J. and Weir, N. (1995) 'Canadian approaches to the promotion of health and safety in small workplaces', *Canadian Journal of Public Health*, 2: 109–13.

Eakin, J., Cava, M., and Smith, T. (2001) 'From theory to practice: a determinants approach to workplace health promotion in small businesses', *Health Promotion Practice*, 2: 172–181.

EASHW (European Agency for Safety and Health at Work) (2002) http://osha.europa.eu/en/sub/sme/publications/assistance_scheme/2002/index_16.htm (accessed 9 March 2011).

EASHW (European Agency for Safety and Health at Work) (2003) 'Improving occupational safety and health in SMEs'. Available at: http://osha.europa.eu/en/publications/factsheets/37 (accessed 2 April 2009).

EFIWLC (European Foundation for the Improvement of Working and Living Conditions) (2007) *Fourth European Working Conditions Survey*. Dublin: European Foundation for the Improvement of Working and Living Conditions.

ENWHP (European Network for Workplace Health Promotion) (1998) *Cardiff Memorandum on Workplace Health Promotion in Small and Medium Sized Enterprises*. Available at: www.ver.is/whp/en/cardiffmemorandum.html (accessed 7 March 2010).

ENWHP (European Network for Workplace Health Promotion) (2001a) *Small Healthy and Competitive – new strategies for improved health in small and medium enterprises*. Available at: www.enwhp.org/enwhp-initiatives/2nd-initiative-small-healthy-and-competitive.html (accessed 11 March 2011).

ENWHP (2001b) *Criteria and Models of Good Practice for Workplace Health Promotion in Small and Medium-Sized Enterprises (SMEs)*. Available at: www.enwhp.org/publications.html (accessed 7 March 2011).

ENWHP (European Network for Workplace Health Promotion) (2002) *Barcelona Declaration on Developing Workplace Health Promotion Practice in Europe*. Available at: www.enwhp.org/publications.html (accessed 7 March 2011).

ENWHP (European Network of Workplace Health Promotion) (2005) *Luxembourg Declaration on Workplace Health Promotion in the European Union*. Available at: www.enwhp.org/fileadmin/downloads/press/Luxembourg_Declaration_June2005_final.pdf (accessed 7 March 2010).

European Commission (2003) Recommendation 2003/361/EC. Available at: http://ec.europa.eu/enterprise/policies/sme/facts-figures-analysis/sme-definition/index_en.htm (accessed 7 March 2010).

Fine, A., Ward, M., Burr, M., Tudor-Smith, C, and Kingdon, A. (2004) 'Health Promotion in small workplaces – a feasibility study', *Health Education Journal*, 63: 334–46.

Gee, D., Hunt, R. and Sayers, M. (1997) *Health Update: Workplace Health*. London: Health Education Authority, cited in B. Griffin, N. Hall and N. Watson (2005) 'Health at work in small and medium sized enterprises', *Health Education*, 105: 126–41.

Griffin, B., Hall, N. and Watson, N. (2005) 'Health at work in small and medium sized enterprises', *Health Education*, 105: 126–41.

Harvey, H.D. and Fleming, P. (2004) *Impacting Health at Work*. London: Chadwick House Publishing.

Health and Safety Authority (2008) *Workplace Health and Well-Being Strategy. Report of the Expert Group*. Dublin: Health and Safety Authority.

Health and Safety Executive (2010) *Evaluation of Workplace Health Connect February 2010 – Final Report*. Available at: www.hse.gov.uk/workplacehealth/evaluation.htm (accessed 3 March 2011).

Hodgins, M. and Swinburne, L. (2008) '"It sort of widens the Health word": evaluation of a health promotion intervention in the youth work setting', *Youth Studies Ireland*, 3: 30–44.

Institute of Employment Studies (2007) *Workplace Health Connect January 2007 Progress Report*. Available at: www.employment-studies.co.uk/policy/summary.php?id=hse_whc_07 (accessed 3 March 2011).

Lansdown, T., Deighan, C. and Brotherton, C. (2007) *Health and Safety in the Small to Medium-sized Enterprise: Psychosocial Opportunities for Intervention*. HSE RR578. Norwich: HSE/TSO.

MacEachen, E., Kosney, A., Scott-Dixon, K., Facey, M., Chambers, L. Breslin, C., Kyle, N., Irvin, E. and Mahmood, Q. (2010) 'Workplace health understandings and processes in small businesses: a systematic review of the qualitative literature', *Journal of Occupational Rehabilitation*, 20: 180–98.

WAG (Welsh Assembly Government) (2011) The Corporate Health Standard. An initiative for employers to improve the health of the workforce and their organisation. http://wales.gov.uk/topics/health/improvement/work/corporate/?lang=en (accessed 3 March 2011).

Subject Index